Advanced Soft Electronics in Biomedical Engineering

The book presents the latest advances in soft electronics in biomedical engineering and its potential applications in various biomedical fields.

The contributors provide comprehensive coverage of how soft electronics are used in diagnostics and monitoring, medical therapy, neural engineering, and wearable and implantable systems. In particular, some emerging research areas such as advanced soft robotics, fiber sensing technologies, and power optimization strategies are explored. In addition, the book highlights international standardization activities in wearable technologies and implantable bioelectronics.

The book will benefit researchers, engineers, and advanced students in biomedical engineering, electrical and computer engineering, and materials science.

Mengxiao Chen is an assistant professor at the College of Biomedical Engineering & Instrument Science, Zhejiang University, Hangzhou. She received her doctoral degree in physics from the Chinese Academy of Sciences. She then worked at the School of Electrical and Electronic Engineering, Nanyang Technological University, Singapore. Dr. Chen's research interests include soft electronics, wearable bioelectronics, and novel multifunctional sensing devices.

Advanced Soft Electronics in Biomedical Engineering

Materials, Manufactures, and Applications

Edited by
Mengxiao Chen

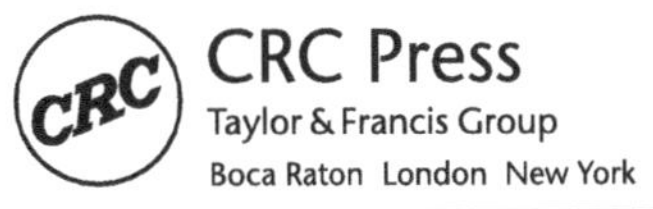

CRC Press
Taylor & Francis Group
Boca Raton London New York

CRC Press is an imprint of the
Taylor & Francis Group, an **Informa** business

Designed cover image: @Mengxiao Chen

First edition published 2025
by CRC Press
2385 NW Executive Center Drive, Suite 320, Boca Raton FL 33431

and by CRC Press
4 Park Square, Milton Park, Abingdon, Oxon, OX14 4RN

CRC Press is an imprint of Taylor & Francis Group, LLC

ISBN: 978-1-032-79744-1 (hbk)
ISBN: 978-1-032-79747-2 (pbk)
ISBN: 978-1-003-49363-1 (ebk)

DOI: 10.1201/9781003493631

Typeset in Minion
by SPi Technologies India Pvt Ltd (Straive)

Contents

Contributors

Yuhan Bian is a PhD student at Zhejiang University, China. Her research interest is in the field of flexible electronics.

Xiahua Cui is a PhD student at Jilin University, China. Her research interest is on the development of bionic tactile sensors.

Tiantian Dai is an assistant research fellow at Zhejiang Lab, China. Her research interest is on developing soft actuators.

Shurong Dong is a professor at Zhejiang University, China. His research interests encompass flexible electronics, sensors, microelectromechanical systems (MEMS), and microelectronics reliability.

Qilin Hua is an associate professor at the Beijing Institute of Technology, China. His research interests focus on flexible/stretchable electronics for artificial sensory systems.

Kaiwei Li is an associate professor at Jilin University, China. His research interests include fiber-optic sensors and robotic tactile sensors.

Yanting Liu is a research fellow at Nanyang Technological University, Singapore. Her research interests include soft robotics and artificial muscles.

Zhiyuan Meng is a PhD student at Zhejiang University, China. His research interest include neuroelectronic devices.

Miao Qi is an assistant research fellow at Zhejiang Lab, China. Her research interests include polymer materials, multifunctional fibers, and soft electronics.

Lei Ren is a professor at Jilin University (P.R. China) and University of Manchester (UK). His research interests include biorobotics, biomechanics, and bionic healthcare.

Guozhen Shen is a professor at the Beijing Institute of Technology, China. His research focuses on flexible electronics and their applications in healthcare, printable electronics and monitoring, smart robots, and related areas.

Bojing Shi is an associate professor at Beihang University, China. His research interest include wearable biosensors and diagnosis and treatment techniques for cardiovascular diseases.

Meng Wang is a postdoctoral researcher at Zhejiang Lab, China. His research interest includes flexible sensing systems.

Xiandi Wang is a professor at Zhejiang University. His research interest includes soft electronics.

Zhe Wang is a professor at Jilin University, China. His research interest includes wearable devices for biorobotics.

Ruilai Wei is a PhD candidate at the Beijing Institute of Technology, China. His research focuses on flexible electronics and their applications in healthcare, printable electronics, and monitoring.

Fan Zhang is a PhD candidate at Zhejiang University, China. Her research focuses on bio-electronics and multimodal neural interfaces.

Shaomin Zhang is a professor at Zhejiang University, China. His research interests include neuroscience, neural engineering, neurorehabilitation, brain–machine interfaces, and implantable medical devices.

Preface

The advent of soft electronics marks a transformative leap from rigid designs to structures that are flexible, stretchable, and biocompatible. The inception leaned heavily on flexible substrates, while material innovations like functional elastomers and conductive polymers catalyzed the production of conformable and deformable electronics. The introduction of multiple modern fabrication techniques further broadened its breadth of functionality, allowing devices to bend without losing integrity. Upheld by continuous research into materials and manufacturing methodologies, soft electronics hold a bright future in diverse applications.

In biomedical engineering, specifically, soft electronics have carved a niche for their distinct flexibility, adaptability, and comfort, which have paved the way for the creation of wearable and implantable devices, revolutionizing healthcare. Capturing this cutting-edge field, this book explores these recent advancements across ten organized chapters, with each chapter presenting a unique facet of the topic. A brief description of each of the chapters is as follows:

- Chapter 1 "Advanced Soft Electronic Materials and Structures for Biomedical Engineering" provides a comprehensive review of materials innovations and structural designs in soft bioelectronics, including conductive elements such as liquid metals and nanomaterials, polymer-based materials such as hydrogels and conductive polymers, and deformable structures like waves, interconnections, origami, kirigami, fabrics, etc.

- Chapter 2 "Advanced Fabrication Technology for Soft Electronics" reviews typical advanced fabrication technologies used in soft electronics, including soft lithography, soft transferring, 3D printing, textile techniques, and other novel techniques.

- Chapter 3 "Soft Electronics for Monitoring and Diagnostics" presents the corresponding soft electronic devices for the monitoring and diagnosis of vascular diseases, respiratory diseases, skeletal muscles and posture, and biochemical indicators.

- Chapter 4 "Soft Electronics for Medical Treatment" discusses the latest developments in soft electronic devices in medical treatment, including smart wound dressings, bioelectronic patch for transdermal and epidermal treatments, soft actuators for drug delivery, and other soft electronics for medical treatment.

- Chapter 5 "Soft Electronics for Neural Engineering" reviews recent advances in soft electronics in multimodal neural interfaces, such as high-resolution neural electrode arrays, transient electronics, etc., and their potential in advancing spatial coverage, resolution, integration, and overall safety within neural interfaces.

- Chapter 6 "Soft Electronics for Wearable and Implantable Systems" reports the latest developments in soft electronics for wearable and implantable systems, including the working principles and structure designs of disparate soft e-skins, diverse applications of soft implantable sensors, and energy storage strategies comprising supercapacitors and batteries for wearable and implantable systems.

- Chapter 7 "Advanced Soft Robotics for Biomedical Applications" reviews the actuating mechanism of soft robots and biomedical applications in surgery, drug delivery, artificial muscle technologies, and microrobots.

- Chapter 8 "Advanced Fiber Sensing Technologies in Bio-Integrated Systems" discusses both materials selection principles and fabrication methods utilized in advanced bio-integrated fiber sensing systems.

- Chapter 9 "Optimizing Power Strategies and Circuit Designs for Soft Electronics in Bio-Integrated systems" presents newly developed energy optimization strategies for soft electronics in bio-integrated systems from the perspectives of self-power technologies, flexible solar cells, and flexible wireless energy transmission.

- Chapter 10 "International Standardization Activities" summarizes international standard activities on soft electronics used in biomedical engineering, including IEEE conferences, IEC standards, and ISO standards, referring to wearable electronics, and implantable electronics and systems.

I would like to thank all the chapters' authors for their excellent contributions. Also, I would like to thank Zhejiang University and Zhejiang Lab for the constant support. Finally, I would like to express my sincere gratitude to my family and friends for their understanding, encouragement, and support.

Mengxiao Chen
Hangzhou

CHAPTER 1

Advanced Soft Electronic Materials and Structures for Biomedical Engineering

Miao Qi

1.1 OVERVIEW OF ADVANCED SOFT ELECTRONIC MATERIALS AND STRUCTURES

With the pressing demand for soft electronics, extensive research has been conducted on materials exhibiting flexibility and stretchability (J. Chen et al., 2021c; Fang et al., 2020; Lim et al., 2020; S. Zhang et al., 2020a). The materials employed in electronic devices are primarily categorised into three groups: Conductors, semiconductors, and insulators (Wang et al., 2018). Conductive materials are commonly utilised as electrodes, encompassing metals and metal compounds, conductive polymers, and carbon-based materials and ionic conductors (Chen et al., 2023; Park et al., 2021; Yue Zhao et al., 2019a). Metals exhibit high conductivity (10^6–10^7 S/m) and can be easily integrated into conventional fabrication processes. Moreover, many metals possess excellent biocompatibility and long-term stability (Babatain et al., 2023; Li et al., 2018). Conductive polymers have a lower Young's modulus compared to metals and are thus suitable for stretchable electrode applications (Herbert et al., 2018; Tian et al., 2020). Carbon-based materials, such as graphene and carbon nanotubes (CNTs), are commonly utilised as dopants or surface coatings on flexible substrates to enhance their properties (Llerena Zambrano et al., 2021; Yao et al., 2020). Ionic conductors are usually made from small molecular or polymer gels swollen with ionic liquids, which function similarly to biological systems by utilising the same transport mechanism (Kim et al., 2016; Yuk et al., 2019). Insulators serve as encapsulation layers to prevent the penetration of ions from biofluids into active layers, typically composed of polymers and elastomers (M. Chen et al., 2021b; S. Wang et al., 2022b). Semiconductors, both inorganic and organic in nature, play a crucial role in fabricating integrated circuits (ICs) (Oh et al., 2016, 2019). This chapter will provide an introduction to typical inorganic conductors, such as liquid metals and nanomaterials, as well as organic functional materials, including hydrogels, conductive polymers, and elastomers.

DOI: 10.1201/9781003493631-1

In addition to the utilisation of flexible and stretchable materials, it is imperative to incorporate structural designs that can effectively absorb mechanical deformation and strain (Rao et al., 2020; Sunwoo et al., 2021; Wang et al., 2017). Various innovative structures have been implemented in advanced soft electronic devices, such as waves (Xu et al., 2012), cracks (Han et al., 2014), origami and kirigami (Guo et al., 2014), textiles (Lee et al., 2013), etc. The rational design of these structures enables them to release strain through geometric changes, effectively preventing physical damage to the materials (Liu et al., 2020, 2017; Niu et al., 2020). A comprehensive elucidation of these structures will be provided subsequently. Furthermore, this chapter will present several exemplary biomedical electronics including self-healing devices capable of recovering their physical properties after damage, adhesive electronics that can adhere to human skin, and biodegradable components that can dissolve, resorb, or physically disintegrate in physiological or environmental solutions. Finally, potential approaches for enhancing the performance of soft electronics will be thoroughly discussed.

1.2 LIQUID METALS

Liquid metals specifically refer to metallic elements and low-melting-point alloys (LMPAs) that are in a liquid state near or below room temperature. Pioneering research on liquid metals dates back to the 1960s (Chen et al., 2020; Kim et al., 2023; Yan et al., 2018). Currently, the most extensively studied liquid metals are non-toxic gallium-based alloys, which have unique properties such as high conductivity, low melting point, fluidity, and biocompatibility (Aukarasereenont et al., 2022; Ren et al., 2020; Yang et al., 2022). Liquid metals exhibit excellent bonding capabilities with various soft materials including elastomers or hydrogels, enabling seamless integration with flexible substrates and making them suitable for fabricating stretchable or flexible electronic devices (Dickey, 2017; Guo et al., 2019; Hao et al., 2021; Hirsch et al., 2019). In recent years, there has been extensive research on the application of liquid metals in biomedical engineering fields such as biosensors (Chen & Pei, 2017), biomedical implants (Sun et al., 2020), and microfluidic pumps (Cole et al., 2021). Section 2.1 will provide a concise overview of the characteristics, fabrication techniques, and diverse biomedical applications associated with liquid metals.

1.2.1 Properties of Liquid Metals

Amongst several metals with low melting points, mercury is known for its toxicity, while rubidium, caesium, and francium are highly reactive and prone to oxidation (Yan et al., 2018). On the other hand, gallium (Ga) demonstrates exceptional stability and biocompatibility, rendering it an optimal choice for biomedical electronic applications. By alloying Ga with other metals such as indium (In) or tin (Sn), lower melting point liquid metals can be obtained. The performance of liquid metal is compared to that of common soft materials (Chen et al., 2020). Notably, liquid metals possess superior electrical conductivity at room temperature comparable to traditional conductive metals like copper and silver. In contrast to conventional soft materials like polydimethylsiloxane (PDMS), rubber, and conductive polymers, they possess an extremely low Young's modulus, thereby demonstrating excellent tensile properties. Furthermore, their volumetric viscosity is only twice that of water, endowing them with superior fluidity. Finally, Ga-based liquid metals readily form thin oxide layers upon exposure to oxygen, thereby facilitating the adhesion of the liquid metal to diverse surfaces and overcoming its high inherent surface tension. This unique property enables the realisation of electronic devices on flexible and stretchable substrates.

1.2.2 Approaches for the Fabrication of Liquid Metal–based Bioelectronics

Using the adhesion of the liquid metal facilitated by the oxide layer and its inherent mobility, electronic devices can be fabricated through precise patterning techniques. The preparation methods for liquid metal bioelectronics can be categorised into two main approaches: 2D and 3D patterning.

2D patterning encompasses various techniques such as microchannel imprinting, screen printing, selective wetting, and direct laser patterning. Microchannel imprinting involves pressing an elastomeric mould with microchannels onto the liquid metal, where the oxide layer adheres to the grooves while avoiding other areas of the mould. Screen printing utilises a stencil mask to apply liquid metal onto a substrate, which is then dispersed using rolling or scraping methods. Selective wetting creates distinct patterns on a substrate by controlling areas of wetting and dewetting during spreading of the liquid metal. Direct laser patterning involves coating both metallic and liquid metal layers on a substrate followed by selective removal of the latter using laser irradiation.

On the other hand, 3D patterning exploits the thin surface oxide layer present in liquid metals to overcome their low viscosity and high surface energy challenges in stabilising complex 3D structures. This includes techniques like direct writing, 3D printing microchannels, and suspension 3D printing. The direct writing method employs a syringe or similar device to spray liquid metal onto surfaces with precision control. In the 3D printing microchannels approach, liquid metal is injected into pre-designed microscopic channels within a 3D printed structure with minimum diameters reaching down to 150 nm. Suspension 3D printing employs an injection needle to introduce liquid metal into the gel medium. The close proximity between the needle tip and the gel results in shear stress that influences the fluidisation of the gel, facilitating the precise deposition of liquid metal into diverse 3D structures.

1.2.3 Application of Liquid Metals in Bioelectronics

By embedding liquid metal circuits into flexible substrates, researchers have developed bioelectronics for applications like interconnections for healthcare devices, biosensors, neural interfaces, and implantable electrodes (Pu et al., 2023; Xu et al., 2023; C. Zhang et al., 2023b). Liquid metal can be used for interconnections, enabling devices to be repositioned without interrupting the operating process. Gu et al. employed liquid metal wires as back contacts for nanowire photoelectric sensors, mimicking human nerve fibres located behind the retina and fabricating a bionic eye with a high degree of structural resemblance to the human eye (Figure 1.1a) (2020). First, a PDMS mould featuring a 10 × 10 hole array was cast, followed by injecting eutectic Ga–In liquid metal into a slender tube to form liquid metal lines. Subsequently, 100 tubes were inserted into the holes in the PDMS mould to create a 10 × 10 photodetector array. Liquid metal wires serve as signal conduits

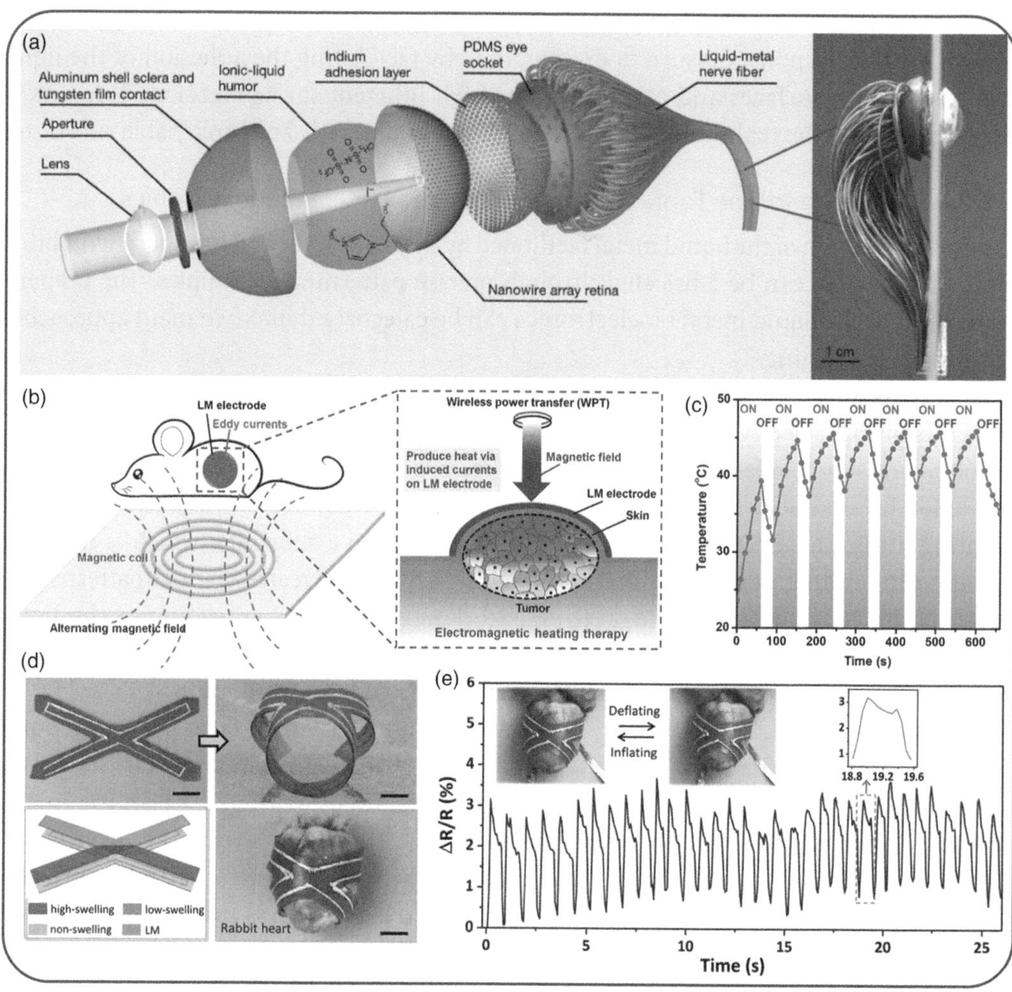

FIGURE 1.1 (a) Schematic diagram of the biomimetic eye. (b) Schematic diagram of the structure of a bioelectrode used for heating tumours in vivo. (c) Temperature changes during switching on and off of the alternating magnetic field. (d) An X-shaped device capable of deforming into a 3D structure for attachment to the rabbit heart. (e) Relative resistance change during heartbeat. ([a] Adapted with permission (Gu et al., 2020). Copyright 2020, Springer Nature; [c] Adapted with permission (X. Wang et al., 2019a). Copyright 2019, Wiley-VCH; [e] Adapted with permission (Hao et al., 2021). Copyright 2021, Wiley-VCH.)

between the nanowires and external circuits. Individual photodetectors can be addressed and measured by selecting corresponding liquid metal wires, akin to how the human retina functions.

Liquid metals possess excellent thermal and electrical properties, enabling them to generate heat when exposed to alternating magnetic fields. Building upon this principle, Wang et al. developed a bioelectrode utilising an oxidised Ga–In mixture that was printed into various customised patterns (X. Wang et al., 2019a). As illustrated in Figure 1.1b, this electronic skin exhibits conformability and can be employed as a versatile tool for tumour treatment in mice. By subjecting the liquid metal electrode to an alternating magnetic field, eddy currents are induced due to its remarkable magnetocaloric effect, facilitating non-invasive wireless multi-site tumour therapy. The repeatability and controllability of temperature rise and fall produced by the liquid metal under alternating magnetic field exposure are demonstrated in Figure 1.1c.

Moreover, liquid metals have shown promising potential in biosensors to detect physiological signals like temperature, pulse, electrocardiogram, and electromyogram. These sensors can be incorporated into clothing, gloves, or even implanted directly into the body to monitor health conditions or aid in rehabilitation. Hao et al. fabricated a conformable biosensor by printing Ga-based liquid metal doped with nickel particles onto a tough hydrogel substrate (2021). The incorporation of nickel particles enhances printability, shape fidelity, and interfacial bonding with hydrogels, enabling intricate patterning of the liquid metals as conductive and sensing elements. The resulting biosensor based on hydrogel exhibits exceptional mechanical properties and remarkable sensitivity to mechanical strain and human movement. It possesses the ability to self-deform into complex 3D configurations, facilitating secure fixation of hydrogel devices onto biological organs for implantable applications. As depicted in Figure 1.1d, an X-shaped device was manufactured with varying gradient structures in its front and rear branches, which subsequently deformed into arch shapes with distinct curvatures. This device autonomously conformed to the rabbit's heart surface, while maintaining excellent interface contact. To simulate cardiac contractions, air circulation was employed; remarkably, the device successfully detected these beating movements (Figure 1.1e). Such self-shaping biosensors hold great promise as implantable devices for healthcare monitoring.

1.3 CONDUCTIVE NANOMATERIALS

Nanostructured electronic materials play a crucial role in the development of soft electronics due to their outstanding electrical conductivity, large surface area, and biocompatibility (Baig et al., 2021). They can be integrated into electrodes for neural interfaces (Chiang et al., 2020), biosensors (Rajeev et al., 2018), and biofuel cells (Mishra et al., 2021), enabling high-performance signal detection and stimulation in biological systems (Cho et al., 2022). Elastic polymers and hydrogels can be doped with conductive nanomaterials, resulting in stretchable conductive nanocomposites that exhibit exceptional thermal, electrical, and mechanical characteristics (Zhang & Lieber, 2016). Conductive nanomaterials can be categorised into two primary groups: Metallic nanomaterials such as gold nanoparticles and silver nanowires and carbon-based nanomaterials including graphene and CNTs (Ehrenfreund & Foing, 2010; Wang et al., 2018). Furthermore, nanostructured materials can be classified based on their morphology ranging from zero-dimensional (0D) to 3D (Song et al., 2022). This section will encompass aspects from material selection to preparation techniques, methods for incorporating nanomaterials into polymers, as well as potential applications.

1.3.1 Metal- and Carbon-based Nanomaterials

Figure 1.2a illustrates a range of metal- and carbon-based nanomaterials, spanning from 0D to 3D structures. Au nanoparticles consist of gold atoms and possess distinctive properties attributed to their small size and high surface-to-volume ratio. The surface chemistry

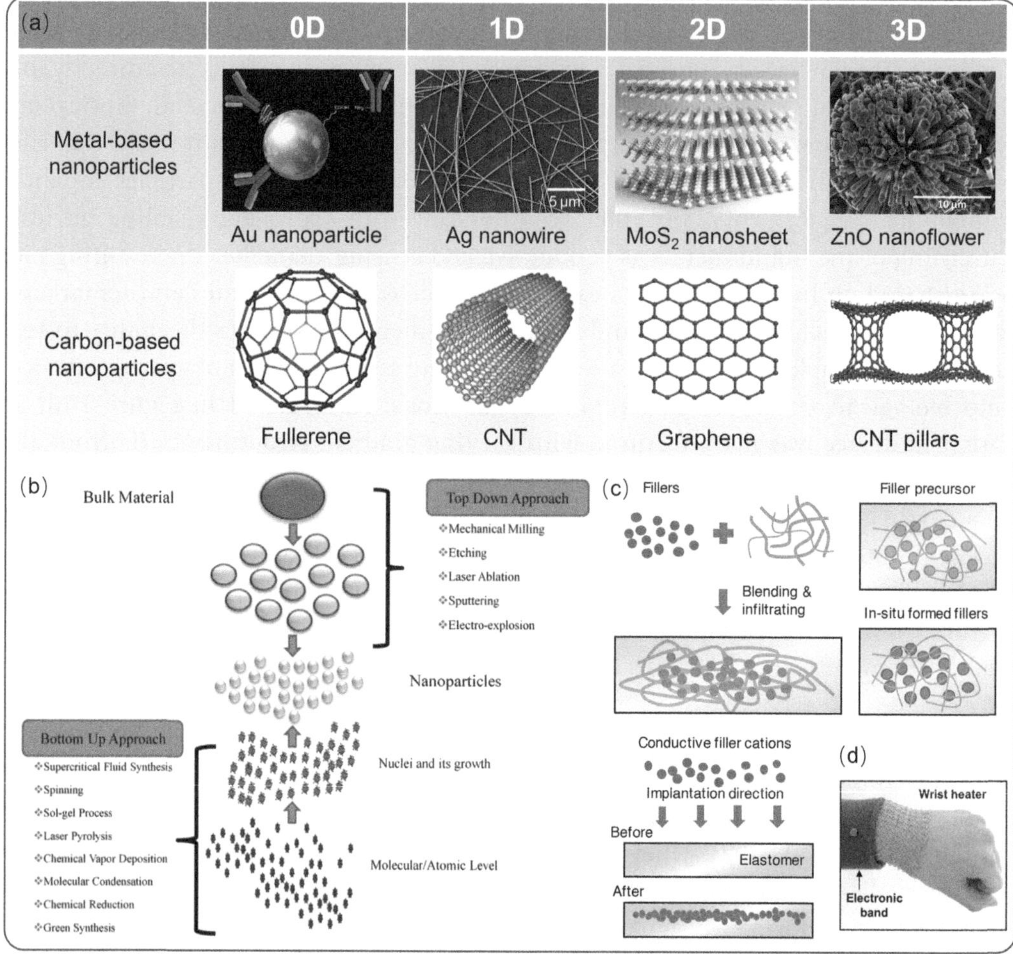

FIGURE 1.2 (a) Metal- and carbon-based nanomaterials from 0D to 1D. (b) Synthesis methods of nanomaterials. (c) Approaches for incorporating nanomaterials into polymers. (d) Ag Nanowires doped heater for wearable articular thermotherapy. ([a] Adapted with permission (Di Nardo et al., 2019). Copyright 2019, American Chemical Society. Adapted with permission (Kou et al., 2017). Copyright 2017, AAAS. Adapted with permission (Sapkota et al., 2020). Copyright 2020, Springer Nature. Adapted with permission (Tang et al., 2015). Copyright 2015, Royal Society of Chemistry. Adapted with permission (Liu et al., 2021). Copyright 2021, De Gruyter. Adapted with permission (Duan et al., 2017). Copyright 2017, AAAS; [b] Adapted with permission (Baig et al., 2021). Copyright 2021, Royal Society of Chemistry; [c] Adapted with permission (Wang et al., 2018). Copyright 2018, Wiley-VCH; [d] Adapted with permission (Choi et al., 2015). Copyright 2015, American Chemical Society.)

of Au nanoparticles can be tailored through modification with molecules or functional groups, enabling manipulation of their properties, stability, and reactivity for targeted applications and interactions with biological systems (Di Nardo et al., 2019). Ag nanowires are 1D structures composed of silver atoms arranged in a wire-like configuration. Typically exhibiting diameters ranging from tens to hundreds of nanometres, these wires can vary in length from micrometres to millimetres (Kou et al., 2017). MoS_2 represents an innovative 2D material that holds great promise for flexible electronics applications. Each layer of MoS_2 nanosheets comprises one molybdenum atom sandwiched between two sulphur atoms (Sapkota et al., 2020). ZnO nanoflowers exhibit ultra-small dimensions and possess a significantly large surface area-to-volume ratio due to their petal-like structure, rendering them superior compared to other nanoparticle shapes (Tang et al., 2015).

Fullerenes are a class of carbon molecules characterised by closed-cage structures containing varying numbers of carbon atoms. The most renowned fullerene is buckminsterfullerene (C60), which exhibits a soccer ball–like arrangement of interlocking hexagons and pentagons, composed of 60 carbon atoms (Ehrenfreund & Foing, 2010). CNTs are cylindrical carbon structures that exhibit excellent electrical conductivity and mechanical flexibility. Graphene, on the other hand, is a single-layer hexagonal lattice of carbon atoms with exceptional electrical conductivity, high carrier mobility, and mechanical strength. These properties make graphene an ideal material for flexible electrodes, transparent conductive films, and energy storage devices in soft electronics (Liu et al., 2021). A notable advantage of graphene over CNTs lies in its sheet-like structure which provides a larger surface area for efficient interaction with the surroundings and enables highly effective detection of incoming mass fluxes. To achieve enhanced mass resolution and increased detection surface area, columnar graphene structures supported by vertically aligned CNTs (referred to as CNT pillars) were fabricated (Duan et al., 2017).

1.3.2 Synthesis of Nanomaterials

The synthesis of nanomaterials employs two primary approaches (Figure 1.2b): The top–down method and the bottom–up method (Khanna et al., 2019).

In top–down approaches, bulk materials are segmented to produce nanostructured materials. Mechanical grinding is a cost-effective method for synthesising nanoscale materials from bulk materials. Laser ablation synthesis involves utilising a powerful laser beam to irradiate a target material and generate nanoparticles. The utilisation of laser ablation for the production of noble metal nanoparticles can be considered an environmentally friendly technology as it eliminates the need for stabilisers or other chemicals. The arc discharge method offers a versatile approach to generate various nanostructured materials, particularly carbon-based ones such as fullerenes, CNTs, few-layer graphene, and amorphous spherical carbon nanoparticles.

Nanomaterials can also be synthesised de novo from their atomic and molecular precursors. The bottom–up approach encompasses solution phase synthesis and gas phase synthesis. In the solution phase synthesis, such as the hydrothermal method, nanostructured materials are prepared through heterogeneous reactions in an aqueous medium within a sealed vessel at high pressure and temperature near the critical point. Solvothermal methods share similarities with hydrothermal methods, except that they are conducted in a non-aqueous medium. Hydrothermal and solvothermal methods represent exciting and valuable techniques for fabricating materials with diverse nanogeometries, including nanowires, nanorods, nanosheets, and nanoflowers. The sol–gel method is commonly employed to develop various high-quality metal oxide–based nanomaterials. Chemical vapour deposition (CVD) plays a significant role in generating carbon-based nanomaterials. Atomic layer deposition (ALD) is capable of creating thinner films than CVD even on the sub-nanometre scale while depositing various materials like metals, insulators, and semiconductors. The hard template method (also known as nanocasting) and soft template method can both produce ordered mesoporous materials.

1.3.3 Preparation of Bioelectronics by Incorporating Nanomaterials into Soft Substrates

To prepare soft bioelectronics, conductive nanomaterials need to be integrated into stretchable matrices. Figure 1.2c depicts three methods for achieving this: Hybrid, in situ formation, and implantation (Wang et al., 2018). The blending method involves directly doping polymers with nanomaterials to create conductivity while maintaining tensile properties by adjusting the filler volume fraction; however, this method needs to overcome the problem of nanomaterial aggregation. Synthesising these nanofillers directly within the polymer matrix can help solve this problem by taking advantage of the good miscibility between nanofiller precursors and elastomers. Another effective technology is ion implantation, which embeds conductive nanofillers directly into the surface area of the polymer matrix. By modulating the acceleration voltage, ions penetrate through porous polymer chains and the total implantation depth can be controlled between 10 nm and 1 μm.

Soft bioelectronic devices utilising nanomaterials exhibit a wide range of applications, including wearable and implantable biosensors and stimulators, information displays, power supply devices, and data storage systems. Diverse biosensors have been developed for the detection of electrophysiological signals, electrochemical signals, strain, and pressure, amongst others. Additionally, there have been advancements in implantable sensors and stimulators for brain monitoring, peripheral nerve stimulation as well as cardiac monitoring. For more comprehensive details on these applications, please refer to the subsequent chapters within this publication. Figure 1.2d illustrates a flexible heater fabricated using nanocomposites composed of Ag nanowires and thermoplastic elastomers (Choi et al., 2015). This heater possesses attributes such as softness, thinness, and stretchability enabling effective heat transfer during physical exercise while facilitating long-term continuous joint heat therapy.

1.4 HYDROGELS, CONDUCTIVE POLYMERS, AND ELASTOMERS

Unlike typical metals or inorganic conductors, polymer-based materials such as hydrogels, conductive polymers, and elastomers are organic and can be customised for specific applications, forming the key to soft bioengineered electronics. These materials exhibit mechanical properties akin to those of biological tissues, such as human skin and muscle, and find applications in healthcare management, disease diagnosis, human–machine interfaces, implantable devices, etc.

1.4.1 Hydrogels

Hydrogels are gel-like materials composed primarily of water and a polymer network (Cong et al., 2021; Xu et al., 2018; Yao et al., 2017). Due to their similarity to biological tissues, hydrogels find extensive applications in the field of bioelectronics (Yuk et al., 2019). By incorporating conductive fillers, hydrogels can be rendered conductive (W. Zhang et al., 2023a). The nanocomposite conductive hydrogel, prepared by a one-pot method in the presence of Laponite ® XLG nanosheets (XLG) nanosheet-stabilised CNTs was reported by Shen et al. XLG sheets were utilised as surfactants to uniformly disperse CNTs in an aqueous solution (Shen et al., 2023). P(AM-APBA)XLG/CNTs were obtained through the polymerisation reaction of 3-acrylamide phenylboronic acid and acrylamide with the presence of XLG-dispersed CNTs. The resulting hydrogel exhibited remarkable elasticity and fatigue resistance due to the formation of B–N coordination, hydrogen bonds, and polymer chain entanglements within its network structure. Moreover, the incorporation of XLG and CNT not only significantly enhanced the mechanical properties but also endowed the conductive hydrogel with high sensitivity, excellent sensing accuracy, and rapid response time. Consequently, this multifunctional wearable sensor based on hydrogels can be employed for wound healing process monitoring. The disparity in electrical resistance between the hydrogel-treated wound group and the control group was evident by the third day. By the seventh day, it was observed that the electrical resistance of the wound group had reached parity with that of the control group, suggesting a partial recovery of surface skin wounds within a 7-day timeframe.

In order to enhance the compatibility between conductive fillers and hydrogel matrices, Zhang et al. employed cellulose nanofibre-stabilised liquid metal droplets as initiators for polymerisation while simultaneously serving as solid conductive fillers to fabricate polyacrylamide/MXene/glycerol hydrogels (Figure 1.3a) (2023a). As shown in Figure 1.3c, 2D MXene nanosheets possess abundant functional groups, large lateral dimensions, and excellent conductivity, enabling them to bridge adjacent droplets and establish more efficient conductive pathways. The hydrogel is endowed with exceptional electrical conductivity, temperature sensitivity, photothermal properties, and strain-sensing capabilities through the incorporation of liquid metal and MXene. At the same time, glycerol is used to replace the water in the hydrogel, which can significantly inhibit the formation of ice crystals at low temperatures and reduce the evaporation of water in the open-air environment to a certain extent. The fabricated hydrogel exhibits versatile applications in triboelectric nanogenerators (TENGs), temperature and deformation sensing, as well as photothermal antibacterial materials (Figure 1.3b).

Ionic hydrogels are fabricated by swelling small molecules or polymers with ionic liquids. Despite the generally higher resistance of ionic conductors compared to electronic conductors, they are extensively utilised in research due to the prevalence of ion movement in biological systems. Liu et al. have developed a novel pressure-resistant zwitterionic hydrogel skin sensor for real-time monitoring and promotion of healing in pressure injuries through

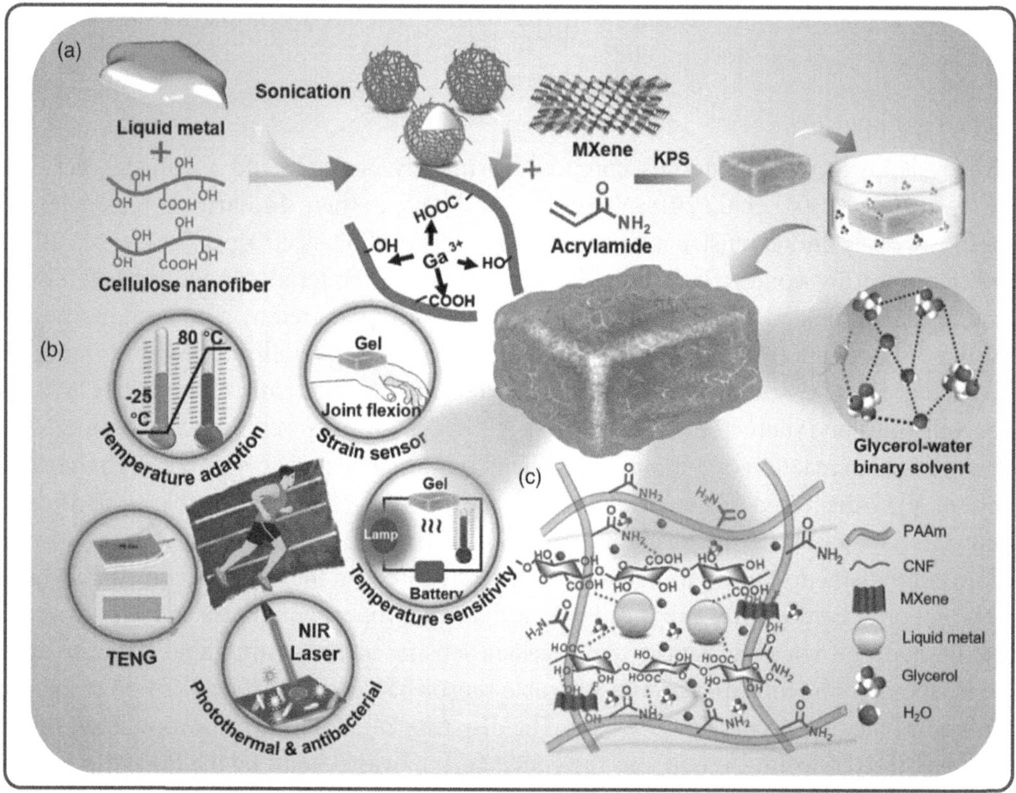

FIGURE 1.3   (a) Preparation of the liquid metal/MXene hydrogel. (b) Supramolecular interaction between the components of the hydrogel. (c) Application of the hydrogel. (Adapted with permission (W. Zhang et al., 2023a). Copyright 2023, Elsevier.)

continuous assessment of temperature, pressure, and exudate indicators (2022). In the zwitterionic hydrogel, silicone nanoparticles (OSNPs) were designed to cross-link copolymers consisting of carboxybetaine methacrylate (CBMA) and 2-hydroxyethyl methacrylate (HEMA). The resulting hydrogel exhibits remarkable pressure resistance owing to the abundance of hydrogen bonds present. This zwitterionic skin sensor demonstrates significant potential for application in domestic health monitoring and care.

1.4.2 Conductive Polymer

Conductive polymers are a class of materials that possess the properties of traditional polymers, such as flexibility and processability, while also exhibiting electrical conductivity (Sekine et al., 2010; S. Wang et al., 2022b; Yuk et al., 2020). This conductivity arises from the presence of conjugated π-bonds or alternating single and double (or triple) covalent bonds within their polymer chains (H. He et al., 2019b; Prunet et al., 2021; Zhao et al., 2021). As depicted in Figure 1.4a, an energy gap (E_g) exists between the top of the valence band and the bottom of the conduction band, resulting in insulating behaviour (Guo & Facchetti, 2020). However, doping polymers can reduce this energy gap and increase carrier density

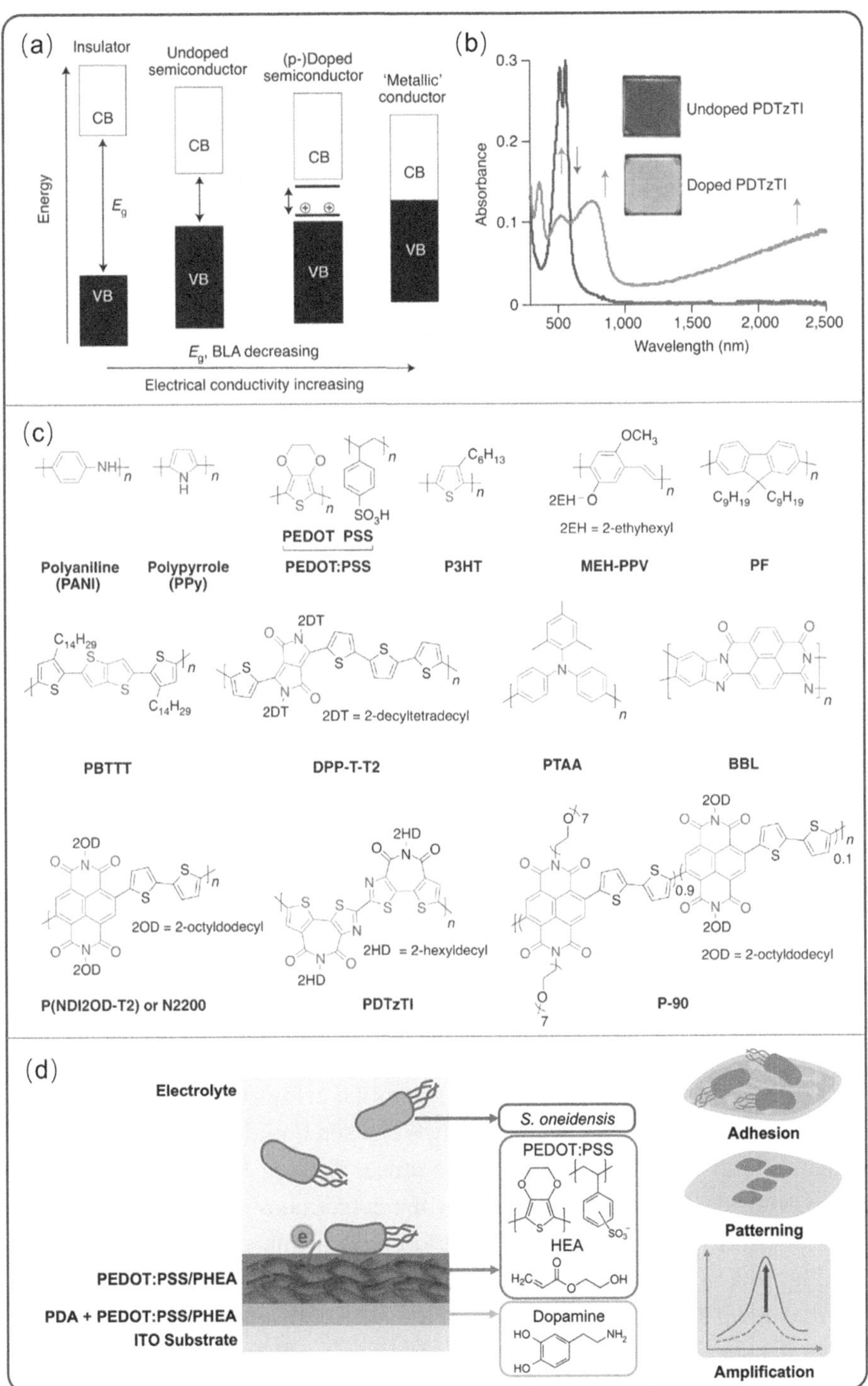

FIGURE 1.4 (a) Mechanism of conductive polymers. (b) Absorption of doped and undoped polymers. (c) Chemical structures of common conducting polymers. (d) Schematic illustration of conductive polymer electrodes for microbial bioelectronics. ([a–c] Adapted with permission (Guo & Facchetti, 2020). Copyright 2020, Springer Nature; [d] Adapted with permission (Tseng et al., 2022). Copyright 2022, Wiley-VCH.)

to achieve varying degrees of semiconducting (or even metallic) behaviour (Figure 1.4a), as well as tune the material's colour (Figure 1.4b). The structures of typically conducting polymers are shown in Figure 1.4c. Polyaniline (PANI) is a well-known example of a conductive polymer, which demonstrates excellent electrical conductivity when appropriately doped. Other conductive polymers include polythiophene, polyacetylene, polypyrrole (PPy), amongst others. These polymers are typically synthesised through chemical processes that enable precise control over their molecular structure and properties. Unlike inorganic semiconductors, where atoms are bound by strong covalent bonds, conductive polymers consist of discrete macromolecules held together by weaker supramolecular π–π interactions, van der Waals forces, and dipolar interactions to form supermolecular assemblies. The arrangement of these assemblies governs the processing performance, optoelectronic properties, and film morphology of the device.

Conductive polymers have garnered significant attention across various disciplines, encompassing electronics, energy storage, sensors, and actuators. Figure 1.4d showcases a novel conductive polymer coating comprising a cross-linked blend of poly(3,4-ethylenedioxythiophene)-poly(styrenesulphonate) (PEDOT:PSS) and poly(2-hydroxyethylacrylate) (PHEA), with an underlying In–Sn oxide (ITO) electrode adhered by a thin layer of polydopamine (PDA) (Tseng et al., 2022). The application of this coating resulted in a substantial increase in current density compared to the unmodified electrode. This innovative coating holds promise for utilisation in microbial fuel cells, multichannel bioelectronic devices, and microbial sensors.

1.4.3 Elastomer

Elastomers are a class of polymer materials that possess rubber-like elasticity and can undergo significant deformation under stress, yet recover their original shape upon the removal of said stress. They exhibit exceptional resilience, efficiently absorbing and dissipating mechanical energy (S. Wang et al., 2022b). The distinctive mechanical properties of elastomers stem from their molecular structure, characterised by highly coiled and entangled long polymer chains that enable them to stretch and recoil akin to springs (Huang et al., 2023). Zhang et al. fabricated a micropyramidal array on the surface of double-sided PDMS elastomer as a dielectric layer, utilising Ga-based liquid metal as an electrode for the development of a flexible capacitive pressure sensor (Figure 1.5b) (2023b). The sensor can be wrapped around the wrist to enable real-time detection of radial artery pressure, facilitating precise control over balloon air injection and ultimately preventing post-operative bleeding (Figure 1.5a). This approach ensures accurate attachment, expeditious haemostasis, and enhanced patient comfort (Figure 1.5c).

Soft hybrid materials that combine the advantages of elastomers and hydrogels have potential applications in areas such as stretchable and biointegrated electronics. Yuk et al. fabricated hybrid materials by assembling preformed elastomers and hydrogels, resulting in strong interfaces and functional microstructures (Figure 1.5d) (2016). First, the shape and microstructure of the tough hydrogel were set through physical cross-linking of its dissipative polymer network. Second, benzophenone modification was applied to the cured elastomer surface to mitigate oxygen inhibition effects and activate it for hydrogel polymer grafting. Third, a mixture of preformed hydrogels and elastomers was assembled, followed

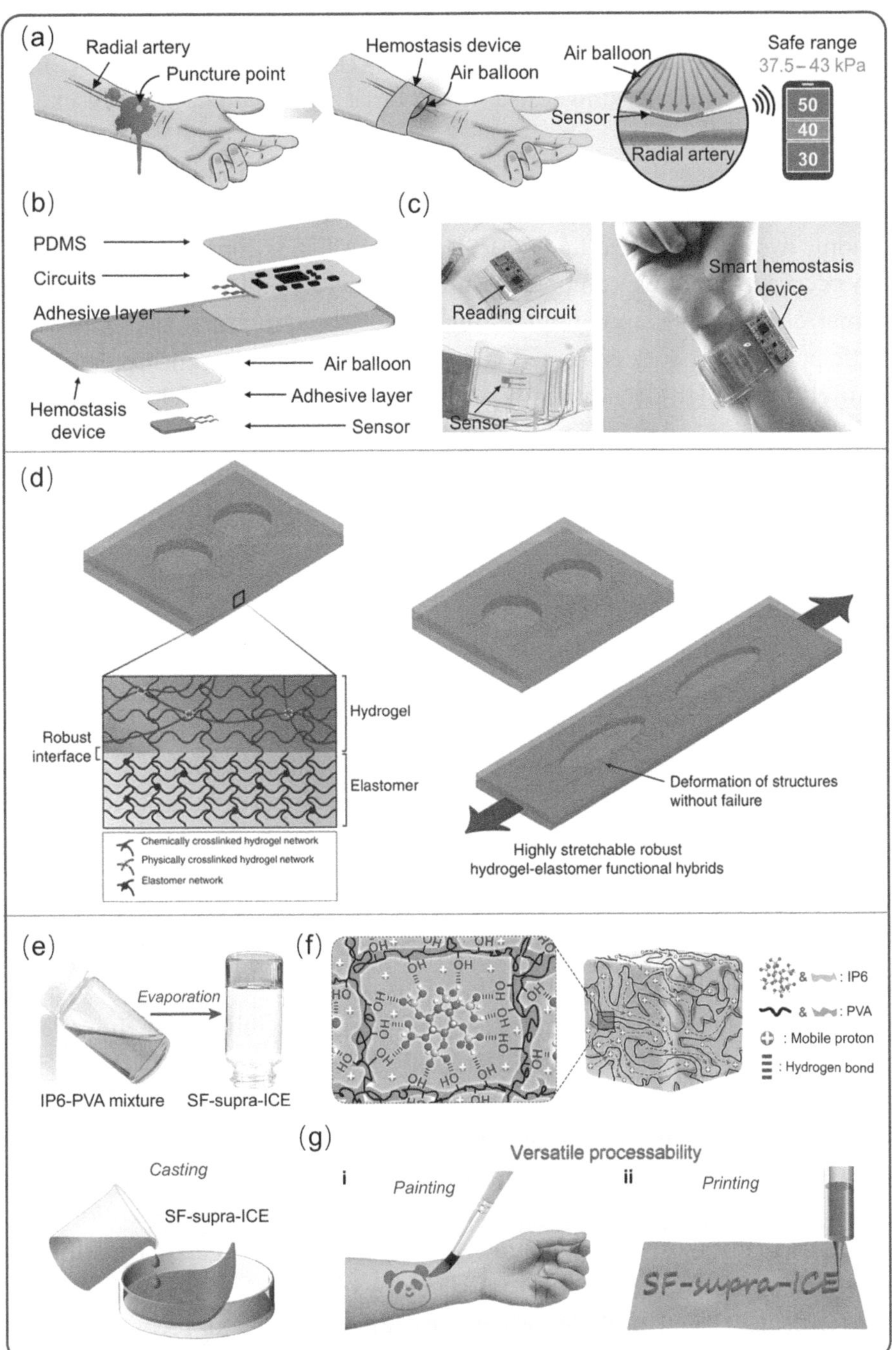

FIGURE 1.5   (a) Schematic diagram of the intelligent haemostasis device. (b) Exploded schematic diagram of the haemostatic device. (c) Image of a smart haemostatic device worn on the wrist. (d) Schematic of a hydrogel–elastomer hybrid with extremely robust interfaces. (e) Preparation of the SF-supra-ICE. (f) Structural diagram of the SF-supra-ICE. (g) Multifunctional processability of the SF-supra-ICE. ([a–c] Adapted with permission (C. Zhang et al., 2023b). Copyright 2023, Wiley-VCH; [d] Adapted with permission (Yuk et al., 2016). Copyright 2016, Springer Nature; [e–g] Adapted with permission (Niu et al., 2023). Copyright 2023, Wiley-VCH.)

by cross-linking and grafting of the elastic polymer network onto the elastomer surface to form an exceptionally robust microstructured interface. The resulting hybrid materials exhibited high stretchability and resistance to large deformations without experiencing microstructural failure.

Niu et al. have developed a solvent-free and biocompatible supramolecular ion-conducting elastomer (SF-supra-ICE) with high ionic conductivity, which overcomes the dehydration issue of ionic hydrogels (Figure 1.5e) (2023). SF-supra-ICE is composed of phytate (IP6), a naturally occurring ionisable compound, and polyvinyl alcohol (PVA), a biocompatible linear polymer, obtained by evaporating/casting a water-based mixture. The solid, dehydrated, and elastic polymer network is formed due to the supramolecular encapsulation of IP6 by PVA chains through high-density hydrogen bonding (Figure 1.5f). High-resolution I-tattoos produced by drawing and printing methods can serve as ultraconformable and stable skin electrodes for long-term recording of various electrophysiological signals with high fidelity (Figure 1.5g).

1.5 ADVANCED STRUCTURES OF SOFT ELECTRONICS FOR BIOMEDICAL ENGINEERING

In addition to the selection of flexible materials, rational structural design can also be employed to fabricate soft electronics, thereby enhancing the stretchability of inherently soft materials and conferring stretchability upon rigid materials. This section will present various structures utilised in bioengineered electronics, including wavy, serpentine, porous, interconnected, origami and kirigami patterns, metasurfaces, as well as 3D architectures (Xu et al., 2015). Furthermore, unique woven and wearable structures such as fibres and textiles will be introduced.

1.5.1 Wavy Structure

The wavy structures, resembling the undulations observed in skin or fabric, possess the ability to undergo out-of-plane bending for strain release, thereby conferring stretchability upon the rigid electrode array (Qi, Liu, Yu, et al., 2015b; Xu et al., 2012; Xu & Zhu, 2012; Xue et al., 2020). Xu et al. ingeniously integrated corrugated CNT strips into an elastomer substrate to fabricate a remarkably stretchable conductor (Xu et al., 2012). Qi, Liu, Liu, et al., on the other hand, employed a tripod-structured PDMS substrate as a platform for transferring graphene microstrips and successfully devised an exceptionally flexible micro-supercapacitor (2015a). The polymer electrode array in Figure 1.6a exhibits a wavy structure, facilitating excellent conformal matching of the electrode–tissue interface with the brain (Qi et al., 2017). This design was successfully employed for recording electrocorticogram signals in rats under normal and epileptic conditions. In this study, the researchers developed a PPy electrode material by integrating PPy nanowires onto a highly conductive PPy electrode array. The incorporation of nanowires introduces a transition layer between the electrodes and substrates, enhancing adhesion, while the PPy films ensure high conductivity and low resistance. The wavy structure not only imparts exceptional stretchability to the electrodes but also reduces the Young's modulus of the entire device compared to flat electrode structures. Consequently, polymer electrode arrays based on wave-structured electrodes are more easily stretched. Moreover, due to their corrugated configuration, these electrodes experience less strain during the stretching/relaxation processes, thereby exhibiting enhanced cycling stability.

1.5.2 Serpentine Structure

The serpentine interconnect features a layout with a serpentine-shaped pattern, comprising numerous periodically distributed unit cells that consist of two semicircles connected by straight lines (Xu et al., 2013). In response to applied strain, the serpentine interconnects can exhibit in-plane rotation or out-of-plane bending, resulting in significantly reduced strain within the serpentine material itself and lower effective stiffness at the system level (Yeo et al., 2013). Figure 1.6b illustrates a graphene-based electrochemical device designed for diabetes monitoring and treatment (Lee et al., 2016). This device comprises three main components: A sweat control component (including a sweat-absorbent layer and waterproof membrane), a sensing component (consisting of humidity, glucose, pH, and tremor sensors), and a treatment component (comprising microneedles, heater, and temperature sensor). The adoption of the serpentine structure ensures mechanical reliability as well as large-area deformability.

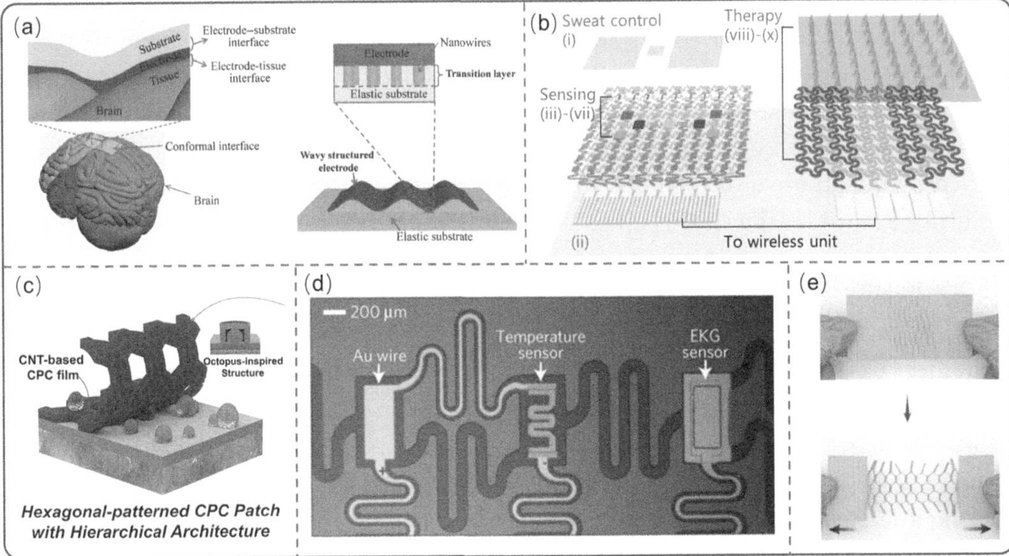

FIGURE 1.6 Structures of soft bioengineering electronics. (a) Wave-like structure. (b) Serpentine structure. (c) Porous structure. (d) Interconnect structure. (e) Kirigami structure. [a] Adapted with permission (Qi et al., 2017). Copyright 2017, Wiley-VCH; [b] Adapted with permission (Lee et al., 2016). Copyright 2016, Springer Nature; [c] Adapted with permission (Min et al., 2020). Copyright 2020, American Chemical Society; [d] Adapted with permission (Kim et al., 2011). Copyright 2011, Springer Nature; [e] Adapted with permission (W. Chen et al., 2021a). Copyright 2021, American Chemical Society.)

1.5.3 Porous Structure

Porous structures composed of flexible materials capable of adapting to strain through volumetric geometric changes within the cartilage scaffold have been introduced to confer flexibility and stretchability to functional materials and substrates, enabling the realisation of flexible devices (Chen et al., 2019; Someya et al., 2005; Wu et al., 2013). Min et al. presented a stretchable conductive polymer composite patch featuring octopus sucker-inspired structures that facilitate conformal contact with biological skin (2020). The patch exhibits a hexagonal mesh structure pattern that ensures both water resistance and breathability (Figure 1.6c). Due to its piezoresistive response being controllable by adjusting the concentration of conductive fillers in the polymerised polyurethane matrix, the patch film is suitable for applications as strain sensors or stretchable electrodes. Specifically, a conductive polymer composite patch incorporating a hexagonal mesh pattern can be easily stretched for use as strain sensors while remaining insensitive to tensile strain, thereby making it an ideal candidate for deployment as a stretchable electrode.

1.5.4 Interconnection Structure

By employing patterning or buckling strategies, individually patterned rigid devices can be interconnected through stretchable electrodes to form integrated systems with stretchable circuits. During stretching, 'soft' interconnects with in-plane or out-of-plane structures can adapt to the applied strain, effectively isolating relatively 'rigid' structures from physical forces that could potentially cause functional failure of delicate components (Ko et al., 2008). Figure 1.6d illustrates the interconnection design featuring a snake-shaped structure composed of gold electrodes connecting micro-LEDs, sensor electrodes, temperature detectors, and other components (Kim et al., 2011). Through an optimised configuration guided by quantitative mechanical modelling, the grid layout demonstrates remarkable resilience against tensile strains up to 200% without fracturing.

1.5.5 Origami and Kirigami Structures

Origami, an ancient art of paper folding that transforms flat sheets into complex 3D structures based on defined patterns of hinged creases, has diverse applications in soft electronics (Guo et al., 2014; Meng et al., 2022; Won et al., 2019). These range from lithium-ion batteries to solar cells, photodetectors, and thermoelectric generators (Guo et al., 2016; Song et al., 2014). Similarly, kirigami is an art that combines paper folding and cutting to create artistic models and has recently emerged as a promising avenue for stretchable electronics. Figure 1.6e displays the most popular stretchable kirigami patterns where patterned slits open to dissipate tensile energy allowing the planar sheet to bend out of the plane perpendicular to the slits (W. Chen et al., 2021a). In this research study, highly stretchable conductive devices are prepared by introducing kirigami patterns into conductive films via laser beam cutting or photolithography resulting in devices suitable for electromagnetic interference (EMI) shielding and pressure sensing.

1.5.6 Cracks

The presence of cracks in materials is typically regarded as a defect resulting from increased induction resistance or potential device failure. However, in the realm of stretchable electronics, strategically controlling the distribution of cracks can yield a percolating conductive mesh that retains its electrical properties even when subjected to stretching (Liu et al., 2014; Yang Zhao et al., 2019b). Zhao et al. reported an interface between bioelectronics and tissue for stimulation and sensing purposes (Zhao et al., 2022). This device employs a three-layer design wherein a strain-induced rupture membrane is coupled with a strain-isolating conductive pathway. Upon reaching an initial pre-strain level of 100%, the brittle solid film on top fractures to dissipate the accumulated strain energy. Nevertheless, this crack facilitates parallel and interconnected charge transport, enabling charge carriers to traverse between layers and bypass the crack.

1.5.7 Metasurface

Metasurfaces are artificial 2D materials comprising subwavelength structures, which facilitate precise control over the electromagnetic fields surrounding the human body (Gollub et al., 2017). This enables the seamless integration of bioelectronic systems with the human body through radio-frequency wireless components (Li et al., 2021). Schmidt et al. fabricated a thin, compact, and flexible metasurface that can be conveniently positioned between the patient and a snugly-fitted array of receiving coils (2017). Such a metasurface exhibits remarkable flexibility and stretchability to ensure comfortable connectivity with the body.

1.5.8 3D Structure

By employing compression buckling, the 2D micro/nanostructure geometry can be transformed into an extended 3D layout, enabling the construction of artificial devices that resemble complex biological structures (Park et al., 2016). These devices hold great potential for diverse bioelectronic applications (Yan et al., 2017). Wang et al. designed a flexible 3D electronic scaffold formed through the geometric transformation of a 2D precursor via compressive buckling (2020a). This scaffold exhibits controlled geometric transformations and allows for various architectures and configurations in virtually any material class, with dimensions ranging from nanometres to centimetres in length. Integration of this scaffold into a thermoresponsive extracellular matrix–based hydrogel could provide structural support for cardiac tissue.

1.5.9 Fibre and Textile

Textiles, being naturally stretchable and indispensable to human life, offer opportunities for the development of wearable devices in soft electronics (W. He et al., 2019a; Liu et al., 2015; H. Wang et al., 2020b). They are typically produced from yarns through weaving or knitting processes, with yarns being prepared from fibres through techniques such as twisting or wrapping (Y. Zhou et al., 2022a). Stretchable conductive fibres can be created using spinning, coating, printing, and thermal drawing methods (Gibson et al., 2021;

Li et al., 2023; Pu et al., 2023; Tat et al., 2022; T. Zhou et al., 2022b). Figure 1.7a illustrates functionalised fibres in various configurations including coaxial structures, twisted arrangements, or parallel alignments (Libanori et al., 2022). For instance, TENG-based coaxial structures can incorporate electrode layers and triboelectric layer encapsulation layers sequentially. In a twisted configuration, the electrode layer can serve as a second fibre entangled with the triboelectric fibre at a specific winding angle. This twisted arrangement enhances interaction between active materials and facilitates the creation of external interfaces. The aforementioned types of fibres can be organised into woven, knitted, or

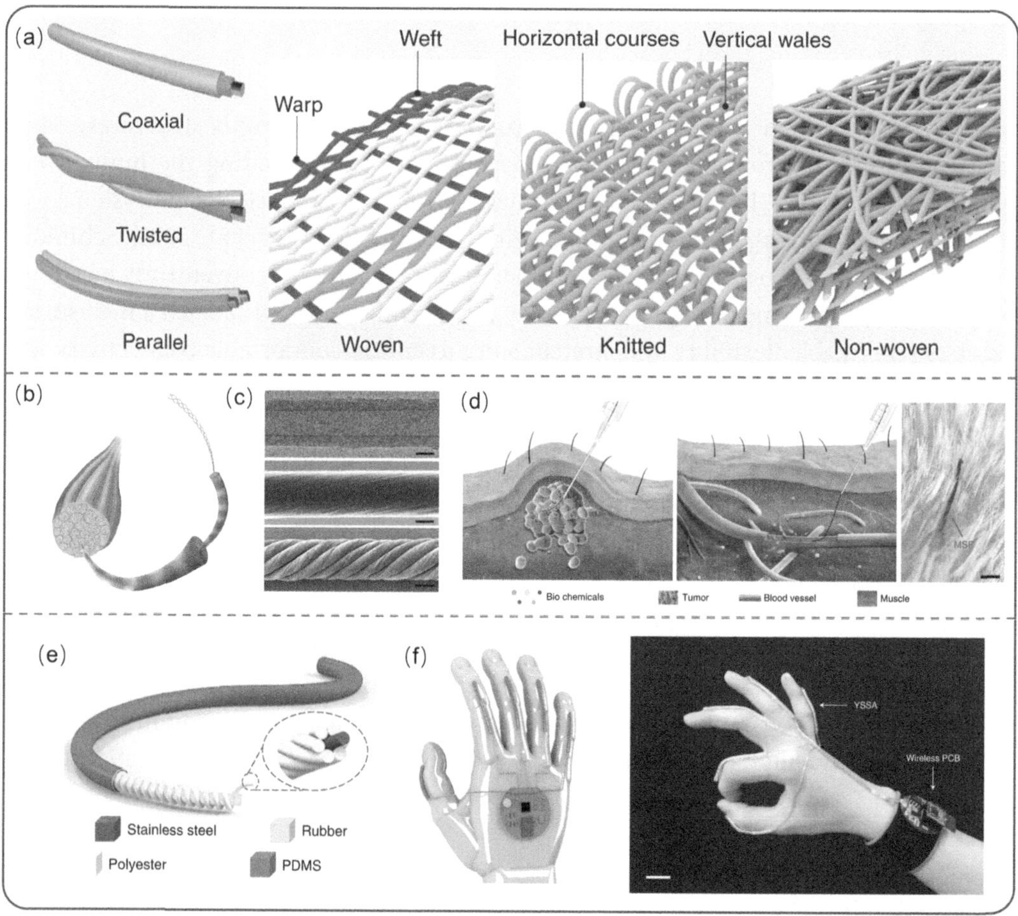

FIGURE 1.7 (a) Structural diagram of fibres and textiles. (b) Schematic of the hierarchical structure of human muscle. (c) SEM images of CNTs and fibre bundles. (d) Schematics showing the injection of the fibre into a human body. (e) Structure of the fibre-based sign language translation system. (f) Diagram and photograph of the system attached to a human hand. Scale bar: 2 cm. ([a] Adapted with permission (Libanori et al., 2022). Copyright 2022, Springer Nature; [b–d] Adapted with permission (L. Wang et al., 2020c). Copyright 2020, Springer Nature; [e, f] Adapted with permission (Zhou et al., 2020). Copyright 2020, Springer Nature.)

non-woven structures to mimic desired traditional textile properties like breathability and flexibility for diverse applications (Figure 1.7a).

Wang et al. fabricated spiral fibre bundles by twisting functionalised multi-walled CNTs, mimicking the layered structure of muscle, enabling monitoring of various disease biomarkers in vivo (Figure 1.7b) (Wang et al., 2020c). The multi-walled CNTs were synthesised via CVD and possessed a diameter ranging from 8 to 15 nanometres (Figure 1.7c). The flexible fibre bundles produced exhibited injectability, low bending stiffness, and demonstrated ultra-low stress under compression (Figure 1.7d). Jeong et al. developed a wearable textile ionic TENG consisting of organic gel and elastomer microtubule structures, which were utilised to promote wound healing (2021). The individual ionic fibres were fabricated by filling the organic gel into microtubules, which could be interwoven to form a single entity resembling satin fabric. The ionic conductivity was achieved by incorporating lithium chloride (LiCl) salt into the organogel. Zhou et al. employed fibre-based stretchable sensor arrays and wireless printed circuit board fibres to construct a wearable sign language translation system (2020). The structural depiction of the fibre is illustrated in Figure 1.7e. The sensing unit's core comprises conductive yarns enveloping rubber microfibres, while the entire structure is encased by a PDMS sleeve. By virtue of its distinctive structural design and utilisation of soft materials, this device can conform to the skin of human fingers during both stretching and releasing motions. Mechanically applied force is converted into periodic electrical signals within the sensing unit, ultimately translating gesture movements into linguistic output (Figure 1.7f).

1.6 SELF-HEALING ELECTRONICS

With the rapid advancement of biomedical electronics, novel structures exhibiting distinctive properties have been developed, including self-healing capabilities, enhanced adhesion, and biodegradable electronics (Baik et al., 2019; Jia et al., 2021; Kang et al., 2019; Kim et al., 2010; Li et al., 2016). These advancements will be discussed individually in subsequent sections. Conventional man-made electronic devices are prone to degradation over time due to factors such as fatigue, corrosion, or operational damage, ultimately leading to device failure (Qi et al., 2023; C. Wang et al., 2022a). To address this issue, self-healing materials have emerged as a promising strategy for constructing mechanically robust and self-repairing soft electronics (Kim et al., 2019; Oh & Bao, 2019). The process of self-healing involves dynamic bond exchange or supramolecular interactions within polymer segments or the controlled release of encapsulated repair agents (Li et al., 2022). In this section, several exemplary self-healing electronic architectures along with their respective applications will be presented.

Tee et al. incorporated micron-sized nickel (μNi) particles into supramolecular polymers, enabling a self-healing mechanism through the dynamic association and dissociation of weak hydrogen bonds within the supramolecular polymer's hydrogen bond network at room temperature (Figure 1.8a) (2012). This passive healing capability is preferentially activated upon mechanical damage events, allowing for fracture surface recovery. The resulting composite material can serve as an electronic skin for pressure and flexion sensing.

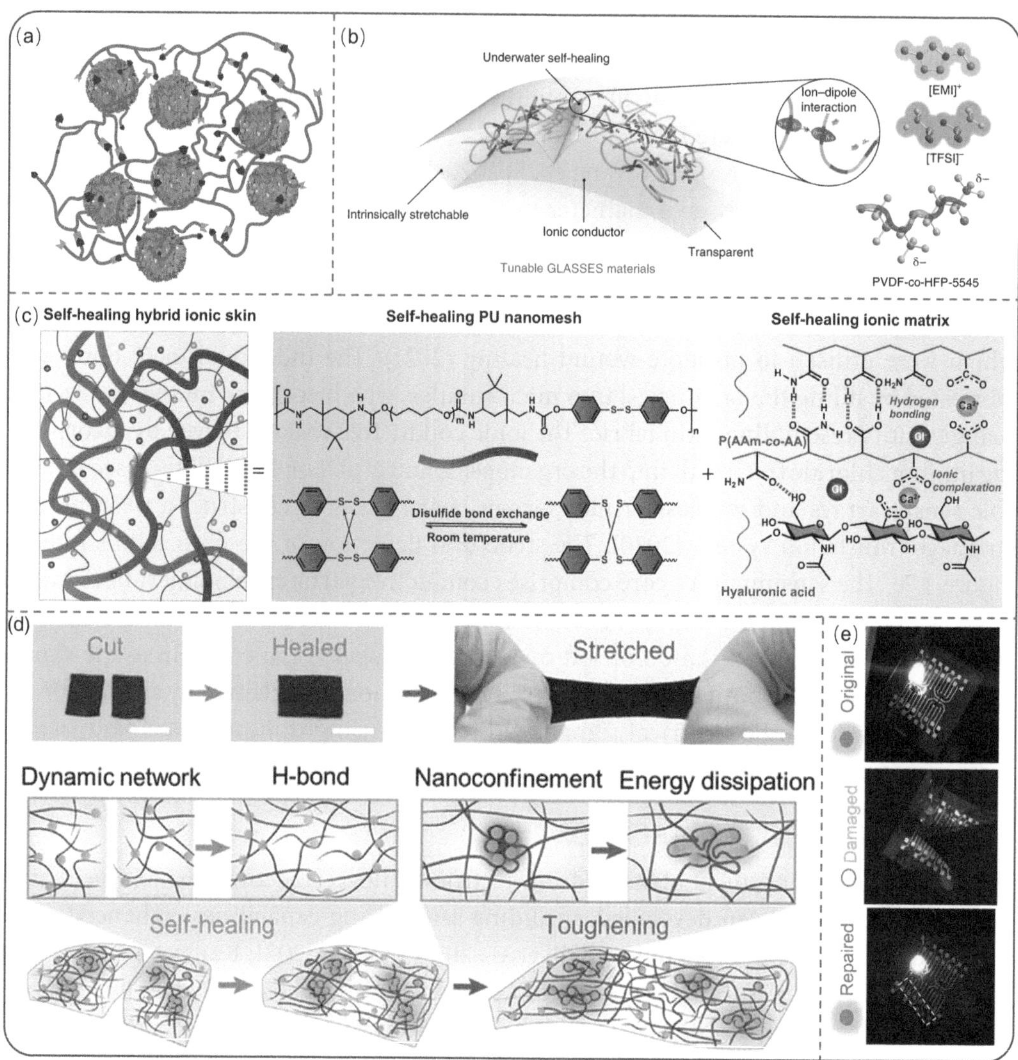

FIGURE 1.8 (a) Schematic diagram of μNi particles doped self-healing conductive polymer. (b) Structure of the self-healing ionic hydrogel for aquatic environments. (c) Schematic illustrations of the fatigue-resistant hybrid ionic hydrogel. (d) Photos and schematics of hydrogel cutting, self-healing, and stretching. (e) Demonstration of functional self-healing of a Ga–In-based flexible circuit. ([a] Adapted with permission (Tee et al., 2012). Copyright 2012, Springer Nature; [b] Adapted with permission (Cao et al., 2019). Copyright 2019, Springer Nature; [c] Adapted with permission (J. Wang et al., 2022c). Copyright 2022, Springer Nature; [d] Adapted with permission (Park et al., 2023). Copyright 2023, Wiley-VCH; [e] Adapted with permission (Fang et al., 2023). Copyright 2023, Wiley-VCH.)

Previous approaches to utilising dynamic bonds for the creation of self-healing materials have predominantly relied on hydrogen bonding and metal–ligand coordination, amongst other strategies. However, these methods face challenges when operating in aquatic conditions due to the versatile nature of water molecules, which can serve as both hydrogen donors/acceptors and ligands. Additionally, polar solvents possess a propensity to bind with most hydrogen bonding sites or metal–ligand coordination sites, thereby diminishing their binding strength. Consequently, this self-healing polymer experiences swelling and a subsequent loss of its repair capability within a water environment. Cao et al. have recently reported on an innovative biomimetic electronic skin that exhibits autonomous self-healing properties in both dry and moist conditions (Cao et al., 2019). This remarkable material comprises a fluorocarbon elastomer combined with a fluorine-rich ionic liquid that facilitates rapid and repeatable electromechanical self-repair even in humid environments characterised by acidic or alkaline conditions owing to ion–dipole interactions (Figure 1.8b).

By incorporating a highly elastic and structurally deformable nanomesh scaffold into a self-healing soft ionic matrix, Wang et al. have successfully developed a fatigue-resistant and fully repairable hybrid ionic hydrogel. The schematic representation of the hydrogel structure is depicted in Figure 1.8c (2022c). The newly prepared nanomesh, fabricated via electrospinning, exhibits remarkable elasticity and forms a flexible fibre network. The self-healing polyurethane (PU) consists of polytetramethylene ether glycol as the soft segment and isophorone diol with an isocyanate/bis(4-hydroxyphenyl)disulphide composition functions as the hard segment. This innovative hybrid design not only enhances fracture energy and fatigue threshold to unprecedented levels but also retains skin-like self-healing ability, softness, stretchability, and strain-hardening behaviour. These materials faithfully replicate the exceptional combination of properties found in natural skin, thereby opening up new avenues for designing durable ion-conducting materials.

In order to confer reliable conductivity to hydrogels, extensive research has been conducted on the incorporation of conductive nanomaterials such as CNTs, graphene, and metallic nanoparticles into hydrogel matrices. However, this approach restricts the dynamic network formation due to weak interactions between the conductive nanomaterials and polymer matrix. To address this limitation, Park et al. have developed a monolithic hydrogel that is inherently non-swellable and incorporates both hydrophilic polymers and functionalised CNTs (2023). Figure 1.8d illustrates a schematic diagram of this multifunctional hydrogel with intrinsic non-swellability. The introduction of carboxyl- and hydroxyl-functionalised CNTs ensures exceptional electrical conductivity in the hydrogel, which can be maintained even under stretching or rupture conditions.

The development of a self-healing bioelectronic patch (iMethy) based on field-effect transistor (FET) technology enables dynamic monitoring of methylated circulating DNA as a prognostic approach for cancer risk management. This innovative approach involves selective wetting of patterned microchannels, mechanical sintering of Ga–In microchannels on the affinity layer, and the utilisation of projection microstereolithography (PµSL) 3D patterning to construct self-healing eutectic Ga–In microfluidic circuits (Fang et al., 2023). Encapsulation of liquid metal within the microchannel networks ensures conductivity even under 100% strain. Additionally, a multilayer composite was fabricated comprising structural, oxide, and Ga–In circuit layers to showcase the inherent self-healing properties of iMethy. Upon being cut and subsequently mechanically reassembled, the circuit undergoes an autonomous healing process to reinstate its normal electrical functionality (Figure 1.8e).

1.7 ADHESIVE ELECTRONICS

Numerous electronics exhibit significant appeal due to their wide-ranging applications in various fields, including electronic skins, wound dressings, and wearable devices. However, the fabrication of electronic materials with both strong adhesion and excellent mechanical properties remains a formidable challenge (Cheng et al., 2022; Han, Lu, Wang, et al., 2017b; Tan et al., 2022; Yamagishi et al., 2021). Mussels possess the ability to secrete adhesive proteins for forming robust adhesive patches that tightly adhere to foreign surfaces in seawater (Liao et al., 2017; Shao et al., 2018; C. Zhang et al., 2020b). Through a combination of non-covalent and covalent chemical interactions with the substrate, mussels can firmly adhere to almost all surfaces regardless of their roughness (Choi et al., 2023). Due to its structural similarity to mussel self-adhesive proteins, PDA with catechol groups exhibits exceptional adhesion to a wide range of surfaces, including both organic and inorganic substrates (Karolina Pierchala et al., 2021). By incorporating a mussel-inspired self-adhesive PDA material into a conductive hydrogel-based soft strain sensor, direct attachment of the strain sensor onto human skin without the need for additional tape is enabled, thereby simplifying practical monitoring processes during surgical procedures.

Han et al. have developed an adhesive and tough polydopamine-clay-polyacrylamide (PDA-clay-PAM) hydrogel using a two-step approach (Figure 1.9a) (2017). Dopamine is incorporated into clay nanosheets and undergoes limited oxidation between layers, resulting in PDA-embedded clay nanosheets containing free catechol groups. Acrylamide monomer is then added and polymerised in situ to form a hydrogel. The resulting hydrogel exhibits reproducible and long-lasting adhesion as well as exceptional toughness, making it an outstanding dressing. A novel biomimetic photonic ion skin (PI-skin) with exceptional adhesion, stability, and elasticity was developed, drawing inspiration from chameleon skin (Sun et al., 2022). This PI-skin is capable of generating synchronised electrical and optical signals under strain (Figure 1.9b). To construct the covalently cross-linked network, a zwitterionic monomer called sulphobetaine methacrylate was employed due to its abundant non-covalent interactions provided by sulphonic acid groups and ammonium cations, which impart appropriate substrate adhesion to the PI-skin. By precisely adjusting the lattice spacing of the photonic crystal, sensitive structural colour changes are exhibited by the PI-skin in tandem with electrical responses. Liao et al. presented a healable adhesive wearable human motion sensor, fabricated using mussel-inspired network hydrogels composed of conductive functionalised single-walled carbon nanotubes (FSWCNTs) and biocompatible PVA (Figure 1.9c) (2017). They successfully prepared a self-adhesive, self-healing, and conductive hybrid hydrogel by controlling the conformal immobilisation of FSWCNT networks through dynamic supramolecular cross-linking between FSWCNTs, PVA, and PDA (Figure 1.9d). Bonded dry electrodes were developed using tannic acid, PVA, and

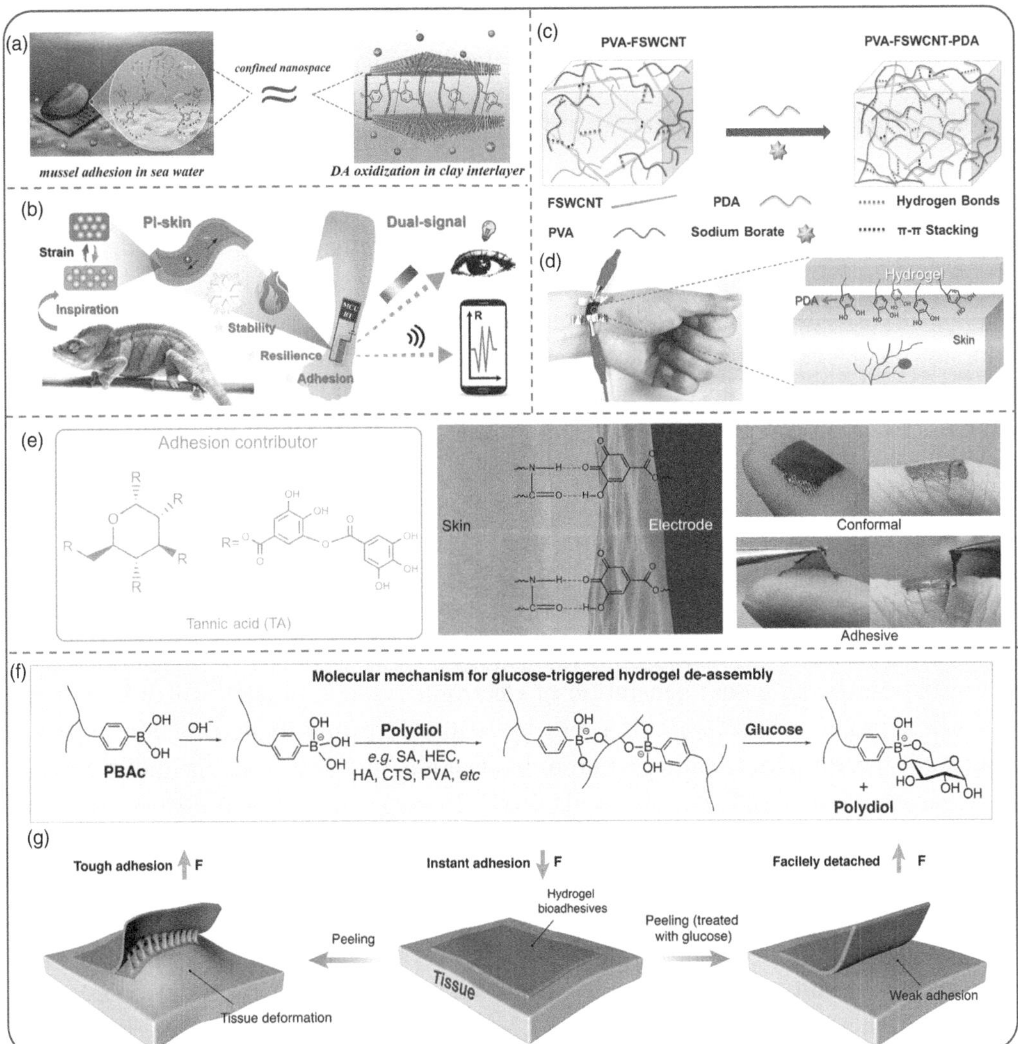

FIGURE 1.9 (a) Schematic of the PDA-clay-PAM hydrogel. (b) Diagram of the biomimetic PI-skin. (c) Schematic of the FSWCNTs-based conductive hybrid hydrogel framework. (d) The hydrogel adheres to the wrist. (e) Chemical structure and photo of the stretchable surface electromyography electrode patch. (f) Mechanisms that trigger removable hydrogel adhesives. (g) Schematic diagram of the trigger-detachable hydrogel adhesive. ([a] Adapted with permission (Han, Lu, Liu, et al., 2017a). Copyright 2017, American Chemical Society; [b] Adapted with permission (Sun et al., 2022). Copyright 2022, Wiley-VCH; [c, d] Adapted with permission (Liao et al., 2017). Copyright 2017, Wiley-VCH; [e] Adapted with permission (Yang et al., 2023). Copyright 2023, Springer Nature; [f, g] Adapted with permission (Xue et al., 2021). Copyright 2021, Wiley-VCH.)

PEDOT:PSS to enhance their performance for long-term usage (Yang et al., 2023). The incorporation of PVA significantly enhances the flexibility of the PEDOT:PSS film, ensuring a better fit on the skin. Additionally, doping TA imparts adhesiveness to the film while further improving its stretchability and compliance (Figure 1.9e).

The separation of reversible adhesion electronics is a critical issue that requires further investigation. Current adhesion layers typically rely on metal ions, heating, ultraviolet irradiation, hydrogen peroxide, or ethylenediaminetetraacetic acid to induce detachment, which may lead to inevitable biological complications. Considering this concern, Xue et al. developed and fabricated a hydrogel bioadhesive capable of instantaneous and robust adhesion as well as triggered detachment upon demand (Xue et al., 2021). The structural depiction of this hydrogel is presented in Figure 1.9f, where hydrogen bonding and chemical cross-linking synergistically contribute to the rapid establishment of strong adhesive properties. By dissociating the boronic acid ester-diol complex from glucose molecules, the overall interface toughness is significantly reduced, enabling benign separation. As illustrated in Figure 1.9g, these bioelectronic devices can be effortlessly detached without causing any harm, trauma, or discomfort to the skin tissues or organs.

1.8 BIODEGRADABLE ELECTRONICS

Given the escalating global generation of electronic waste (e-waste), which is projected to reach approximately 74.7 million tons by 2030, addressing its detrimental impact on ecosystems necessitates the integration of biodegradability as a fundamental attribute in novel electronic materials (Ghosh et al., 2022). In response to this pressing issue, there is an urgent demand for transient electronics composed of ingestible and biodegradable substances, such as cellulose, silk, gelatin, or other natural polymers that exhibit biocompatibility (Hwang et al., 2014; Song et al., 2023; C. Wang et al., 2019b). These materials are selected based on their capacity to undergo decomposition in response to moisture, heat, or enzymes present in the surrounding environment. Biodegradable electronics exhibit promising potential in the field of medicine, as exemplified by implantable medical devices crafted from biodegradable materials that could obviate the necessity for subsequent surgical removal (Lei et al., 2017). Biodegradable electronics also prove particularly advantageous for temporary applications where short-term electronic functionality is required, such as environmental monitoring systems, agricultural sensors, or disposable consumer electronics.

Hwang et al. presented a suite of silicon-based complementary metal oxide semiconductor devices and implantable transient devices for programmable non-antibiotic biocides, which exhibit a medically useful lifespan before undergoing complete absorption by the body (Hwang et al., 2012). All materials utilised in transient electronics consist of Si, Mg, MgO/SiO_2, and Silk. Porous Si and Si nanoparticles have been widely acknowledged as promising candidates for bioabsorbable drug delivery applications. Mg and Mg alloys have demonstrated utility in biodegradable stents, while silk is approved for clinical use in absorbable surgical sutures and soft tissue scaffolds. All components including inductors, capacitors, resistors, substrates, and packages decompose and dissolve upon immersion in deionised (DI) water.

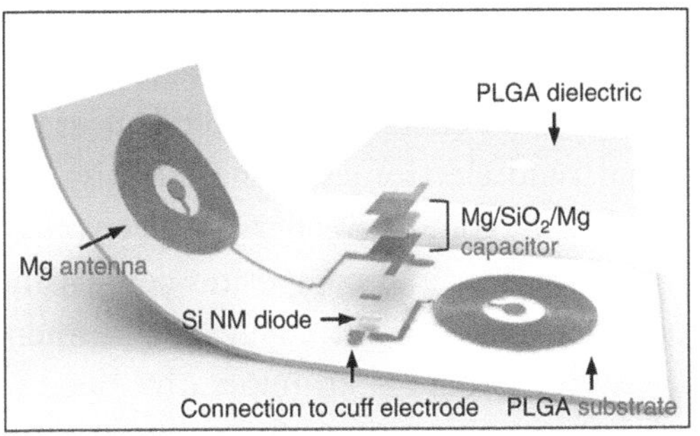

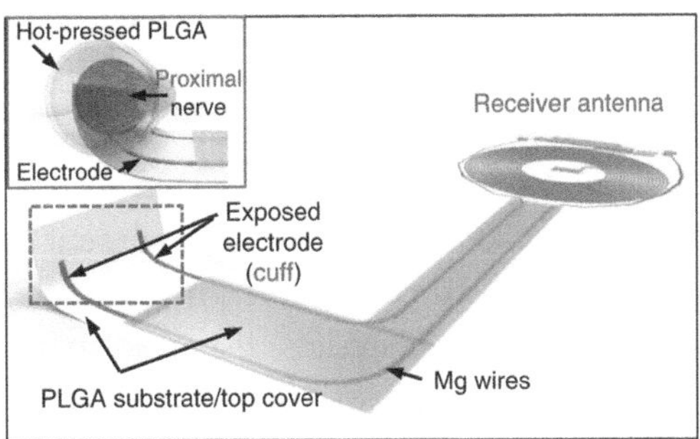

FIGURE 1.10 Structure design of the wireless bioresorbable electronic system. (Adapted with permission (Koo et al., 2018). Copyright 2018, Springer Nature.)

MacEwan presented a wireless, programmable electrical peripheral nerve stimulation platform composed of fully bioabsorbable and biocompatible circuit components and substrates (Koo et al., 2018). Figure 1.10 illustrates the device structure, comprising a Mg loop antenna and a polylactic glycolic acid (PLGA) dielectric sandwich, a doped Si nanofilm-based radio-frequency diode with Mg electrodes, as well as silicon dioxide dielectric above and parallel plate capacitors below utilising Mg conductive planes. When exposed to biological fluids in the subcutaneous tissue vicinity, the constituent materials undergo controlled bioresorption within a defined timeframe.

Ghosh et al. developed a high-performance ionic biogel device with a three-dimensional (3D) microstructure design using ionically cross-linked gelatin derived from biomass resources (2022). Due to their cost-effectiveness, rapid degradation, and edible properties, gelatin-based hydrogels are considered promising candidates for biodegradable electronics. By incorporating ionic liquids into gelatin, stretchable hydrogels known as ionic biogels were prepared. To enhance stretchability while maintaining modulus, the researchers employed a 3D microstructural design in the fabrication of the ionic biogels. The resulting 3D microstructured ion biogel featured interlocking micropyramidal layers covered by microdomed layers. The TENG based on this 3D ion biogel exhibited exceptional power output, superior energy conversion efficiency, and high-resolution mechanical force sensing capabilities. Furthermore, when used as an electronic skin in a phosphate-buffered saline (PBS) solution at 37°C, the ionic biogel degraded within one hour to support ecological balance.

1.9 ENHANCING PROPERTY AND PERFORMANCE THROUGH MATERIAL- AND STRUCTURE-BASED APPROACHES

Enhanced property and performance of bioelectronics necessitate improvements in sensitivity, specificity, stability, biocompatibility, and integration with biological systems. Achieving this objective demands a substantial interdisciplinary endeavour encompassing advancements in materials science, bioengineering, electronic device/system manufacturing, and chemistry. Herein lie several strategies and techniques that can be employed to accomplish these enhancements.

From a chemical perspective, there exist numerous opportunities to enhance the bio-compatibility, biomechanical properties, and electronic/optoelectronic characteristics of bioelectronics devices. First, the conductivity of stretchable conductors in soft devices has remained relatively low compared to conventional rigid electronics. Consequently, it is imperative to explore the development of more highly conductive flexible electronics, including doped conductive polymers. Second, the patterning of composites comprising functional filler materials dispersed in a soft polymer matrix at extremely small dimensions may give rise to non-uniformity issues. Therefore, there is an imperative need to further advance nanoscale materials and optimise their uniform dispersion within polymer matrices. Third, surface treatments have the potential to enhance the quality of the device–tissue interface by mitigating fouling, minimising immune responses, and facilitating seamless integration with biological tissues. Additionally, soft bioelectronics can be endowed with other therapeutic functionalities such as controlled drug delivery.

Another approach involves optimising the selection of materials. For instance, combining materials with similar chemical compositions but distinct functionalities can be employed to create devices that surpass the capabilities of any single material. Additionally, incorporating a combination of materials with diverse chemistries can either mitigate weaknesses or provide multiple functions in the resulting device. For example, by employing periodic space-filling convex polyhedra interconnected by elastic hinges on rigid substrates, 3D reconfigurable building materials capable of manifesting diverse responses can be realised. Through adjusting the composition of the infill units, these adaptable materials exhibit distinct responses and degrees of freedom in various deformation modes, enabling them to effectively adapt to dynamic environments.

From a structural design perspective, the performance of bioengineered electronics can be further enhanced. For instance, conventional flexible stretchable materials often fail to withstand significant deformations under extreme conditions due to inherent structural limitations. However, by leveraging metamaterials with exceptional properties that surpass those achievable through material design alone, such challenges can be overcome. The integration of advanced manufacturing techniques at the micro/nanoscale enables the creation of complex metamaterials tailored for specific functionalities and facilitates the miniaturisation of electronic devices. Additionally, origami or kirigami-inspired approaches allow for transforming 2D flat paper into predefined 3D sculptures, thereby yielding stretchable platforms capable of enduring substantial deformations. Drawing inspiration from biological systems empowers designers to mimic natural structures, processes, and functions in order to enhance the performance of bioelectronic devices. For instance, biomimetic strategies inspired by various natural structures like octopus suckers, gecko feet, beetle pads, and slug foot pads provide robust adhesion even on wet surfaces – a characteristic that holds promise for developing resilient adhesives adaptable to rapid environmental changes when combined with material modification and thoughtful structural design.

1.10 CONCLUSION

In this chapter, we provide a comprehensive overview of the materials and structures employed in bioengineered soft electronics. From a materials perspective, we present liquid metals, nanomaterials, hydrogels, conductive polymers, and elastomers in terms of their fundamental concepts, unique properties, and diverse applications. Regarding the structural aspects, we introduce various architectures including waves, cracks, porous structures, serpentine patterns, origami and kirigami-inspired designs, metasurfaces composed of engineered nanostructures as well as fibres and textiles. Additionally highlighted are advanced bioelectronic structures such as self-healing devices with intrinsic repair capabilities along with adhesive and biodegradable electronics that offer promising solutions for biomedical applications. Finally, this chapter discusses strategies for enhancing the performance of soft bioelectronics through materials and structural design.

There are still several pressing challenges in the development of soft bioelectronics. First, it is crucial to develop optimised manufacturing techniques for soft materials due to their inherent incompatibility with traditional methods. For instance, many elastomers and hydrogels tend to swell or degrade when exposed to organic solvents and etchants. Additionally, plasma-based thin film deposition can cause damage to delicate organic materials through ion bombardment during plasma treatment. Therefore, novel dry patterning methods, low-temperature deposition techniques, and plasma-free manufacturing processes that are compatible with soft materials need to be developed. Second, reinforcing the interfaces between device components is essential to prevent slipping and separation during stretching. It is imperative that the mechanical compatibility of different component materials is ensured. Third, power supply remains a major challenge for soft electronic systems as it serves as a common bottleneck for all power-dependent devices. Current solutions for providing power in soft electronics do not yet meet the long-term power requirements necessary for their operation. Finally, further optimisation of system performance and integration of devices are required by leveraging cutting-edge scientific and technological advancements such as algorithms, machine learning, and wireless charging technologies. This will enhance the advanced capabilities of implantable bioelectronics enabling them to adapt effectively to complex microenvironments inside the human body. Overall, the field of bioengineering electronics is experiencing significant growth, and this chapter foresees an imminent shift in electronic engineering from rigid to stretchable electronics.

REFERENCES

Aukarasereenont, P., Goff, A., Nguyen, C. K., McConville, C. F., Elbourne, A., Zavabeti, A., & Daeneke, T. (2022). Liquid metals: An ideal platform for the synthesis of two-dimensional materials. *Chemical Society Reviews, 51*(4), 1253–1276.

Babatain, W., Kim, M. S., & Hussain, M. M. (2023). From droplets to devices: Recent advances in liquid metal droplet enabled electronics. *Advanced Functional Materials*, 2308116. https://doi.org/10.1002/adfm.202308116

Baig, N., Kammakakam, I., & Falath, W. (2021). Nanomaterials: A review of synthesis methods, properties, recent progress, and challenges. *Materials Advances, 2*(6), 1821–1871.

Baik, S., Lee, H. J., Kim, D. W., Kim, J. W., Lee, Y., & Pang, C. (2019). Bioinspired adhesive architectures: From skin patch to integrated bioelectronics. *Advanced Materials, 31*(34), 1803309.

Cao, Y., Tan, Y. J., Li, S., Lee, W. W., Guo, H., Cai, Y., Wang, C., & Tee, B. C. K. (2019). Self-healing electronic skins for aquatic environments. *Nature Electronics, 2*(2), 75–82.

Chen, D., & Pei, Q. (2017). Electronic muscles and skins: A review of soft sensors and actuators. *Chemical Reviews, 117*(17), 11239–11268.

Chen, J., Zhu, Y., Chang, X., Pan, D., Song, G., Guo, Z., & Naik, N. (2021c). Recent progress in essential functions of soft electronic skin. *Advanced Functional Materials, 31*(42), 2104686.

Chen, M., Wang, Z., Li, K., Wang, X., & Wei, L. (2021b). Elastic and stretchable functional fibers: A review of materials, fabrication methods, and applications. *Advanced Fiber Materials, 3*, 1–13.

Chen, S., Fan, S., Qi, J., Xiong, Z., Qiao, Z., Wu, Z., Yeo, J. C., & Lim, C. T. (2023). Ultrahigh strain-insensitive integrated hybrid electronics using highly stretchable bilayer liquid metal based conductor. *Advanced Materials, 35*(5), 2208569.

Chen, S., Jiang, J., Xu, F., & Gong, S. (2019). Crepe cellulose paper and nitrocellulose membrane-based triboelectric nanogenerators for energy harvesting and self-powered human-machine interaction. *Nano Energy, 61*, 69–77.

Chen, S., Wang, H.-Z., Zhao, R.-Q., Rao, W., & Liu, J. (2020). Liquid metal composites. *Matter, 2*(6), 1446–1480.

Chen, W., Liu, L.-X., Zhang, H.-B., & Yu, Z.-Z. (2021a). Kirigami-inspired highly stretchable, conductive, and hierarchical Ti3C2T x MXene films for efficient electromagnetic interference shielding and pressure sensing. *ACS Nano, 15*(4), 7668–7681.

Cheng, J., Shang, J., Yang, S., Dou, J., Shi, X., & Jiang, X. (2022). Wet-adhesive elastomer for liquid metal-based conformal epidermal electronics. *Advanced Functional Materials, 32*(25), 2200444.

Chiang, C.-H., Won, S. M., Orsborn, A. L., Yu, K. J., Trumpis, M., Bent, B., Wang, C., Xue, Y., Min, S., & Woods, V. (2020). Development of a neural interface for high-definition, long-term recording in rodents and nonhuman primates. *Science Translational Medicine, 12*(538), eaay4682.

Cho, K. W., Sunwoo, S.-H., Hong, Y. J., Koo, J. H., Kim, J. H., Baik, S., Hyeon, T., & Kim, D.-H. (2022). Soft bioelectronics based on nanomaterials. *Chemical Reviews, 122*(5), 5068–5143.

Choi, H., Kim, Y., Kim, S., Jung, H., Lee, S., Kim, K., Han, H.-S., Kim, J. Y., Shin, M., & Son, D. (2023). Adhesive bioelectronics for sutureless epicardial interfacing. *Nature Electronics, 6*, 779–789.

Choi, S., Park, J., Hyun, W., Kim, J., Kim, J., Lee, Y. B., Song, C., Hwang, H. J., Kim, J. H., & Hyeon, T. (2015). Stretchable heater using ligand-exchanged silver nanowire nanocomposite for wearable articular thermotherapy. *ACS Nano, 9*(6), 6626–6633.

Cole, T., Khoshmanesh, K., & Tang, S.-Y. (2021). Liquid metal enabled biodevices. *Advanced Intelligent Systems, 3*(7), 2000275.

Cong, J., Fan, Z., Pan, S., Tian, J., Lian, W., Li, S., Wang, S., Zheng, D., Miao, C., & Ding, W. (2021). Polyacrylamide/Chitosan-based conductive double network hydrogels with outstanding electrical and mechanical performance at low temperatures. *ACS Applied Materials & Interfaces, 13*(29), 34942–34953.

Di Nardo, F., Cavalera, S., Baggiani, C., Giovannoli, C., & Anfossi, L. (2019). Direct vs mediated coupling of antibodies to gold nanoparticles: The case of salivary cortisol detection by lateral flow immunoassay. *ACS Applied Materials & Interfaces, 11*(36), 32758–32768.

Dickey, M. D. (2017). Stretchable and soft electronics using liquid metals. *Advanced Materials, 29*(27), 1606425.

Duan, K., Li, L., Hu, Y., & Wang, X. (2017). Pillared graphene as an ultra-high sensitivity mass sensor. *Scientific Reports, 7*(1), 14012.

Ehrenfreund, P., & Foing, B. H. (2010). Fullerenes and cosmic carbon. *Science, 329*(5996), 1159–1160.

Fang, P., Ji, X., Zhao, X., Yan-Do, R., Wan, Y., Wang, Y., Zhang, Y., & Shi, P. (2023). Self-healing electronics for prognostic monitoring of methylated circulating tumor DNAs. *Advanced Materials, 35*(5), 2207282.

Fang, Y., Meng, L., Prominski, A., Schaumann, E. N., Seebald, M., & Tian, B. (2020). Recent advances in bioelectronics chemistry. *Chemical Society Reviews, 49*(22), 7978–8035.

Ghosh, S. K., Kim, M. P., Na, S., Lee, Y., Park, J., Cho, S., Cho, J., Kim, J. J., & Ko, H. (2022). Ultra-stretchable yet tough, healable, and biodegradable triboelectric devices with microstructured and ionically crosslinked biogel. *Nano Energy, 100*, 107438.

Gibson, U. J., Wei, L., & Ballato, J. (2021). Semiconductor core fibres: Materials science in a bottle. *Nature Communications, 12*(1), 3990.

Gollub, J., Yurduseven, O., Trofatter, K. P., Arnitz, D., F.M. Imani, Sleasman, T., Boyarsky, M., Rose, A., Pedross-Engel, A., & Odabasi, H. (2017). Large metasurface aperture for millimeter wave computational imaging at the human-scale. *Scientific Reports, 7*(1), 42650.

Gu, L., Poddar, S., Lin, Y., Long, Z., Zhang, D., Zhang, Q., Shu, L., Qiu, X., Kam, M., & Javey, A. (2020). A biomimetic eye with a hemispherical perovskite nanowire array retina. *Nature, 581*(7808), 278–282.

Guo, C. F., Sun, T., Liu, Q., Suo, Z., & Ren, Z. (2014). Highly stretchable and transparent nanomesh electrodes made by grain boundary lithography. *Nature Communications, 5*(1), 3121.

Guo, H., Yeh, M.-H., Lai, Y.-C., Zi, Y., Wu, C., Wen, Z., Hu, C., & Wang, Z. L. (2016). All-in-one shape-adaptive self-charging power package for wearable electronics. *ACS Nano, 10*(11), 10580–10588.

Guo, R., Sun, X., Yuan, B., Wang, H., & Liu, J. (2019). Magnetic liquid metal (Fe-EGaIn) based multifunctional electronics for remote self-healing materials, degradable electronics, and thermal transfer printing. *Advanced Science, 6*(20), 1901478.

Guo, X., & Facchetti, A. (2020). The journey of conducting polymers from discovery to application. *Nature Materials, 19*(9), 922–928.

Han, B., Huang, Y., Li, R., Peng, Q., Luo, J., Pei, K., Herczynski, A., Kempa, K., Ren, Z., & Gao, J. (2014). Bio-inspired networks for optoelectronic applications. *Nature Communications, 5*(1), 5674.

Han, L., Lu, X., Liu, K., Wang, K., Fang, L., Weng, L.-T., Zhang, H., Tang, Y., Ren, F., & Zhao, C. (2017a). Mussel-inspired adhesive and tough hydrogel based on nanoclay confined dopamine polymerization. *ACS Nano, 11*(3), 2561–2574.

Han, L., Lu, X., Wang, M., Gan, D., Deng, W., Wang, K., Fang, L., Liu, K., Chan, C. W., & Tang, Y. (2017b). A mussel-inspired conductive, self-adhesive, and self-healable tough hydrogel as cell stimulators and implantable bioelectronics. *Small, 13*(2), 1601916.

Hao, X. P., Li, C. Y., Zhang, C. W., Du, M., Ying, Z., Zheng, Q., & Wu, Z. L. (2021). Self-shaping soft electronics based on patterned hydrogel with stencil-printed liquid metal. *Advanced Functional Materials, 31*(47), 2105481.

He, H., Zhang, L., Guan, X., Cheng, H., Liu, X., Yu, S., Wei, J., & Ouyang, J. (2019b). Biocompatible conductive polymers with high conductivity and high stretchability. *ACS Applied Materials & Interfaces, 11*(29), 26185–26193.

He, W., Wang, C., Wang, H., Jian, M., Lu, W., Liang, X., Zhang, X., Yang, F., & Zhang, Y. (2019a). Integrated textile sensor patch for real-time and multiplex sweat analysis. *Science Advances, 5*(11), eaax0649.

Herbert, R., Kim, J.-H., Kim, Y. S., Lee, H. M., & Yeo, W.-H. (2018). Soft material-enabled, flexible hybrid electronics for medicine, healthcare, and human-machine interfaces. *Materials, 11*(2), 187.

Hirsch, A., Dejace, L., Michaud, H. O., & Lacour, S.P. (2019). Harnessing the rheological properties of liquid metals to shape soft electronic conductors for wearable applications. *Accounts of Chemical Research, 52*(3), 534–544.

Huang, Y., Peng, C., Li, Y., Yang, Y., & Feng, W. (2023). Elastomeric polymers for conductive layers of flexible sensors: Materials, fabrication, performance, and applications. *Aggregate, 4*(4), e319.

Hwang, S. W., Song, J. K., Huang, X., Cheng, H., Kang, S. K., Kim, B. H., Kim, J. H., Yu, S., Huang, Y., & Rogers, J. A. (2014). High-performance biodegradable/transient electronics on biodegradable polymers. *Advanced Materials, 26*(23), 3905–3911.

Hwang, S.-W., Tao, H., Kim, D.-H., Cheng, H., Song, J.-K., Rill, E., Brenckle, M. A., Panilaitis, B., Won, S. M., & Kim, Y.-S. (2012). A physically transient form of silicon electronics. *Science, 337*(6102), 1640–1644.

Jeong, S.-H., Lee, Y., Lee, M.-G., Song, W. J., Park, J.-U., & Sun, J.-Y. (2021). Accelerated wound healing with an ionic patch assisted by a triboelectric nanogenerator. *Nano Energy, 79*, 105463.

Jia, Z., Lv, X., Hou, Y., Wang, K., Ren, F., Xu, D., Wang, Q., Fan, K., Xie, C., & Lu, X. (2021). Mussel-inspired nanozyme catalyzed conductive and self-setting hydrogel for adhesive and antibacterial bioelectronics. *Bioactive Materials, 6*(9), 2676–2687.

Kang, J., Tok, J. B.-H., & Bao, Z. (2019). Self-healing soft electronics. *Nature Electronics, 2*(4), 144–150.

Karolina Pierchala, M., Kadumudi, F. B., Mehrali, M., Zsurzsan, T.-G., Kempen, P. J., Serdeczny, M. P., Spangenberg, J., Andresen, T. L., & Dolatshahi-Pirouz, A. (2021). Soft electronic materials with combinatorial properties generated via mussel-inspired chemistry and halloysite nanotube reinforcement. *ACS Nano, 15*(6), 9531–9549.

Khanna, P., Kaur, A., & Goyal, D. (2019). Algae-based metallic nanoparticles: Synthesis, characterization and applications. *Journal of Microbiological Methods, 163*, 105656.

Kim, C.-C., Lee, H.-H., Oh, K. H., & Sun, J.-Y. (2016). Highly stretchable, transparent ionic touch panel. *Science, 353*(6300), 682–687.

Kim, D.-H., Lu, N., Ghaffari, R., Kim, Y.-S., Lee, S. P., Xu, L., Wu, J., Kim, R.-H., Song, J., Liu, Z., Viventi, J., de Graff, B., Elolampi, B., Mansour, M., Slepian, M. J., Hwang, S., Moss, J. D., Won, S.-M., Huang, Y., … Rogers, J. A. (2011). Materials for multifunctional balloon catheters with capabilities in cardiac electrophysiological mapping and ablation therapy. *Nature Materials, 10*(4), 316–323.

Kim, D.-H., Viventi, J., Amsden, J. J., Xiao, J., Vigeland, L., Kim, Y.-S., Blanco, J. A., Panilaitis, B., Frechette, E. S., & Contreras, D. (2010). Dissolvable films of silk fibroin for ultrathin conformal bio-integrated electronics. *Nature Materials, 9*(6), 511–517.

Kim, M., Lim, H., & Ko, S. H. (2023). Liquid metal patterning and unique properties for next-generation soft electronics. *Advanced Science, 10*(6), 2205795.

Kim, S. H., Seo, H., Kang, J., Hong, J., Seong, D., Kim, H.-J., Kim, J., Mun, J., Youn, I., & Kim, J. (2019). An ultrastretchable and self-healable nanocomposite conductor enabled by autonomously percolative electrical pathways. *ACS Nano, 13*(6), 6531–6539.

Ko, H. C., Stoykovich, M. P., Song, J., Malyarchuk, V., Choi, W. M., Yu, C.-J., Geddes, J. B., Xiao, J., Wang, S., Huang, Y., & Rogers, J. A. (2008). A hemispherical electronic eye camera based on compressible silicon optoelectronics. *Nature, 454*(7205), 748–753.

Koo, J., MacEwan, M. R., Kang, S.-K., Won, S. M., Stephen, M., Gamble, P., Xie, Z., Yan, Y., Chen, Y.-Y., & Shin, J. (2018). Wireless bioresorbable electronic system enables sustained nonpharmacological neuroregenerative therapy. *Nature Medicine, 24*(12), 1830–1836.

Kou, P., Yang, L., Chang, C., & He, S. (2017). Improved flexible transparent conductive electrodes based on silver nanowire networks by a simple sunlight illumination approach. *Scientific Reports, 7*(1), 42052.

Lee, H., Choi, T. K., Lee, Y. B., Cho, H. R., Ghaffari, R., Wang, L., Choi, H. J., Chung, T. D., Lu, N., Hyeon, T., Choi, S. H., & Kim, D.-H. (2016). A graphene-based electrochemical device with thermoresponsive microneedles for diabetes monitoring and therapy. *Nature Nanotechnology, 11*(6), 566–572.

Lee, Y.-H., Kim, J.-S., Noh, J., Lee, I., Kim, H. J., Choi, S., Seo, J., Jeon, S., Kim, T.-S., & Lee, J.-Y. (2013). Wearable textile battery rechargeable by solar energy. *Nano Letters, 13*(11), 5753–5761.

Lei, T., Guan, M., Liu, J., Lin, H.-C., Pfattner, R., Shaw, L., McGuire, A. F., Huang, T.-C., Shao, L., & Cheng, K.-T. (2017). Biocompatible and totally disintegrable semiconducting polymer for ultrathin and ultralightweight transient electronics. *Proceedings of the National Academy of Sciences, 114*(20), 5107–5112.

Li, B., Cao, P.-F., Saito, T., & Sokolov, A. P. (2022). Intrinsically self-healing polymers: From mechanistic insight to current challenges. *Chemical Reviews, 123*(2), 701–735.

Li, C.-H., Wang, C., Keplinger, C., Zuo, J.-L., Jin, L., Sun, Y., Zheng, P., Cao, Y., Lissel, F., & Linder, C. (2016). A highly stretchable autonomous self-healing elastomer. *Nature Chemistry, 8*(6), 618–624.

Li, H., Qu, R., Ma, Z., Zhou, N., Huang, Q., & Zheng, Z. (2023). Permeable and patternable super-stretchable liquid metal fiber for constructing high-integration-density multifunctional electronic fibers. *Advanced Functional Materials*, 2308120. https://doi.org/10.1002/adfm.202308120

Li, R., Wang, L., & Yin, L. (2018). Materials and devices for biodegradable and soft biomedical electronics. *Materials*, *11*(11), 2108.

Li, Z., Tian, X., Qiu, C.-W., & Ho, J. S. (2021). Metasurfaces for bioelectronics and healthcare. *Nature Electronics*, *4*(6), 382–391.

Liao, M., Wan, P., Wen, J., Gong, M., Wu, X., Wang, Y., Shi, R., & Zhang, L. (2017). Wearable, healable, and adhesive epidermal sensors assembled from mussel-inspired conductive hybrid hydrogel framework. *Advanced Functional Materials*, *27*(48), 1703852.

Libanori, A., Chen, G., Zhao, X., Zhou, Y., & Chen, J. (2022). Smart textiles for personalized healthcare. *Nature Electronics*, *5*(3), 142–156.

Lim, H. R., Kim, H. S., Qazi, R., Kwon, Y. T., Jeong, J. W., & Yeo, W. H. (2020). Advanced soft materials, sensor integrations, and applications of wearable flexible hybrid electronics in healthcare, energy, and environment. *Advanced Materials*, *32*(15), 1901924.

Liu, C., Huang, X., Wu, Y.-Y., Deng, X., Zheng, Z., Xu, Z., & Hui, D. (2021). Advance on the dispersion treatment of graphene oxide and the graphene oxide modified cement-based materials. *Nanotechnology Reviews*, *10*(1), 34–49.

Liu, R., Zhao, S., & Liu, J. (2020). From lithographically patternable to genetically patternable electronic materials for miniaturized, scalable, and soft implantable bioelectronics to interface with nervous and cardiac systems. *ACS Applied Electronic Materials*, *3*(1), 101–118.

Liu, X., Tian, S., Xu, S., Lu, W., Zhong, C., Long, Y., Ma, Y., Yang, K., Zhang, L., & Yang, J. (2022). A pressure-resistant zwitterionic skin sensor for domestic real-time monitoring and pro-healing of pressure injury. *Biosensors and Bioelectronics*, *214*, 114528.

Liu, Y., He, K., Chen, G., Leow, W. R., & Chen, X. (2017). Nature-inspired structural materials for flexible electronic devices. *Chemical Reviews*, *117*(20), 12893–12941.

Liu, Z., Fang, S., Moura, F., Ding, J., Jiang, N., Di, J., Zhang, M., Lepró, X., Galvao, D., & Haines, C. (2015). Hierarchically buckled sheath-core fibers for superelastic electronics, sensors, and muscles. *Science*, *349*(6246), 400–404.

Liu, Z., Yu, M., Lv, J., Li, Y., & Yu, Z. (2014). Dispersed, porous nanoislands landing on stretchable nanocrack gold films: Maintenance of stretchability and controllable impedance. *ACS Applied Materials & Interfaces*, *6*(16), 13487–13495.

Llerena Zambrano, B., Renz, A. F., Ruff, T., Lienemann, S., Tybrandt, K., Vörös, J., & Lee, J. (2021). Soft electronics based on stretchable and conductive nanocomposites for biomedical applications. *Advanced Healthcare Materials*, *10*(3), 2001397.

Meng, K., Xiao, X., Liu, Z., Shen, S., Tat, T., Wang, Z., Lu, C., Ding, W., He, X., & Yang, J. (2022). Kirigami-inspired pressure sensors for wearable dynamic cardiovascular monitoring. *Advanced Materials*, *34*(36), 2202478.

Min, H., Jang, S., Kim, D. W., Kim, J., Baik, S., Chun, S., & Pang, C. (2020). Highly air/water-permeable hierarchical mesh architectures for stretchable underwater electronic skin patches. *ACS Applied Materials & Interfaces*, *12*(12), 14425–14432.

Mishra, A., Bhatt, R., Bajpai, J., & Bajpai, A. (2021). Nanomaterials based biofuel cells: A review. *International Journal of Hydrogen Energy*, *46*(36), 19085–19105.

Niu, W., Tian, Q., Liu, Z., & Liu, X. (2023). Solvent-Free And Skin-Like Supramolecular ion-conductive elastomers with versatile processability for multifunctional ionic tattoos and on-skin bioelectronics. *Advanced Materials*, *35*, 2304157.

Niu, Y., Liu, H., He, R., Li, Z., Ren, H., Gao, B., Guo, H., Genin, G. M., & Xu, F. (2020). The new generation of soft and wearable electronics for health monitoring in varying environment: From normal to extreme conditions. *Materials Today*, *41*, 219–242.

Oh, J. Y., & Bao, Z. (2019). Second skin enabled by advanced electronics. *Advanced Science, 6*(11), 1900186.

Oh, J. Y., Rondeau-Gagné, S., Chiu, Y.-C., Chortos, A., Lissel, F., Wang, G.-J. N., Schroeder, B. C., Kurosawa, T., Lopez, J., & Katsumata, T. (2016). Intrinsically stretchable and healable semiconducting polymer for organic transistors. *Nature, 539*(7629), 411–415.

Oh, J. Y., Son, D., Katsumata, T., Lee, Y., Kim, Y., Lopez, J., Wu, H.-C., Kang, J., Park, J., & Gu, X. (2019). Stretchable self-healable semiconducting polymer film for active-matrix strain-sensing array. *Science Advances, 5*(11), eaav3097.

Park, J., Choi, S., Janardhan, A. H., Lee, S.-Y., Raut, S., Soares, J., Shin, K., Yang, S., Lee, C., & Kang, K.-W. (2016). Electromechanical cardioplasty using a wrapped elasto-conductive epicardial mesh. *Science Translational Medicine, 8*(344), 344ra386.

Park, J., Kim, J. Y., Heo, J. H., Kim, Y., Kim, S. A., Park, K., Lee, Y., Jin, Y., Shin, S. R., & Kim, D. W. (2023). Intrinsically nonswellable multifunctional hydrogel with dynamic nanoconfinement networks for robust tissue-adaptable bioelectronics. *Advanced Science, 10*(12), 2207237.

Park, Y. G., Lee, G. Y., Jang, J., Yun, S. M., Kim, E., & Park, J. U. (2021). Liquid metal-based soft electronics for wearable healthcare. *Advanced Healthcare Materials, 10*(17), 2002280.

Prunet, G., Pawula, F., Fleury, G., Cloutet, E., Robinson, A. J., Hadziioannou, G., & Pakdel, A. (2021). A review on conductive polymers and their hybrids for flexible and wearable thermoelectric applications. *Materials Today Physics, 18*, 100402.

Pu, J., Cao, Q., Gao, Y., Wang, Q., Geng, Z., Cao, L., Bu, F., Yang, N., & Guan, C. (2023). Liquid metal-based stable and stretchable Zn-ion battery for electronic textiles. *Advanced Materials, 36*, 2305812.

Qi, D., Liu, Z., Liu, Y., Jiang, Y., Leow, W. R., Pal, M., Pan, S., Yang, H., Wang, Y., & Zhang, X. (2017). Highly stretchable, compliant, polymeric microelectrode arrays for in vivo electrophysiological interfacing. *Advanced Materials, 29*(40), 1702800.

Qi, D., Liu, Z., Liu, Y., Leow, W. R., Zhu, B., Yang, H., Yu, J., Wang, W., Wang, H., & Yin, S. (2015a). Suspended wavy graphene microribbons for highly stretchable microsupercapacitors. *Advanced Materials, 27*(37), 5559–5566.

Qi, D., Liu, Z., Yu, M., Liu, Y., Tang, Y., Lv, J., Li, Y., Wei, J., Liedberg, B., & Yu, Z. (2015b). Highly stretchable gold nanobelts with sinusoidal structures for recording electrocorticograms. *Advanced Materials, 27*(20), 3145–3151.

Qi, M., Yang, R., Wang, Z., Liu, Y., Zhang, Q., He, B., Li, K., Yang, Q., Wei, L., & Pan, C. (2023). Bioinspired self-healing soft electronics. *Advanced Functional Materials, 33*, 2214479.

Rajeev, G., Prieto Simon, B., Marsal, L. F., & Voelcker, N. H. (2018). Advances in nanoporous anodic alumina-based biosensors to detect biomarkers of clinical significance: A review. *Advanced Healthcare Materials, 7*(5), 1700904.

Rao, Z., Ershad, F., Almasri, A., Gonzalez, L., Wu, X., & Yu, C. (2020). Soft electronics for the skin: From health monitors to human–machine interfaces. *Advanced Materials Technologies, 5*(9), 2000233.

Ren, Y., Sun, X., & Liu, J. (2020). Advances in liquid metal-enabled flexible and wearable sensors. *Micromachines, 11*(2), 200.

Sapkota, B., Liang, W., VahidMohammadi, A., Karnik, R., Noy, A., & Wanunu, M. (2020). High permeability sub-nanometre sieve composite MoS_2 membranes. *Nature Communications, 11*(1), 2747.

Schmidt, R., Slobozhanyuk, A., Belov, P., & Webb, A. (2017). Flexible and compact hybrid metasurfaces for enhanced ultra high field in vivo magnetic resonance imaging. *Scientific Reports, 7*(1), 1678.

Sekine, S., Ido, Y., Miyake, T., Nagamine, K., & Nishizawa, M. (2010). Conducting polymer electrodes printed on hydrogel. *Journal of the American Chemical Society, 132*(38), 13174.

Shao, C., Wang, M., Meng, L., Chang, H., Wang, B., Xu, F., Yang, J., & Wan, P. (2018). Mussel-inspired cellulose nanocomposite tough hydrogels with synergistic self-healing, adhesive, and strain-sensitive properties. *Chemistry of Materials, 30*(9), 3110–3121.

Shen, K., Liu, Z., Xie, R., Zhang, Y., Yang, Y., Zhao, X., Zhang, Y., Yang, A., & Cheng, Y. (2023). Nanocomposite conductive hydrogels with Robust elasticity and multifunctional responsiveness for flexible sensing and wound monitoring. *Materials Horizons, 10*, 2096–2108.

Someya, T., Kato, Y., Sekitani, T., Iba, S., Noguchi, Y., Murase, Y., Kawaguchi, H., & Sakurai, T. (2005). Conformable, flexible, large-area networks of pressure and thermal sensors with organic transistor active matrixes. *Proceedings of the National Academy of Sciences, 102*(35), 12321–12325.

Song, H., Wang, H., Gan, T., Shi, S., Zhou, X., Zhang, Y., & Handschuh-Wang, S. (2023). Gelatin biogel–liquid metal composite transient circuits for recyclable flexible electronics. *Advanced Materials Technologies*, 2301483. https://doi.org/10.1002/admt.202301483

Song, S., Kim, K. Y., Lee, S. H., Kim, K. K., Lee, K., Lee, W., Jeon, H., & Ko, S. H. (2022). Recent advances in 1D nanomaterial-based bioelectronics for healthcare applications. *Advanced NanoBiomed Research, 2*(3), 2100111.

Song, Z., Ma, T., Tang, R., Cheng, Q., Wang, X., Krishnaraju, D., Panat, R., Chan, C. K., Yu, H., & Jiang, H. (2014). Origami lithium-ion batteries. *Nature Communications, 5*(1), 3140.

Sun, X., Yuan, B., Sheng, L., Rao, W., & Liu, J. (2020). Liquid metal enabled injectable biomedical technologies and applications. *Applied Materials Today, 20*, 100722.

Sun, Y., Wang, Y., Liu, Y., Wu, S., Zhang, S., & Niu, W. (2022). Biomimetic chromotropic photonic-ionic skin with robust resilience, adhesion, and stability. *Advanced Functional Materials, 32*(33), 2204467.

Sunwoo, S.-H., Ha, K.-H., Lee, S., Lu, N., & Kim, D.-H. (2021). Wearable and implantable soft bioelectronics: Device designs and material strategies. *Annual Review of Chemical and Biomolecular Engineering, 12*, 359–391.

Tan, P., Wang, H., Xiao, F., Lu, X., Shang, W., Deng, X., Song, H., Xu, Z., Cao, J., & Gan, T. (2022). Solution-processable, soft, self-adhesive, and conductive polymer composites for soft electronics. *Nature Communications, 13*(1), 358.

Tang, J.-F., Su, H.-H., Lu, Y.-M., & Chu, S.-Y. (2015). Controlled growth of ZnO nanoflowers on nanowall and nanorod networks via a hydrothermal method. *CrystEngComm, 17*(3), 592–597.

Tat, T., Chen, G., Zhao, X., Zhou, Y., Xu, J., & Chen, J. (2022). Smart textiles for healthcare and sustainability. *ACS Nano, 16*(9), 13301–13313.

Tee, B. C. K., Wang, C., Allen, R., & Bao, Z. (2012). An electrically and mechanically self-healing composite with pressure- and flexion-sensitive properties for electronic skin applications. *Nature Nanotechnology, 7*(12), 825–832.

Tian, B., Liu, Q., Luo, C., Feng, Y., & Wu, W. (2020). Multifunctional ultrastretchable printed soft electronic devices for wearable applications. *Advanced Electronic Materials, 6*(2), 1900922.

Tseng, C. P., Liu, F., Zhang, X., Huang, P. C., Campbell, I., Li, Y., Atkinson, J. T., Terlier, T., Ajo-Franklin, C. M., & Silberg, J. J. (2022). Solution-deposited and patternable conductive polymer thin-film electrodes for microbial bioelectronics. *Advanced Materials, 34*(13), 2109442.

Wang, C., Liu, Y., Qu, X., Shi, B., Zheng, Q., Lin, X., Chao, S., Wang, C., Zhou, J., & Sun, Y. (2022a). Ultra-stretchable and fast self-healing ionic hydrogel in cryogenic environments for artificial nerve fiber. *Advanced Materials, 16*, 34.

Wang, C., Wang, C., Huang, Z., & Xu, S. (2018). Materials and structures toward soft electronics. *Advanced Materials, 30*(50), 1801368.

Wang, C., Xia, K., Zhang, Y., & Kaplan, D. L. (2019b). Silk-based advanced materials for soft electronics. *Accounts of Chemical Research, 52*(10), 2916–2927.

Wang, H., Wang, H., Wang, Y., Su, X., Wang, C., Zhang, M., Jian, M., Xia, K., Liang, X., & Lu, H. (2020b). Laser writing of janus graphene/kevlar textile for intelligent protective clothing. *ACS Nano, 14*(3), 3219–3226.

Wang, J., Wu, B., Wei, P., Sun, S., & Wu, P. (2022c). Fatigue-free artificial ionic skin toughened by self-healable elastic nanomesh. *Nature Communications, 13*(1), 4411.

Wang, L., Chen, D., Jiang, K., & Shen, G. (2017). New insights and perspectives into biological materials for flexible electronics. *Chemical Society Reviews, 46*(22), 6764–6815.

Wang, L., Xie, S., Wang, Z., Liu, F., Yang, Y., Tang, C., Wu, X., Liu, P., Li, Y., Saiyin, H., Zheng, S., Sun, X., Xu, F., Yu, H., & Peng, H. (2020c). Functionalized helical fibre bundles of carbon nanotubes as electrochemical sensors for long-term in vivo monitoring of multiple disease biomarkers. *Nature Biomedical Engineering*, 4(2), 159–171.

Wang, S., Nie, Y., Zhu, H., Xu, Y., Cao, S., Zhang, J., Li, Y., Wang, J., Ning, X., & Kong, D. (2022b). Intrinsically stretchable electronics with ultrahigh deformability to monitor dynamically moving organs. *Science Advances*, 8(13), eabl5511.

Wang, X., Fan, L., Zhang, J., Sun, X., Chang, H., Yuan, B., Guo, R., Duan, M., & Liu, J. (2019a). Printed conformable liquid metal e-skin-enabled spatiotemporally controlled bioelectromagnetics for wireless multisite tumor therapy. *Advanced Functional Materials*, 29(51), 1907063.

Wang, X., Feiner, R., Luan, H., Zhang, Q., Zhao, S., Zhang, Y., Han, M., Li, Y., Sun, R., & Wang, H. (2020a). Three-dimensional electronic scaffolds for monitoring and regulation of multifunctional hybrid tissues. *Extreme Mechanics Letters*, 35, 100634.

Won, P., Park, J. J., Lee, T., Ha, I., Han, S., Choi, M., Lee, J., Hong, S., Cho, K.-J., & Ko, S. H. (2019). Stretchable and transparent kirigami conductor of nanowire percolation network for electronic skin applications. *Nano Letters*, 19(9), 6087–6096.

Wu, X.-L., Wen, T., Guo, H.-L., Yang, S., Wang, X., & Xu, A.-W. (2013). Biomass-derived sponge-like carbonaceous hydrogels and aerogels for supercapacitors. *ACS Nano*, 7(4), 3589–3597.

Xu, F., Wang, X., Zhu, Y., & Zhu, Y. (2012). Wavy ribbons of carbon nanotubes for stretchable conductors. *Advanced Functional Materials*, 22(6), 1279–1283.

Xu, F., & Zhu, Y. (2012). Highly conductive and stretchable silver nanowire conductors. *Advanced Materials*, 24(37), 5117–5122.

Xu, S., Yan, Z., Jang, K.-I., Huang, W., Fu, H., Kim, J., Wei, Z., Flavin, M., McCracken, J., & Wang, R. (2015). Assembly of micro/nanomaterials into complex, three-dimensional architectures by compressive buckling. *Science*, 347(6218), 154–159.

Xu, S., Zhang, Y., Cho, J., Lee, J., Huang, X., Jia, L., Fan, J. A., Su, Y., Su, J., & Zhang, H. (2013). Stretchable batteries with self-similar serpentine interconnects and integrated wireless recharging systems. *Nature Communications*, 4(1), 1543.

Xu, Y., Su, Y., Xu, X., Arends, B., Zhao, G., Ackerman, D. N., Huang, H., Reid, S. P., Santarpia, J. L., & Kim, C. (2023). Porous liquid metal–elastomer composites with high leakage resistance and antimicrobial property for skin-interfaced bioelectronics. *Science Advances*, 9(1), eadf0575.

Xu, Y., Yang, X., Thomas, A., Kuriakose, P., & Panagiotis, A. (2018). Noncovalently assembled electroconductive hydrogel. *ACS Applied Materials & Interfaces*, 10(17), 14418–14425.

Xue, Y., Zhang, J., Chen, X., Zhang, J., Chen, G., Zhang, K., Lin, J., Guo, C., & Liu, J. (2021). Trigger-detachable hydrogel adhesives for bioelectronic interfaces. *Advanced Functional Materials*, 31(47), 2106446.

Xue, Z., Song, H., Rogers, J. A., Zhang, Y., & Huang, Y. (2020). Mechanically-guided structural designs in stretchable inorganic electronics. *Advanced Materials*, 32(15), 1902254.

Yamagishi, K., Zhou, W., Ching, T., Huang, S. Y., & Hashimoto, M. (2021). Ultra-deformable and tissue-adhesive liquid metal antennas with high wireless powering efficiency. *Advanced Materials*, 33(26), 2008062.

Yan, J., Lu, Y., Chen, G., Yang, M., & Gu, Z. (2018). Advances in liquid metals for biomedical applications. *Chemical Society Reviews*, 47(8), 2518–2533.

Yan, Z., Han, M., Shi, Y., Badea, A., Yang, Y., Kulkarni, A., Hanson, E., Kandel, M. E., Wen, X., & Zhang, F. (2017). Three-dimensional mesostructures as high-temperature growth templates, electronic cellular scaffolds, and self-propelled microrobots. *Proceedings of the National Academy of Sciences*, 114(45), E9455–E9464.

Yang, N., Gong, F., Zhou, Y., Yu, Q., & Cheng, L. (2022). Liquid metals: Preparation, surface engineering, and biomedical applications. *Coordination Chemistry Reviews*, 471, 214731.

Yang, S., Cheng, J., Shang, J., Hang, C., Qi, J., Zhong, L., Rao, Q., He, L., Liu, C., & Ding, L. (2023). Stretchable surface electromyography electrode array patch for tendon location and muscle injury prevention. *Nature Communications*, 14(1), 6494.

Yao, B., Wang, H., Zhou, Q., Wu, M., Zhang, M., Li, C., & Shi, G. (2017). Ultrahigh-conductivity polymer hydrogels with arbitrary structures. *Advanced Materials, 29*(28), 1700974.

Yao, G., Yin, C., Wang, Q., Zhang, T., Chen, S., Lu, C., Zhao, K., Xu, W., Pan, T., & Gao, M. (2020). Flexible bioelectronics for physiological signals sensing and disease treatment. *Journal of Materiomics, 6*(2), 397–413.

Yeo, W.-H., Kim, Y.-S., Lee, J., Ameen, A., Shi, L., Li, M., Wang, S., Ma, R., Jin, S. H., & Kang, Z. (2013). Multifunctional epidermal electronics printed directly onto the skin. *Advanced Materials, 25*(20).

Yuk, H., Lu, B., Lin, S., Qu, K., Xu, J., Luo, J., & Zhao, X. (2020). 3D printing of conducting polymers. *Nature Communications, 11*(1), 1604.

Yuk, H., Lu, B., & Zhao, X. (2019). Hydrogel bioelectronics *Chemical Society Reviews, 48*(6), 1642–1667.

Yuk, H., Zhang, T., Parada, G. A., Liu, X., & Zhao, X. (2016). Skin-inspired hydrogel–elastomer hybrids with robust interfaces and functional microstructures. *Nature Communications, 7*(1), 12028.

Zhang, A., & Lieber, C. M. (2016). Nano-bioelectronics. *Chemical Reviews, 116*(1), 215–257.

Zhang, C., Wu, B., Zhou, Y., Zhou, F., Liu, W., & Wang, Z. (2020b). Mussel-inspired hydrogels: From design principles to promising applications. *Chemical Society Reviews, 49*(11), 3605–3637.

Zhang, C., Yang, Q., Meng, X., Li, H., Luo, Z., Kai, L., Liang, J., Chen, S., & Chen, F. (2023b). Wireless, smart hemostasis device with all-soft sensing system for quantitative and real-time pressure evaluation. *Advanced Science, 10*, 2303418.

Zhang, S., Li, S., Xia, Z., & Cai, K. (2020a). A review of electronic skin: Soft electronics and sensors for human health. *Journal of Materials Chemistry B, 8*(5), 852–862.

Zhang, W., Wang, P.-L., Huang, L.-Z., Guo, W.-Y., Zhao, J., & Ma, M.-G. (2023a). A stretchable, environmentally tolerant, and photoactive liquid metal/MXene hydrogel for high performance temperature monitoring, human motion detection and self-powered application. *Nano Energy, 117*, 108875.

Zhao, Y., Kim, A., Wan, G., & Tee, B. C. (2019a). Design and applications of stretchable and self-healable conductors for soft electronics. *Nano Convergence, 6*(1), 1–22.

Zhao, Y., Wang, B., Tan, J., Yin, H., Huang, R., Zhu, J., Lin, S., Zhou, Y., Jelinek, D., & Sun, Z. (2022). Soft strain-insensitive bioelectronics featuring brittle materials. *Science, 378*(6625), 1222–1227.

Zhao, Y., Yu, M., Liu, Z., & Yu, Z. (2019b). Electrical and thermal effects on electromechanical performance of stretchable thin gold films on PDMS substrates for stretchable electronics. *Journal of Applied Physics, 125*(16).

Zhao, Z., Xia, K., Hou, Y., Zhang, Q., Ye, Z., & Lu, J. (2021). Designing flexible, smart and self-sustainable supercapacitors for portable/wearable electronics: From conductive polymers. *Chemical Society Reviews, 50*(22), 12702–12743.

Zhou, T., Yu, Y., He, B., Wang, Z., Xiong, T., Wang, Z., Liu, Y., Xin, J., Qi, M., Zhang, H., Zhou, X., Gao, L., Cheng, Q., & Wei, L. (2022b). Ultra-compact MXene fibers by continuous and controllable synergy of interfacial interactions and thermal drawing-induced stresses. *Nature Communications, 13*(1), 4564.

Zhou, Y., Xiao, X., Chen, G., Zhao, X., & Chen, J. (2022a). Self-powered sensing technologies for human Metaverse interfacing. *Joule, 6*(7), 1381–1389.

Zhou, Z., Chen, K., Li, X., Zhang, S., Wu, Y., Zhou, Y., Meng, K., Sun, C., He, Q., & Fan, W. (2020). Sign-to-speech translation using machine-learning-assisted stretchable sensor arrays. *Nature Electronics, 3*(9), 571–578.

CHAPTER 2

Advanced Fabrication Technology for Soft Electronics

Ruilai Wei, Qilin Hua, and Guozhen Shen

2.1 INTRODUCTION

Soft electronics is a rapidly emerging field dedicated to the development of flexible and stretchable electronic devices and systems, setting them apart from conventional rigid electronics. The unique characteristics of soft electronics, such as flexibility, stretchability, conformability, and lightweight, enable their suitability for a wide range of applications, including wearable devices (Huang et al., 2023), soft robotics (Kim et al., 2018; X. Q. Wang et al., 2020a), medical healthcare (Gao et al., 2016; Li et al., 2023), flexible displays (Choi et al., 2015; C. Wang et al., 2020b), and conformal sensors (Y. S. Kim et al., 2019b; Wang et al., 2018). The increasing demand for versatile applications in soft electronics has stimulated the exploration of advanced fabrication technologies. These techniques leverage the exceptional properties of new materials along with innovative structural designs to achieve flexible and stretchable electronic devices endowed with advantageous characteristics.

Significantly, a range of advanced fabrication technologies, including soft lithography, soft transferring, 3D printing, textile technology, and other novel techniques (the typical ones as illustrated in Figure 2.1), play a pivotal role in shaping the distinctive characteristics of soft electronics. These fabrication techniques demonstrate remarkable capabilities in addressing critical challenges encountered during the development of devices and systems in soft electronics. For instance, soft lithography enables the precise transfer of micro- and nanoscale patterns onto flexible substrates, resolving the challenge of achieving high-precision fabrication. Soft transferring allows the deposition of multiple functional materials/structures into user-defined high-resolution patterns without altering their characteristics, overcoming the material transfer issue in the manufacturing of flexible electronic devices. In addition, 3D printing facilitates the direct processing of soft materials to construct complex structures/systems, providing a solution for rapid prototyping and batch customization of intricate designs. Furthermore, textile technology tackles the

DOI: 10.1201/9781003493631-2

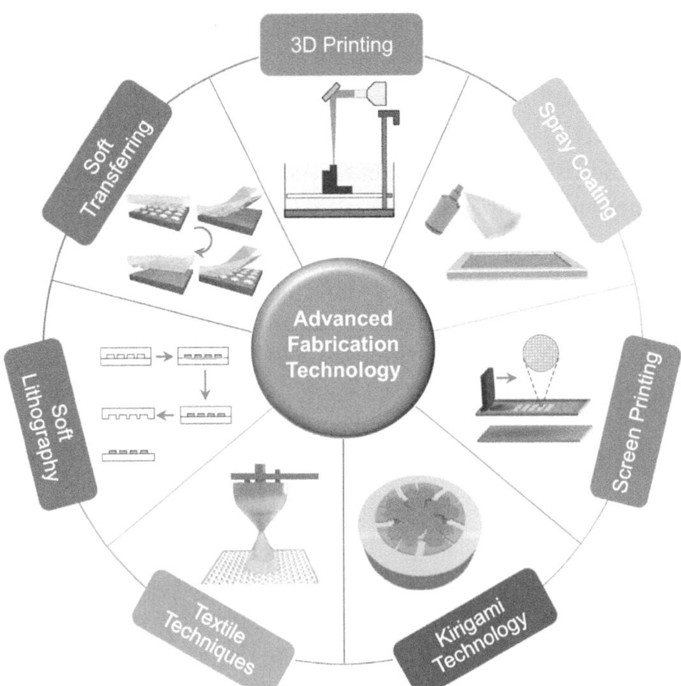

FIGURE 2.1   Illustration of advanced fabrication technology for soft electronics.

integration of electronic components into flexible fibers or fabrics, enabling the production of flexible sensors and wearable devices. Through the application of these advanced fabrication technologies, the development of soft electronics has experienced significant advancement, empowering it to effectively meet the demands of modern electronic devices characterized by their lightweight, bendable, and wearable nature.

This chapter provides a comprehensive review of typical advanced fabrication technologies for soft electronics, encompassing their preparation processes, typical applications, as well as advantages and disadvantages. Additionally, it presents a comparative analysis of these fabrication processes, highlighting their significant impact on device fabrication. This chapter illustrates the existing challenges, proposed solution strategies, and the future application prospects of advanced fabrication techniques in flexible electronics manufacturing.

2.2 SOFT LITHOGRAPHY

Soft lithography emerges as a versatile fabrication technique extensively employed in the field of soft electronics to pattern and structure soft materials like elastomers and polymers, enabling the creation of microscale and nanoscale features. This method offers precise control over pattern shape, size, and placement while remaining compatible with flexible and elastic substrates. Soft lithography encompasses several techniques, including replica molding (REM), microtransfer molding (μTM), microcontact printing (μCP), capillary microforming technology (MIMIC), and solvent-assisted micromolding in capillaries

(SAMIM), all of which find applications in various stages of soft electronics fabrication (Mukherjee, 2019).

These technologies exhibit a certain degree of correlation primarily due to their shared reliance on the properties of elastic materials, namely flexibility, malleability, and the ability to replicate microstructures with ease. As a result, these fabrication methods have the potential to complement one another, allowing for the selection of the most suitable manufacturing approach based on specific application requirements and equipment conditions. While various additional soft lithography methods have been reported, most of them are derived from the aforementioned techniques. Consequently, this section primarily focuses on introducing the principles and highlighting the applications of soft lithography technology.

2.2.1 Replica Molding

Replica molding (REM) is a microfabrication technique used to create micro- and nanoscale patterns, usually the first step in stamp fabrication. The specific process flowchart is schematically illustrated in Figure 2.2a. First, a mold with patterned relief features is fabricated on a Si/SiO$_2$ wafer by using a photolithography process. The mold is usually made from a rigid material like nickel or SU-8 photoresist. Then, the mold is used to shape the features into a substrate. This process involves filling the mold with a liquid precursor material like polydimethylsiloxane (PDMS), polymethyl methacrylate (PMMA), or an ultraviolet (UV) curable polymer. Finally, after the material has cured, the mold is removed, leaving the patterned features on the substrate surface. The molded substrate can serve as a stamp or mold for subsequent processes.

There are some key advantages of REM like high resolution down to sub-100 nm features, ability to produce 3D topography, low-cost and high-throughput process, and applicability to a wide range of materials. Most importantly, REM can be used to fabricate large-area stamps and the rigid mold can be reused many times to generate multiple replica substrates. However, the reused times depend on the durability and chemical stability of the materials of the mold. Despite its obvious advantages, there are also some evident issues, for example, REM requires high precision in mold manufacturing, and it takes a long time to make high-precision molds.

REM is widely used for rapid prototyping and fabrication of microfluidic devices, microelectromechanical systems, and micro/nanoscale structures. Hart et al. reported a glassy crystalline polymer microstructure based on REM (Zhao et al., 2016), as illustrated in Figure 2.2b. They developed a custom apparatus to enable a controlled atmosphere, temperature, light exposure, and magnetic field during the REM process, which was critical for achieving glassy liquid crystalline polymer networks. High fidelity replication was demonstrated down to 10 μm diameter pillars, though limitations existed for structures with very high aspect ratios (>10).

2.2.2 Microtransfer Molding

Microtransfer molding (μTM) is a microfabrication process that uses a PDMS mold, which is created by using the process dictated by REM, to shape liquid prepolymers into

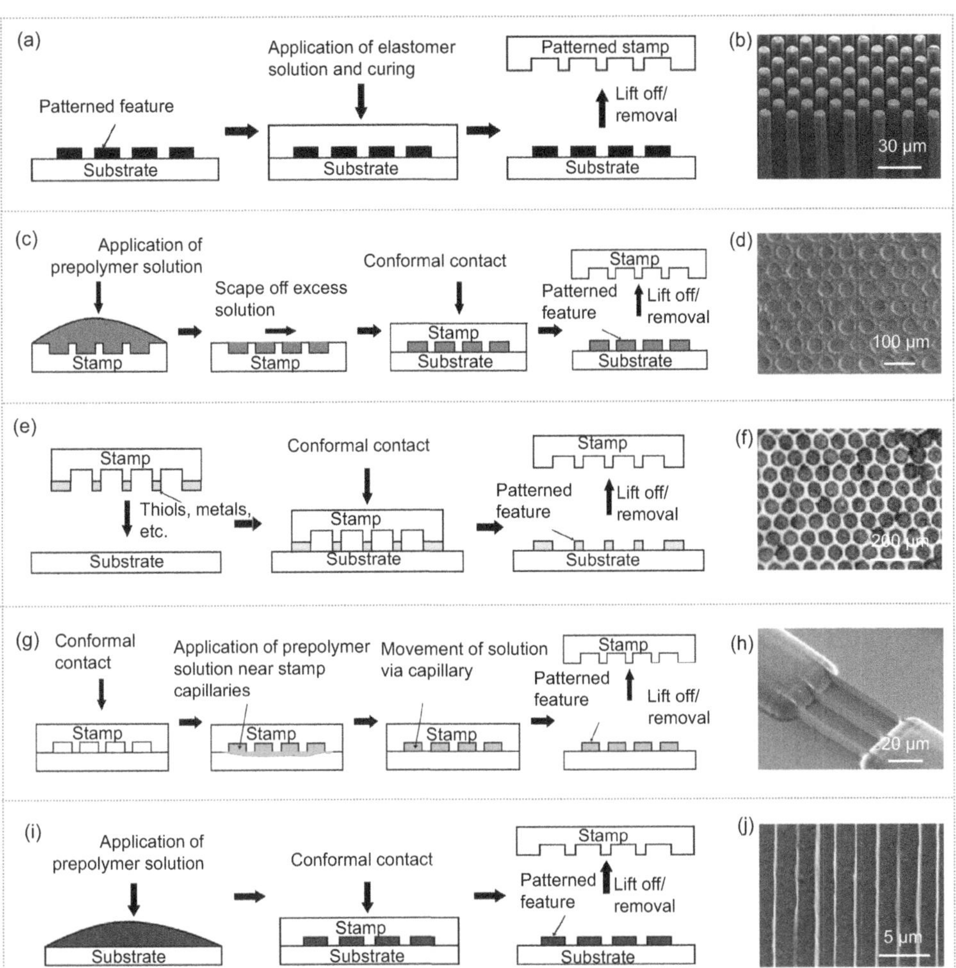

FIGURE 2.2   Soft lithography for the fabrication of soft electronics and its applications (Mukherjee, 2019). (a) Replica molding (REM) is a fabrication technique to obtain a cured patterned stamp. (b) SEM images of large arrays of high aspect ratio microcolumns with circular and square cross-sectional shapes produced by REM. (c) Microtransfer molding (μTM) is a method of filling the REM stamp recesses with a liquid prepolymer, removing the excess liquid, inverting the stamp mold to cure, and then peeling off the mold to leave a positive patterned structure on the substrate. (d) Patterned catalyst inks fabricated by the μTM technique. (e) Microcontact printing (μCP) is employed to selectively pattern a solution (or ink) based on self-assembled monolayers (SAM) based on silanes and thiols onto a substrate. (f) Optical microscopy images of the cathode catalyst layer (CCL) holes and islands obtained using the μCP technique. (g) Capillary microforming technology (MIMIC) patterns the interconnection network of a capillary channel with stamping molds obtained by REM. (h) The design of a submicron structure without the residual layer is realized through MIMIC. (i) Solvent-assisted micromolding in capillaries (SAMIM) is an embossing technique that uses patterned stamps manufactured by REM to imprint features onto a substrate. (j) Schematic cross-section of a vertical MXene line pattern fabricated by the SAMIN. ([a, b] Adapted with permission (Zhao et al., 2016). Copyright 2016, American Chemical Society; [c, d] Adapted with permission (Paul et al., 2020). Copyright 2020, American Chemical Society; [e, f] Adapted with permission (Paul et al., 2020). Copyright 2020, American Chemical Society; [g, h] Adapted with permission (Cadarso et al., 2017). Copyright 2017, Springer Nature; [i, j] Adapted with permission (Song et al., 2020). Copyright 2020, Wiley-VCH.)

microscale structures. The flowchart of the fabrication process is shown in Figure 2.2c. First of all, place the PDMS mold on the substrate and fill the channels in the PDMS mold with a liquid polymer or prepolymer. After the liquid is drawn into the molded channels due to capillary action, dispose the excess liquid with a separate PDMS block. Then, bring the patterned stamp in conformal contact with the substrate. After curing the polymer with heat or UV light, peel off the PDMS mold, leaving cured microstructures.

µTM presents a host of compelling advantages within the realm of advanced microfabrication. Foremost, it leverages a streamlined, expeditious, and cost-efficient process, rendering it an exceptionally effective method for microstructure production. Notably, µTM technology facilitates the creation of intricate 3D microstructures with exceptional resolution, thereby furnishing a superlative tool for micro and nanoscale research and applications. It is also notable for its broad applicability, accommodating various polymers including PMMA, PDMS, and epoxies. Furthermore, µTM seamlessly integrates with diverse microfabrication processes, thereby substantiating its potential for expansive applications within the intricate domain of microstructure manufacturing. However, there can be more material waste associated with µTM, especially during the setup and optimization phases.

µTM provides a straightforward approach to replicating microscale 3D patterns from a master into polymeric materials using an intermediate PDMS mold. The technique is versatile for microfluidic devices, prototyping, and manufacturing microstructures. Gates et al. patterned catalyst inks using the µTM method (Paul et al., 2020), patterning circular holes with a diameter of 50 µm, as shown in Figure 2.2d. Although there is still a problem with membrane deformation, it demonstrates the ability of the µTM technique to accurately prepare micro-sized patterns.

2.2.3 Microcontact Printing

Microcontact printing (µCP) is a soft lithography technique that uses an elastomeric stamp to pattern molecules on a substrate surface. Most commonly uses PDMS stamps. The fabrication process flowchart is illustrated in Figure 2.2e. Based on the PDMS stamp with patterned features fabricated by REM, ink the stamp with the molecules to be transferred, like thiols, metals, and nanoparticles. Bring the stamp into conformal contact with the substrate to transfer the ink. Remove the stamp, leaving behind a molecular ink pattern on the substrate.

µCP provides a straightforward way to pattern molecular inks on surfaces with microscale resolution using an elastomeric stamp. There are numerous obvious advantages to this approach. It can achieve high-resolution patterning of molecular films, with a resolution that can be as high as the submicron level. The process is fast and simple and can be achieved using low-cost methods. µCP can pattern a variety of molecules on various substrates, including glass, silicon, polymers, and other materials. This technique requires minimal equipment, is easy to integrate into existing processes, and is suitable for patterning self-assembled monolayers (SAMs). µCP can be performed under conditions that do not require clean rooms or flat surfaces, making it more flexible and practical for various applications. However, µCP also has some limitations in applications. It is generally suitable for creating micron-scale patterns, but it may be unable to achieve the nanoscale resolution required for some applications. Moreover, μCP relies on using an elastomeric stamp to transfer ink or molecules to a substrate. This limits the compatibility of this technique with certain materials that may interact with or adhere poorly to the stamp, thereby restricting its applicability in some cases.

μCP is versatile and accessible for many applications, including defining regions for selective surface chemistry, manufacturing biosensors, controlling microfluidic surface properties, and depositing nanoparticle structures. Figure 2.2f shows the cylindrical microstructures prepared by the μCP method with a cylindrical diameter of 50 μm (Paul et al., 2020). Similar to μTM, it also confirms that μCP has the ability to prepare micro-sized patterns. It has greater flexibility in transferring micro-sized patterns by applying simpler conditions.

2.2.4 Capillary Microforming Technology

Capillary microforming technology (MIMIC) is a microfabrication technique that uses capillary forces to fill microchannels and mold structures. The fabrication process of MIMIC is illustrated in Figure 2.2g. The PDMS mold with an array of microchannels was created by REM, which was brought into contact with the substrate. Then, fill the channels with liquid via capillary action. After the polymer is cured, remove the PDMS mold to reveal the cured microstructures.

MIMIC offers a range of compelling advantages as a fabrication technique. Notably, it excels in achieving exceptionally high resolution, capable of working at sub-micron scales. Furthermore, it boasts a rapid, self-contained process that eliminates the need for external pumping or pressure, streamlining production. This versatility extends to the creation of intricate, 3D geometries, making it an ideal choice for complex microstructures. Additionally, the self-assembly nature of the process helps minimize defects, ensuring a high level of precision and quality in the final products.

The principle of MIMIC is that the surface tension of the liquid generates the pressure needed to drive flow and filling of the channels, without any external forces. However, it has a limit in large-scale applications, because the longer the capillary the greater the resistance that accumulates as the liquid advances. When the viscosity of the prepolymer is high, it is also difficult to obtain the pattern through MIMIC.

MIMIC utilizes capillary forces for the self-assembly of microstructures within a mold, enabling rapid and versatile fabrication of complex 3D microscale elements. Schift et al. fabricated photonic grating structures with an aspect ratio of up to 17 and trench widths as small as 180 nm using the MIMIC (Cadarso et al., 2017). The opened silicon mold is placed on a glass substrate, forming a closed microfluidic channel. The polymer fills the micro/nanostructures in the mold by capillary action. After curing and peeling off the silicon mold, the obtained polymer product containing micro/nanostructures is shown in Figure 2.2h. This work demonstrates the ability of MIMIC to produce polymer devices on hard substrates in high volume. Complex geometries can be designed and produced in high volume with MIMIC after applying the right combination of methods and materials.

2.2.5 Solvent-Assisted Micromolding in Capillaries

Solvent-assisted micromolding in capillaries (SAMIM) is an embossing technique that uses a solvent to facilitate the filling of a PDMS mold. Figure 2.2i illustrates the SAMIM manufacturing process. The first step in the process of SAMIM is the application of liquid polymer or prepolymer on the substrate. Then, the patterned PDMS mode fabricated by REM was in conformal contact with the substrate. During this process, the mold fills with liquid polymer or prepolymer. After the polymer is cured, remove the PDMS mold to reveal the cured microstructures.

The principle of SAMIM involves using a solvent to temporarily swell the PDMS, facilitating the thorough filling of channels, followed by solvent evaporation and PDMS shrinkage to effectively trap the polymer within the microstructures. SAMIM is a microfabrication technique similar to MIMIC. It significantly enhances the filling capabilities when compared to standard MIMIC, ensuring a more thorough and precise replication of microstructures. SAMIM exhibits adaptability to higher-viscosity prepolymers, expanding its range of applicable materials. Moreover, it excels in filling high aspect ratio channels, making it an ideal choice for microfabrication projects that demand intricate and challenging geometries.

SAMIM leverages a solvent swelling process to enhance capillary filling for the microfabrication of complex 3D microstructures using a PDMS mold. It finds diverse applications in various fields, including the fabrication of microfluidic devices, microoptics, and the templating of carbon microstructures. Lee et al. fabricated MXene microstructures with line widths smaller than 200 nm and a pitch of 2 μm using sophisticated PDMS molds (Song et al., 2020). The SEM image is shown in Figure 2.2j. This technique, which uses PDMS stamping to enable 2D MXene sheets to form patterns and micro/nanostructures without lithography, is also applicable to other 2D materials.

2.3 SOFT TRANSFERRING

Soft transferring is an advanced fabrication technique used in the field of soft electronics to transfer a variety of materials and devices such as sensors, thin-film transistors (TFTs), or interconnects onto flexible or stretchable substrates with high precision, which solves the problems of substrate selection and material transfer during the fabrication of flexible electronics. Soft transferring offers several advantages, including the ability to combine different materials, create complex structures, and enable large-area manufacturing. Soft transferring has low production costs relative to other micro- and nanofabrication technologies, which is conducive to promoting the popularization and application of soft electronics.

Soft transferring utilizes a soft stamp to transfer materials/devices between the donor and receiver substrates, the core principle utilized being the modulation of adhesion between the stamp and the materials/devices interface. It mainly involves two processes: the first step is soft stamp transfer the materials/devices from the donor substrate, in which the adhesion of the materials/devices to the stamp is greater than that to the donor substrate; the second step is to transfer the materials/devices from the soft stamp to the receiving substrate, in which the adhesion of the materials/devices to the receiving substrate is greater than that to the soft stamp. With further research on soft transferring technology, various transfer methods have emerged. Based on the modulation of adhesion, soft transfer technology can be categorized in the following manners: kinetically controlled transfer printing technology, surface protrusions of adhesion-assisted transfer technology, inflatable stamp-assisted transfer technology, glue-assisted and surface chemical transfer technology, laser-based non-contact transfer technology, and adhesion pad-assisted transfer technology.

2.3.1 Kinetically Controlled Transfer Printing

Kinetically controlled transfer printing has proven to be a developed and powerful transfer technique, where the adhesion between the soft stamp and the materials/devices is modulated by a rate-dependent adhesion effect. The rate-dependent adhesion effect refers to the phenomenon that bond strength decreases with increasing loading rate, which is caused by the viscoelastic behavior of the adhesive of the soft stamp. While the stamp is peeled off the donor at a slower rate, the stamp has a stronger adhesion to the materials/devices and can stick the ink off the substrate; as the stamp is peeled off the substrate quickly, the stamp has a weaker adhesion to the materials/devices and transfers the materials/devices to the receiving substrate. A typical schematic of kinetically controlled transfer printing technology is shown in Figure 2.3a (Cavallo & Lagally, 2010). The soft stamp is contacted on a printed ink donor substrate and then peeled off at a high speed (~10 mm/sec or faster), at which time the ink is transferred to the stamp. Next, the stamp with ink is brought into contact with the receiving substrate, and the stamp is peeled off at a slow rate (~1 mm/sec or slower), whereupon the ink is transferred to the receiving substrate.

Kinetically controlled transfer printing technology offers a range of significant advantages in the field of materials integration and nanotechnology. They enable the heterogeneous integration of various materials, including semiconductors, metals, and polymers, onto a variety of substrates. This method allows for precise and deterministic assembly of microscale materials in predefined patterns while causing minimal damage to the materials during the transfer process, due to the kinetic and mechanical release technology involved. Furthermore, it is highly versatile, accommodating a wide variety of materials, including thin films, nanowires, and nanomembranes. Lagally et al. made a breakthrough in the transfer of solid objects by applying kinetically controlled transfer printing technology (Cavallo & Lagally, 2010). They successfully transferred an array containing 24,000 silicon microstructures onto a 100 mm GaAs wafer. The optical photo of the transferred array is shown in Figure 2.3b, with an inset SEM image. This technology allows for the selective release and transfer of materials from their original growth substrates and is adaptable for use on non-conventional substrates, such as plastics, textiles, and curved surfaces. Additionally, it is a scalable process suitable for large-area electronics manufacturing and is compatible with roll-to-roll processing, making it ideal for high-throughput production. However, it still faces challenges, such as tricky to achieve 100% transfer yield, and feature sizes are typically limited to microscale rather than nanoscale.

2.3.2 Surface Protrusions of Adhesion-Assisted Transfer Technique

Surface protrusions-assisted transfer technology, inspired by aphid's adhesive pad, utilizes small protruding structures or pillars on stamp surfaces to enable controlled pickup and printing of materials. This technique relies on changes in the contact area between the stamp and the transfer material to regulate adhesion. Stamp is typically prepared from elastomers. When picking up functional materials, applying pressure increases the contact area between the stamp and materials to increase the bonding force. When the

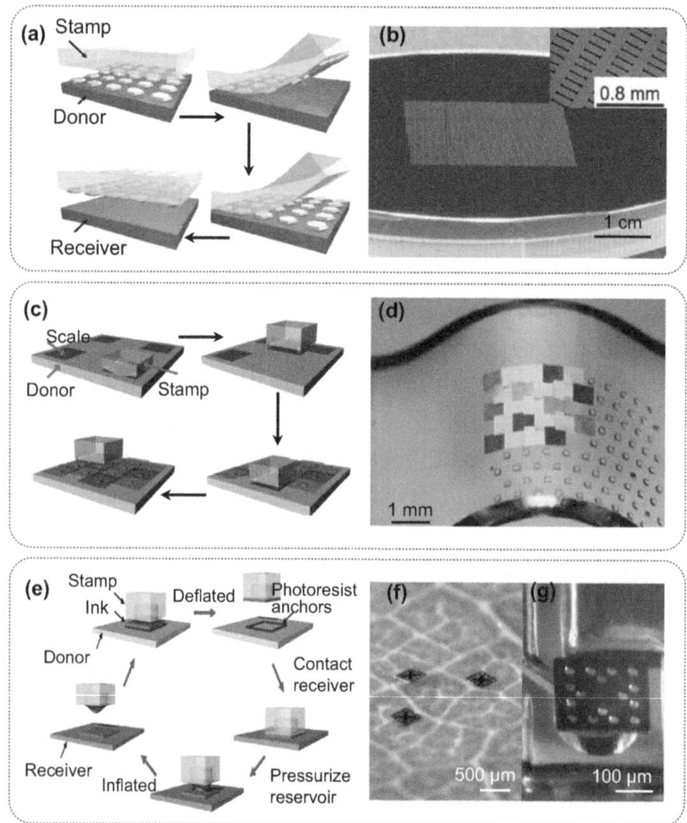

FIGURE 2.3   Soft transferring technologies for the fabrication of soft electronics devices and its applications. (a) Kinetically controlled transfer printing technique (Cavallo & Lagally, 2010). Copyright 2010, Royal Society of Chemistry. (b) Kinetically controlled transfer printing technique. Adapted with permission (Cavallo & Lagally, 2010). Copyright 2010, Royal Society of Chemistry. An array of about 24, 000 silicon microstructures transferred to a 100 mm GaAs wafer. The inset shows the SEM image of silicon microstructures. (c) Surface protrusions of adhesion-assisted transfer technique. Adapted with permission (Kim, Su, et al., 2012b). Copyright 2012, Wiley-VCH. (d) Optical images of a heterogeneous imbricate architecture on a PDMS substrate. Adapted with permission (Kim, Su, et al., 2012b). Copyright 2012, Wiley-VCH. The silicon platelets are transferred by surface protrusions by the adhesion-assisted transfer technique. (e) Inflatable stamp-assisted transfer technique. (f) Optical image of 250 µm × 250 µm silicon wafer transferred by inflatable stamp. (g) The structure of inflatable stamps. Adapted with permission (Carlson et al., 2012). Copyright 2012, Wiley-VCH.

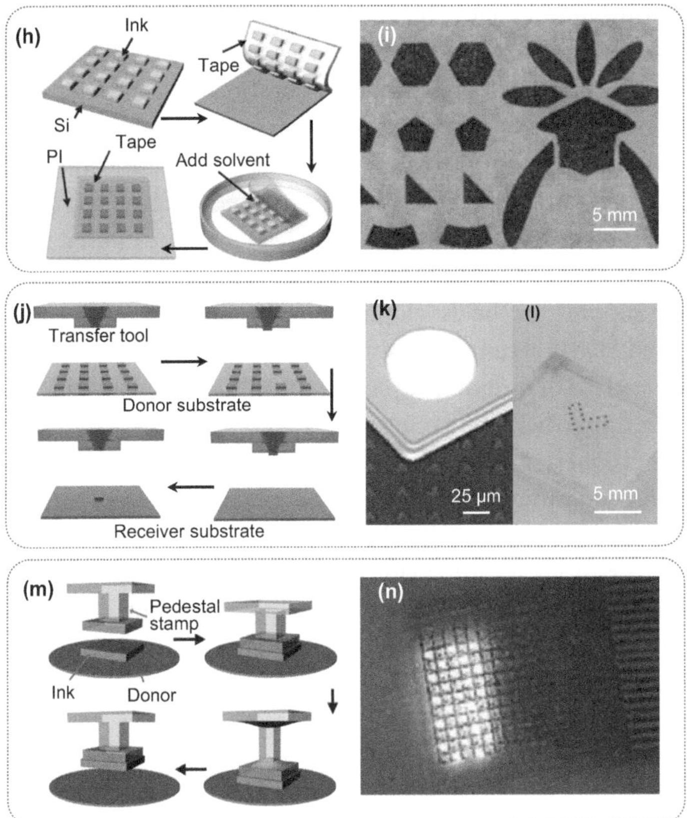

FIGURE 2.3 (Cont.) Soft transferring technologies for the fabrication of soft electronics devices and its applications. (h) Glue-assisted and surface chemical transfer technique. Adapted with permission (Sim et al., 2015). Copyright 2015, Springer Nature. (i) A pattern transferred by surface chemistry on a double-sided tape. Adapted with permission (Dong et al., 2022). Copyright 2022, AAAS. (j) Laser-based non-contact transfer technique. (k) Printing μ-LEDs with a laser-based non-contact transfer technique. (l) μ-LED heart pattern printed onto PDMS substrate. Adapted with permission (Luo et al., 2021). Copyright 2021, Wiley-VCH. (m) Adhesion pad-assisted transfer technique. Adapted with permission (Kim, Carlson, et al., 2012a). Copyright 2012, AIP Publishing. (n) Schematic of a flexible display transferred by using adhesion pad-assisted transfer technique, adhered to a medical tape and mounted on the skin. Adapted with permission (C. Wang et al., 2020b). Copyright 2020, AAAS.

microstructure springs back, the contact area decreases, the bonding force weakens, and the material is transferred to the received substrate. The springback time of the microstructure is adjustable and may vary from a few seconds or a few hours. For transfer success, the material should be transferred as quickly as possible after pickup. The detail of the process is illustrated in Figure 2.3c (Kim, Su, et al., 2012b). First, load the stamp aligned over the donor substrate. Then, pick up the devices and move to the target substrate. Next, materials are printed from the protrusions onto the receiver substrate. Finally, the stamp is detached and withdrawn, leaving behind printed materials.

Compared to conventional flat PDMS stamps, surface protrusions in adhesion-assisted transfer technology offer a multitude of advantages, making it a versatile and powerful tool in the field of micro/nanomaterial assembly and positioning. It provides deterministic control over the placement of these materials, significantly improving pick-up selectivity and the kinetics of material release. One of its key strengths lies in its compatibility with a wide range of materials, including semiconductors, graphene, nanotubes, metals, and polymers. Moreover, this technology enables printing on non-planar and curved surfaces, expanding its applicability to various substrates. Rogers and his research team provided theoretical and experimental support for the development and application of this technology (Kim et al., 2010). They used PDMS stamps with surface protrusions to transfer 100×100 μm silicon platelets onto the surface of different substrates. These silicon platelets can be placed independently or stacked together. The same transfer technique was also used for conventional non-stacked layouts, where silicon wafers were successfully transferred to the PDMS substrate. Figure 2.3d is an optical photo of stacked silicon platelets (Kim, Su, et al., 2012b). Nonetheless, several challenges need to be addressed. These include achieving extremely high-resolution protrusions, ideally below 100 nm in size, extending the lifespan of the stamp, and ensuring a 100% transfer yield over large areas. In summary, surface protrusions in adhesion-assisted transfer technology provide a comprehensive and adaptable solution for precise and efficient assembly, positioning, and mixing of micro/nanomaterials across various surfaces and at different scales.

2.3.3 Inflatable Stamp-Assisted Transfer Technique

Similar to surface protrusions of adhesion-assisted transfer technology, inflatable stamp-assisted transfer technology draws inspiration from the adhesive pad of aphids and relies on alterations in the contact area between the stamp and the transfer material to control adhesion, which utilize inflatable elastomeric stamps to pick up and transfer inks, materials, or structures onto a receiving substrate. Figure 2.3e is a typical fabrication process for transfer printing using inflatable stamps (Carlson et al., 2012). In the deflated state, the stamp makes quick contact with the material/device supported on the donor substrate. At this point, the material/device from the donor substrate transfers to the stamp. Subsequently, the stamp is gently brought into contact with the receiving substrate. Pressure is applied to the reservoir of the stamp, causing localized inflation of the stamp. The gradual inflation of the stamp releases the material/device onto the receiving substrate. Figure 2.3f shows an application example of the inflatable stamp-assisted transfer technology (Carlson et al., 2012). Through this technology, a silicon plate with a size of 250 μm × 250 μm × 3 μm is transferred onto a leaf, demonstrating the ability to transfer objects onto organic surfaces. This technique can also transfer objects onto plastic sheets, glossy cardboards, and photonic crystals. The structure of the inflatable stamp is shown in Figure 2.3g.

Inflatable stamp-assisted techniques utilize soft and expandable stamps as a means of controllably transferring functional materials/devices from the stamp onto a substrate through programmable inflation/deflation cycles. It offers a range of notable advantages for transfer printing. It facilitates conformal contact between the stamp and substrate. This technology offers kinetic control of the transfer process by modulating inflation pressure, making it adaptable to various materials and substrates. In the application of thin films like Si, GaN, GaAs, and plastic, inflatable stamps prove highly useful. Moreover, it excels at printing on non-planar and curved surfaces. However, several disadvantages need to be addressed for wider adoption. These include the requirement for complex systems for pressure regulation and control, the risk of stamp deformation, and pattern collapse during inflation. Addressing these challenges will be crucial for fully realizing the potential of inflatable stamp-based transfer printing. Overall, inflatable stamps offer unique advantages but require the engineering of stamp materials and pressure control systems to become viable for commercial manufacturing.

2.3.4 Glue-Assisted and Surface Chemical Transfer Technique

Glue-assisted and surface chemical transfer techniques utilize intermediate polymer layers or surface functionalization to enable the transfer and printing of materials. Chemical linkages like covalent bonding can also be used instead of polymers to bind materials to stamp surfaces. The polymer layers or chemical moieties act as a dynamic adhesive interface that controls attachment/detachment. Heating or solvent dissolution can be used to help release the materials from the stamp. Materials such as nanowires, carbon nanotubes (CNTs), 2D materials, and thin films have been transferred using this method.

Figure 2.3h is a typical fabrication process for glue-assisted transfer printing using intermediate polymer layers (Sim et al., 2015). A sacrificial polymer layer is applied to the stamp surface and makes conformal contact with the donor substrate carrying the material to be transferred. Picked up functional materials array on the tape and the loaded stamp is aligned over the target substrate. A solvent is used to release the polymer and material from the stamp. Any residual polymer is removed by solvent dissolution or reactive ion etching. Transferred materials may be annealed to improve adhesion to the target substrate. Critical process parameters are surface functionalization, polymer materials and thickness, release kinetics, temperature, and pressure control during pick-up and transfer.

The advantages of this technology include simplicity, the ability to transfer fragile materials, compatibility with non-planar or curved surfaces, and precise kinetic control over release. However, issues with material embedding into polymers and residue formation exist. Zhang et al. successfully demonstrated the use of double-sided tape to peel off a patterned NdFeB/PEI film from the surface of a PEI tape (Dong et al., 2022), which provides a new approach to transfer fragile or dispersed materials. Some NdFeB particles remained on the surface of the PEI tape, which can be attributed to the uneven size of the NdFeB particles, as shown in Figure 2.3i.

2.3.5 Laser-based Non-contact Transfer Technique

Laser-based non-contact transfer technique refers to methods of transferring materials from one substrate to another without physically contacting the substrates. The transfer is induced by focused laser irradiation which is focused on the donor substrate to provide localized heating or ablation to release and transfer material to the receiver substrate. Materials like metals, semiconductors, polymers, and nanostructures can be transferred.

Figure 2.3j provides a concise overview of the typical fabrication process steps for laser-based non-contact transfer technology. The material slated for transfer is first either deposited or grown on the donor substrate. Following this, the donor substrate is carefully mounted and precisely aligned with the receiver substrate, ensuring proximity with only a small gap between them. The pivotal step involves a focused pulsed laser beam that is directed at the donor material. This laser beam induces localized heating, ultimately leading to the release of the material onto the receiver substrate. This process offers a highly controlled and precise means of material transfer in various applications. Key applications are in electronics, photonics, sensors, and biotechnology.

This technology has been applied in the transfer of micro-LED (μ-LED) and Si ink. Song et al. successfully transferred a 280 μm × 280 μm × 8 μm μ-LED and a 90 μm × 90 μm × 2 μm Si ink onto a PDMS substrate with a pyramid microstructure on the surface and a glass substrate, respectively (Luo et al., 2021). Figure 2.3k is an SEM image of the μ-LED transferred onto the PDMS substrate; the LEDs are arranged in a heart-shape pattern (Figure 2.3l). The removable transfer printing of microscale Si ink and μ-LED illustrates the excellent capabilities of laser-based non-contact transfer technology for deterministic assembly.

Laser-based non-contact transfer technique offers several compelling advantages. It enables non-contact, dry transfer without physically contacting substrates, reducing the risk of contamination, and is capable of selectively and precisely transferring micro- and nanoscale materials with minimal mechanical damage or stress to the transferred materials. However, there are certain disadvantages to consider. Laser-based transfer technology is typically a serial process with limited throughput compared to parallel methods. Heat-affected zones and thermal damage can occur in the transferred materials.

Laser transfer enables non-contact integration not feasible with contact printing but has limitations in throughput and resolution compared to lithography which needs further improvement. The optimization of laser parameters, substrate performance, and other factors to improve transfer yield, accuracy, and resolution is the future development trend of this technique.

2.3.6 Adhesion Pad-assisted Transfer Technique

Adhesion pad-assisted transfer technology utilizes controllable adhesion forces to pick up and print materials in a deterministic way. The technology is inspired by the gecko's toe pad, the adhesion is controlled by the mechanical deformation caused by the vertical and lateral loads on the toe pad. Some gecko-inspired methods have been used, mainly using a pedestal stamp and embossing the pattern on the flexible stamp.

A typical process of adhesion pad-assisted transfer technique, employing a pedestal stamp, is depicted in Figure 2.3m (Kim, Carlson, et al., 2012a). The pedestal stamp initially makes contact with the donor substrate containing the functional material. After applying the necessary force for a certain duration, the stamp is retracted at a constant rate. During this retraction, the functional material is brought back along with the stamp. Subsequently, when the stamp makes conformal contact with the receiving substrate, adhesion can be altered by controlling the peeling direction. This step facilitates the printing of the material onto the receiving substrate.

The adhesion pad-assisted transfer technique offers several notable advantages. It excels in high precision and accuracy, leveraging van der Waals forces for the deterministic pickup of nanoscale materials, facilitating precise positioning and assembly. Furthermore, it minimizes surface contamination as it relies solely on adhesion, avoiding the need for disruptive methods like solvents or etching. Its versatility is evident in its capability to pick and place a wide variety of materials, including graphene, nanowires, and more. The approach is scalable and reusable, making it a cost-effective choice, with nanostructured adhesives being fabricated through simple molding processes.

This technique has been successfully used in flexible displays and medical applications (C. Wang et al., 2020a). Figure 2.3n shows a photograph of μ-LEDs transferred to a medical tape and adhered to the surface of human skin, which can be applied in psoriasis photo-therapy. However, there are certain disadvantages to consider. Adhesion pad-assisted transfer technology has limited adhesion strength due to the relatively weak van der Waals forces, which restricts the size and weight of materials that can be picked up.

2.4 3D PRINTING

3D printing has revolutionized the field of soft electronics by enabling the fabrication of complex, customizable, and functional soft electronic devices. The most common materials used for soft electronics are thermoplastics like acrylonitrile butadiene styrene (ABS) and polylactic acid (PLA). Common 3D printing techniques include stereolithography (SLA), inkjet printing technology, selective laser sintering (SLS), direct ink writing (DIW), shape deposition manufacturing (SDM), and fused deposition modeling (FDM) (Gul et al., 2018).

Unlike traditional manufacturing, which relies on subtracting material from a larger block, 3D printing creates objects by depositing material layer-by-layer until the object is complete. The fundamental principles of 3D printing involve a systematic process that transforms digital designs into physical objects through additive manufacturing. It all begins with the creation of a 3D model using CAD software, followed by saving it in the STL file format, which facilitates slicing the model into thin layers. Slicing software further breaks down the design into hundreds or thousands of horizontal layers, generating specific instructions for the 3D printer, such as layer thickness, infill patterns, and print speed. Finally, the 3D printer executes the commands to complete the operation.

2.4.1 Stereolithography

Stereolithography (SLA) is one of the most common 3D printing technologies which utilizes a laser to selectively cure liquid UV curable resin layer-by-layer to solidify an object. A laser source, displacement stage, optical control platform, and resin are necessary for an SLA standard system, as shown in Figure 2.4a.

In the SLA process, each layer is meticulously traced out by a laser on the surface of the liquid resin. Exposure to UV light plays a crucial role in curing and solidifying the resin. Once a layer is fully cured, the build platform lifts, creating space for fresh resin to flow underneath, preparing for the next layer. This repetitive sequence continues until the entire 3D object is meticulously formed. To complete the process, the object is then carefully rinsed in a solvent to remove any excess resin and undergoes further curing under UV light to ensure its structural integrity. Figure 2.4b shows a simplified structural schematic of an SLA 3D printer, which can be used to print hydrogel actuators (Mishra et al., 2020).

Compared to other 3D printing processes, SLA can produce parts with high precision and smooth surfaces. The support structure is required to support overhangs and bridges during the SLA printing process, which can be removed after printing is complete. Commonly used materials are photopolymers such as acrylates or epoxy resins, which offer the advantages of high fineness, high strength, and heat resistance. As a result, SLA is ideal for prototypes, small batches, and parts with complex geometries and is used in a wide range of industries including automotive, aerospace, dental, and healthcare. However, SLA has some limitations, such as smaller manufacturing volumes, potentially brittle materials, and the need for post-processing.

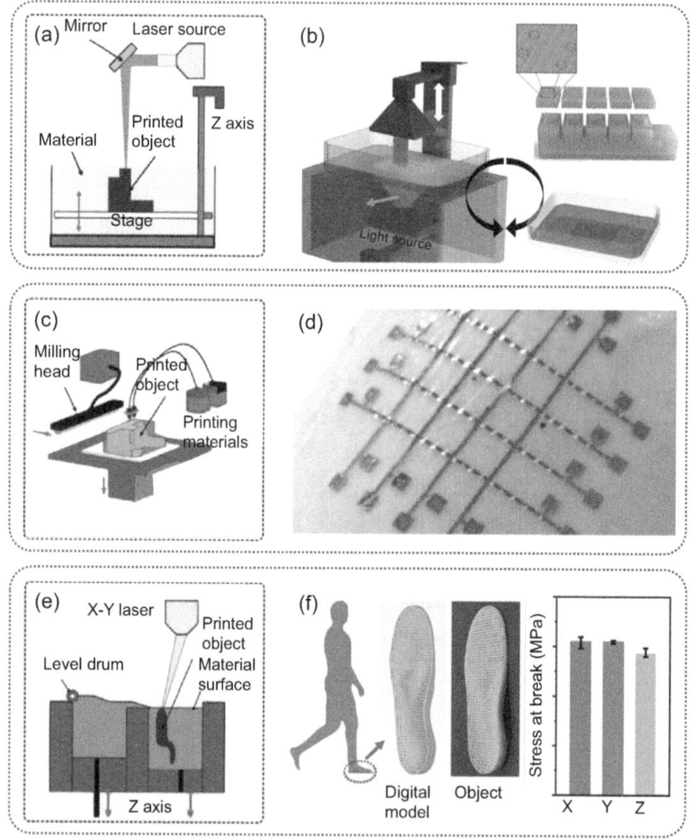

FIGURE 2.4 3D printing technology for fabricating soft electronic devices and its applications. The 3D printing technologies include (a) stereolithography (SLA), (c) inkjet printing technology, (e) selective laser sintering (SLS), (g) direct ink writing (DIW), (i) shape deposition modeling (SDM), and (k) fused deposition modeling (FDM). (b) Simplified architecture of the SLA 3D printer and SLA-printed actuator. (d) The photograph of a multilayer structure circuit attached to human skin. (f) Digital model and SLS print of AtBuPU-PDMS orthotic insole with tensile strength higher than TPU elastomers.

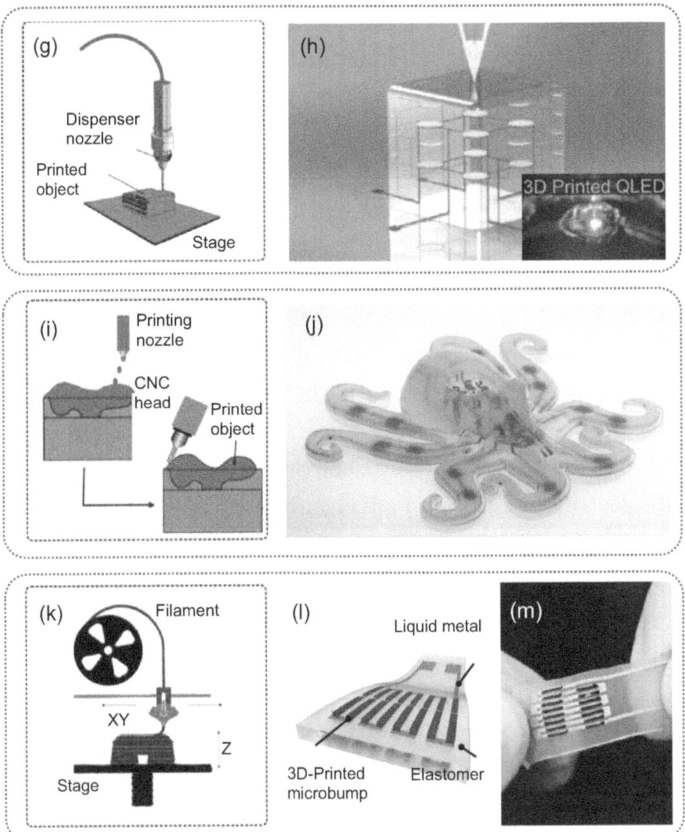

FIGURE 2.4 (Cont.) 3D printing technology for fabricating soft electronic devices and its applications. The 3D printing technologies include (h) Quantum dot light-emitting diodes (QD-LEDs) with pure and tunable color emission characteristics fabricated by the DIW technique. The inset shows an optical photo of DIW-printed QD-LED with orange light. (j) Application of SDM in soft robotics manufacturing. (l) Schematic of FDM-printed microbump with integrated liquid metal pressure sensor. (l and m) The optical photo of an FDM-printed microbump with an integrated liquid metal pressure sensor. ([a, c, e, g, i, k] Adapted with permission (Gul et al., 2018). Copyright 2018, Taylor & Francis; [b] Adapted with permission (Mishra et al., 2020). Copyright 2020, AAAS; [d] Adapted with permission (Mikkonen et al., 2020). Copyright 2020, American Chemical Society; [f] Adapted with permission (Sun et al., 2021). Copyright 2021, Elsevier; [h] Adapted with permission (Kong et al., 2014). Copyright 2014, American Chemical Society; [j] Adapted with permission (Mazzolai & Mattoli, 2016). Copyright 2016, Springer Nature; [m] Adapted with permission (K. Kim et al., 2019a). Copyright 2019, Wiley-VCH.)

2.4.2 Inkjet Printing Technique

The inkjet printing technique is a group of 3D printing processes that work by selectively depositing droplets of material layer-by-layer to build an object. Figure 2.4c is a schematic diagram of the device for inkjet printing technology. This technology uses an inkjet head similar to that of a 2D paper printer, but instead of spraying ink, tiny droplets of material are precisely ejected. These droplets can contain light-curing resins, ceramic suspensions, fused polymers, and more. Depending on each cross-section of the 3D model, the inkjet head deposits the droplets onto the build platform. These materials cure quickly upon contact with the platform, thus maintaining the printed shape.

Some of the common inkjet 3D printing processes include material jetting, drop-on-demand, and nanoparticle jetting. Material jetting involves using a print head to jet liquid resin or metal material in tiny droplets onto a platform and then curing them layer-by-layer through UV light or heat source, thus constructing a 3D object. Drop-on-demand, on the other hand, involves using a print head to jet solid or semi-solid materials in droplets onto a platform when needed, melting or curing them with a heat source layer-by-layer, thus constructing a 3D object. Lastly, nanoparticle jetting involves using a print head to jet droplets containing nanoparticles onto a platform and then solidifying them layer-by-layer through high temperatures, thus constructing a 3D object. Mantysalo et al. proposed a direct digital printing fabrication process in multilayer electronic devices based on inkjet printing technology, which utilizes silicone ink and silver nanoparticles. Figure 2.4d shows an optical schematic of a multilayer circuit printed by inkjet onto human skin (Mikkonen et al., 2020).

Inkjet printing uses an inkjet printhead to accurately eject droplets of material to build objects layer-by-layer at a high resolution. It is capable of printing multicolor, high-resolution, and good surface finish, supports a wide range of materials, and is widely used in the fields of art, medical products, electronic printing, education, and research. However, the current speed is relatively slow, and the choice of materials is limited.

2.4.3 Selective Laser Sintering

Selective laser sintering (SLS) is a 3D printing technique that uses a laser to fuse powdered material and build objects layer-by-layer. The schematic diagram of the device for the SLS technology is shown in Figure 2.4e. It is a powder-based additive manufacturing process that uses a high-power laser to selectively fuse or sinter powdered material layered in a chamber. The powder is spread into thin layers across a build platform and the laser fuses the powder together where required to form that particular cross-section, as guided by a 3D model. After one layer is fused, the platform lowers, a fresh layer of powder is spread over the previous layer, and the process repeats until the complete object is formed through successive layers.

SLS uses a laser to selectively fuse successive layers of powdered material based on a 3D model to create solid objects with good strength and high accuracy. It can utilize a wide range of materials including polymers like thermoplastic urethanes (TPUs) and polyamides (PAs), metals like titanium and aluminum alloys, ceramics like Si_3N_4 and Al_2O_3, and composite materials like carbon fiber and glass fiber. The unfused powder itself provides support for the object as it is being printed, eliminating the need for dedicated internal support structures. With large print sizes, excellent mechanical properties, and relatively high precision, SLS is considered the most suitable 3D printing technology for large-scale industrial production. It is used for rapid prototyping as well as short-run production across automotive, aerospace, dental, and healthcare industries. Some limitations are porosity in the final parts, size constraints based on the build chamber, higher running costs, and requirements for powder removal and cleanup after a build.

With the development of SLS technology, some materials that were once considered difficult to use for 3D printing are becoming possible. Due to the inherent thermosetting nature of PDMS, 3D printing of powder-based PDMS poses significant challenges. Xia et al. achieved SLS 3D printing of powder-based PDMS and successfully printed a complex-structured PDMS insole with strong tensile properties (Sun et al., 2021). Its digital model and physical image are shown in Figure 2.4f. A new powder material that can be used for SLS has been added to this work, driving further development of 3D printing in the field of powder-based elastomer additive manufacturing.

2.4.4 Direct Ink Writing

Direct ink writing (DIW) is an extrusion-based 3D printing technique that works by depositing viscoelastic inks layer-by-layer to fabricate 3D objects. Figure 2.4g shows a schematic of the device for DIW technology. Unlike inkjet printing technology that uses inkjet heads to precisely eject tiny droplets of material, DIW uses computer-controlled syringes or nozzles to precisely extrude viscous ink materials as continuous filaments. The inks are specially formulated viscoelastic materials that can flow through a nozzle under pressure but quickly solidify after deposition. Typical ink materials include hydrogels, ceramics, polymers, composites, and even living cells. By depositing the ink filaments in a layer-by-layer method side-by-side, following digital designs, 3D structures can be built up. The precisely extruded filaments fuse and solidify shortly after deposition to form the designed 3D architecture.

DIW has high material flexibility since it can print a wide range of functional ink materials that can be carefully formulated. It also allows multi-material printing where different inks are combined in one part. No support structures are required, and overhangs can be printed through careful toolpath planning. DIW does not require heat or lasers, making room-temperature extrusion suitable for delicate biomaterials. The DIW process can achieve high resolution down to tens of micrometers and the ability to print tall structures. DIW is relatively low cost, requiring inexpensive equipment and materials compared to other methods. Limitations are mainly slower speed, limited strength depending on the ink, and constraints on ink material development. Extremely complex organic shapes also remain difficult. Overall, material flexibility, resolution, and low cost make DIW suitable for a wide range of applications, ranging from printed electronics, batteries, and bioprinting tissues to chemical sensors.

Seamlessly interweaving materials of different properties into one architecture is an important feature of 3D printing. The more materials there are, the greater the difference in properties between them and the greater the challenges faced in integrating them. McAlpine et al. interwove five different materials into a QD-LED system through DIW, which exhibited pure and tunable color properties (Kong et al., 2014). Figure 2.4h shows a schematic diagram of printing QD-LEDs using DIW technology, with an optical photo of orange-emitting QD-LEDs as an illustration. The emergence of this application further demonstrates the greater versatility of 3D printing in the field of material integration.

2.4.5 Shape Deposition Manufacturing

Shape deposition manufacturing (SDM) is a hybrid additive and subtractive manufacturing process that combines material deposition and CNC machining. The schematic of the device for the SDM is demonstrated in Figure 2.4i. This technique uses a multi-axis robotic arm that alternates between material deposition and precision milling. The robotic arm switches between a material extruder to deposit layers of material and a milling spindle to precisely cut each layer to the final shape and dimensions.

The materials typically deposited by the extruder in SDM are thermoplastics, waxes, ceramics, and metal pastes. The milling helps expose any embedded parts or features. The combination of additive and subtractive technology provides greater geometric freedom and accuracy in the parts produced compared to regular 3D printing alone. Discrete components can be placed during the layering process before milling. This enables the creation of complex internal features like cavities and the assembling of multi-material components. SDM is used for applications like lightweight aerospace parts, integrated circuits with embedded electronics, and medical implants. Key advantages are high-dimensional accuracy, good surface finish, and the ability to produce complex geometries and combine dissimilar materials. Limitations are the relatively slower speed compared to regular 3D printing, higher system complexity, and restrictions on usable materials. Walsh et al. designed and produced a robotic hand using SDM technology, which was used in minimally invasive surgical robots to provide a soft interface between metal laparoscopic forceps and grasping hands (Gafford et al., 2015). It demonstrates the potential of SDM in the field of soft electronics, particularly in the area of soft medical device development, to meet the compliance, consistency, and flexibility requirements of medical devices. As shown in Figure 2.4j (Mazzolai & Mattoli, 2016), a soft octopus robot fabricated by SDM technology. The octopus robot is a minimal system, which may serve as the basis for a new generation of fully soft autonomous robots.

2.4.6 Fused Deposition Modeling

Fused deposition modeling (FDM) is a 3D printing technique that works by depositing and fusing thermoplastic filaments layer-by-layer to build objects. The device schematic for FDM is shown in Figure 2.4k. This technology uses a continuous filament of thermoplastic material such as ABS, PLA, or nylon. This filament is fed into a heated extrusion nozzle that melts the material and deposits it in thin layers onto a build platform. The extruded material quickly hardens after being deposited. The nozzle can move horizontally and vertically, controlled by computer-aided manufacturing (CAM) software. As the model is built up layer-by-layer, the nozzle deposits material only where required for that particular cross-section. Where internal features like cavities or overhangs are needed, temporary support structures are printed from the nozzle and later removed after the print is completed. In this way, FDM selectively deposits melted thermoplastic in successive layers based on a 3D model to construct the physical object.

Key advantages of FDM include lower costs for both printers and materials, minimal material waste, the ability to use engineering thermoplastics, ease of use even for non-experts, and the potential to achieve moderate print speeds and resolution based on factors like layer height and infill density. However, FDM also has some limitations – it offers lower accuracy and more visible layer lines compared to other processes like SLA. The technology is constrained to only thermoplastic materials, lacking the flexibility for other methods. While ideal for more conceptual prototypes, tooling applications, and models, FDM lacks the precision and detailed resolution required for highly detailed parts. It provides an accessible and practical 3D printing method but has limitations in accuracy and materials compared to other processes. Its low cost has fueled the wide adoption of desktop 3D printers aimed at hobbyists, educators, and home users.

The application of FDM in the field of wearable and soft electronics is attracting more and more attention from researchers, which can be attributed to the fact that FDM improves the simplicity and cost-effectiveness of flexible electronic device fabrication. Park's team has previously proposed a highly sensitive wearable liquid metal-based pressure sensor for health detection (K. Kim et al., 2019a). The device structure of the sensor is shown in Figure 2.4l, where an FDM-prepared microbump array with microchannels is used to sense changes in pressure. The optical photo of the device is shown in Figure 2.4m. With the help of FDM technology, this work has significantly simplified the complexity of the microchannel fabrication process.

2.5 TEXTILE TECHNOLOGY

Textile technology plays a crucial role in the development and integration of soft electronics into fabric-based applications. This technique enables the seamless integration of electronic components, sensors, and interconnects into textiles, resulting in wearable technology, smart textiles, and e-textiles. Coating, spinning, and thermal drawing are key textile technologies that allow conductive materials and electronics to be directly integrated into the fabric itself for soft electronics. And their fabrication strategies are shown schematically in Figures 2.5a, c, and f, respectively (Libanori et al., 2022). They enable unique capabilities ranging from flexible circuits to smart sensors.

2.5.1 Coating

Coating is a textile technique that involves applying a layer of a specific material onto the surface of a fabric to impart certain properties. In the context of soft electronics, coating refers to applying conductive materials onto fabric surfaces to create flexible and stretchable electronic components.

The process of coating conductive materials to textiles involves several steps. The process starts with pre-treatment of the fabric to improve the adhesion of the conductive coating. Then a conductive coating material is prepared, including conductive nanoparticles, polymers, binders, and solvents, to optimize its conductivity, flexibility, and printability. Afterward, the conductive coating is applied to the fabric surface through dipping. Then a drying or curing process is carried out to ensure the coating is firmly adhered to the fabric. Finally, the technical parameters of the product such as electrical conductivity and tensile strength are tested to ensure quality. The entire process should be properly controlled, such as coating thickness, softness, adhesion, and pattern clarity, to produce high-quality and reliable conductive textile products.

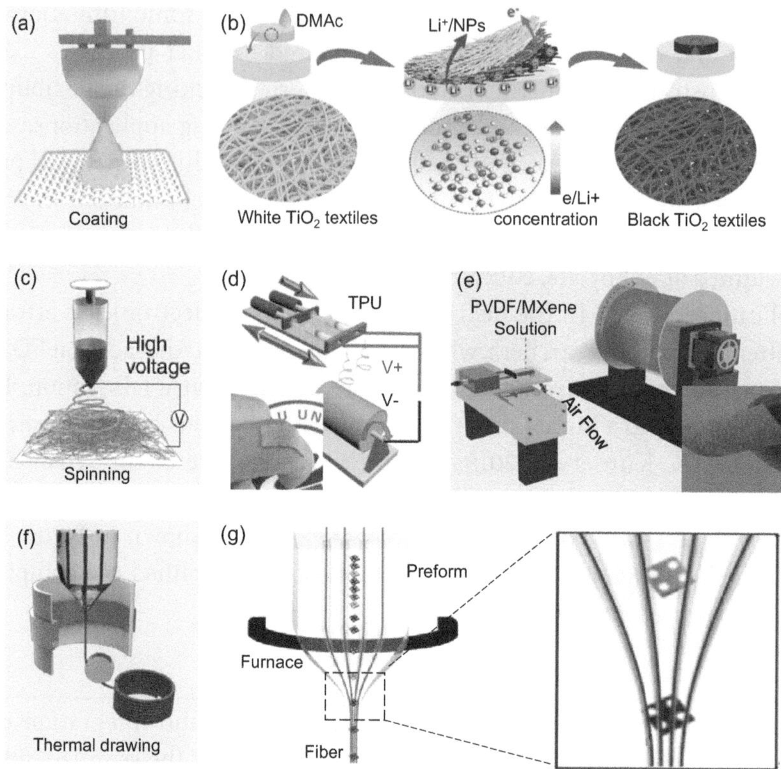

FIGURE 2.5 Fabrication strategies of smart textiles for soft electronics and applications of smart textile technology in functional fabrics. Fabricating functional fibers by using techniques including (a) coating, (c) spinning, and (f) thermal drawing. (b) Flowchart for fabricating TiO_2 fibers by coating technique. (d) Schematic diagram of electrostatic spinning for textile fibers. The inset shows a photograph of a textile fabric on a finger. (e) Schematic diagram of solution blow spinning for textiles. The inset shows the textile fabricated by the solution blow spinning technique. (g) Manufacture of fibers with digital devices by the thermal drawing technique. ([a, c, f] Adapted with permission (Libanori et al., 2022). Copyright 2022, Springer Nature; [b] Adapted with permission (Yan et al., 2020). Copyright 2020, AAAS; [d] Adapted with permission (Zhou et al., 2020). Copyright 2020, Elsevier; [e] Adapted with permission (Xu et al., 2022). Copyright 2022, Wiley-VCH; [g] Adapted with permission (Loke et al., 2021). Copyright 2021, Springer Nature.)

Ding et al. have made an effective practice in turning insulators into conductors by coating and succeeded in producing good electrical conductivity from insulating ceramic nanofiber textiles (Yan et al., 2020). The flowchart of achieving electrically conductive TiO_2 fibers is shown in Figure 2.5b. Insulating TiO_2 was dropped with dimethylacetamide (DMAc) to initiate defects in the TiO_2 interfacial layer to obtain electrical conductivity for insulating TiO_2.

Coating enables the simple integration of electronics onto fabrics, such as soft circuits, wearable devices, and smart textiles. The advantages of coating lie in its simplicity and cost efficiency in adding electronic functionality directly onto textile surfaces while maintaining conformal and lightweight properties. However, its limitations include coatings that may crack or delaminate over time, particularly under stretching. This requires optimal binder/coating thickness and adhesion, while multi-layer coatings can become rigid.

So, it requires careful design and material selection to maximize durability, maintain stretchability, and minimize stiffness.

2.5.2 Spinning

Spinning is a textile technique used to incorporate conductive nanomaterials such as silver, copper, and carbon nanotubes into polymer fiber materials during the fiber spinning process. This is used to produce conductive yarns and fibers suitable for soft electronics applications. Electrospinning and solution blow spinning are two important spinning technologies used to fabricate fibers and membranes for soft electronics applications. Both are versatile techniques to spin nano-microscale fibers with capabilities to incorporate electronics for soft devices.

Electrospinning is a technique that uses electrostatic forces to spin polymer fibers from a solution. In this process, a polymer solution is pumped through a nozzle to which a high voltage is applied. The strong electric field causes the solution to eject from the nozzle as thin charged jets dry into nanofibers as the solvent evaporates. Electrospinning allows the fabrication of nanofibers down to tens of nanometers in diameter. Conductive nanomaterials can also be incorporated into the fibers during electrospinning. This technique is used to produce flexible electrodes, sensors, battery separators, and other nanostructured materials. The fine fiber morphology provides high surface area and porosity. The schematic diagram of the device for producing TPU fiber structure thin films by electrospinning is shown in Figure 2.5d (Zhou et al., 2020). A photograph of the TPU film adhered to the finger is shown in the inset.

Solution blow spinning is a technique that uses compressed air to spin polymer fibers from solution. The polymer solution is extruded out and drawn into fibers by high-velocity air. Compared to electrospinning, it is a simpler setup without the need for voltage. It enables large-scale production of sub-micron fibers, which can be layered into porous membranes for e-textiles. This technique is suitable for low-cost, roll-to-roll production of large-area fabrics, and is often used for textile gas sensors, battery separators, and tissue scaffolds. The schematic diagram of the device for producing a PVDF/MXene fiber structure thin film by solution blow spinning is shown in Figure 2.5e (Xu et al., 2022). As shown in the inset, the fabric sensor made by air spinning has good mechanical properties.

Spinning has some unique advantages and limitations as a fabrication method for conductive fibers in soft electronics. This technique can produce fibers and yarns with intrinsic conductivity, while maintaining the softness, flexibility, and feel of textiles. By adjusting the doping levels, the electrical properties of the fibers can be tuned flexibly. Also, as a continuous process, the spinning technique can enable large-scale production. However, it is relatively difficult to achieve fine patterning of circuits and hard to control the uniform dispersion of nanofillers. If the process parameters are not well controlled, there could be large variations in properties between different batches.

2.5.3 Thermal Drawing

Thermal drawing is an emerging manufacturing technique that produces micro- and nanoscale multilayer fibers by heating and drawing layered thermoplastic and metal sheets, suitable for fabricating conductive fibers and yarns for soft electronics applications.

Thermal drawing involves stacking sheets of predefined geometries and heating them to a molten state, then drawing them under tension to reduce dimensions through viscous flow, forming long conductive fibers. This process allows combining polymer and metal layers together to selectively incorporate metallic conductors. By controlling the initial sheet arrangements, the cross-section of the conductive fibers can be tailored, and fibers with complex geometries (such as core-shell or multi-domain) can be created. Typical materials are combinations of thermoplastics (such as PMMA, PC, and PS) and metals (such as tin, indium, and gold). This technique can manufacture highly flexible and stretchable conductors, and the fibers can be insulated with a polymer jacket and then woven or knitted into electronic textiles. It also enables miniaturization and high-precision patterning not achievable by conventional textile technology.

From the working mechanism perspective, thermal drawing and FDM appear similar, but in fact, there are significant differences between the two. FDM works by additive manufacturing through layer-by-layer extrusion of thermoplastics to build 3D objects, using a variety of thermoplastic materials and being simple and accessible, but with weaker mechanical properties, whereas thermal drawing produces long thin conductive fibers by heating and drawing multilayer sheets, with limited material choices and needing precise control, yet having high strength and miniaturization advantages.

The unique ability of thermal drawing to produce multilayer and multi-material conductive fibers enables high-density integration and miniaturization that is difficult to achieve with conventional textile technology. The highly aligned drawn fibers also exhibit excellent mechanical properties like strength and flexibility. However, the limitations include restricted choices of combinable polymers and metals, challenges in attaining very high uniformity and alignment consistency, as well as difficulty in incorporating stretchability and elasticity into the drawn fibers.

The application of the thermal drawing-based process in integrating digital devices into fibers to enable fabrics to function as digital systems has been demonstrated (Loke et al., 2021). Functional fibers with independently addressable digital devices were prepared by embedding digital chips at a precise angle into a prefabricated rod consisting of a rigid PC and a soft PMMA sandwich, and by thermally pulling the chips to achieve a directional connection with coaxially fed tungsten electrodes under the synergistic effect of the soft and hard polymer interlayers. Figure 2.5g shows the schematic diagram of the device.

2.6 OTHER FABRICATION TECHNOLOGIES

Soft electronics is an emerging field that aims to develop stretchable and flexible electronic devices using novel materials and fabrication technology. In addition to these key technologies, kirigami technology, coating technology, and screen-printing technology have also driven the development of soft electronics.

By using these technologies, researchers can develop fully integrated soft electronic systems, including sensors (Keller et al., 2023), circuits (Gong et al., 2022), power sources (Zheng et al., 2021), and displays (X. Wang et al., 2023b). These technologies enable electronics to be embedded into soft materials for applications ranging from robotics to wearable devices. This section provides an overview of these key technology-advancing soft electronics.

2.6.1 Kirigami Technology

Kirigami is a method of fabricating flexible electronic devices that draws on the concept of traditional paper-cutting art. The process generally uses laser or mechanical cutting techniques to cut metal foils, films, or other thin-film materials into desired shapes, which are then assembled onto a flexible substrate to form a flexible electronic device. It allows for the fabrication of very thin, lightweight materials with good flexibility. The reconfigurability and shape-changing ability of the kirigami structure for devices is realized by folding and unfolding the devices.

The kirigami technique requires going through the key steps of design and modeling, precise cutting, controlled folding, and packaging and assembly in order to optimize the pattern design and achieve the desired electrical performance and mechanical flexibility. This process involves using modeling software to strategically design the kirigami patterns and predict the shapes, folds, and electronic properties. Precise cutting along the designed lines and controlled origami-style folding help form the 3D shapes. Conductive adhesives or solders are used to interconnect electronic components, which are then encapsulated between flexible polymer layers for reliability.

Kirigami can create soft sensors (Zhuo et al., 2023), circuits (Liu et al., 2022), antennas (Zheng et al., 2022), and micro-batteries (Li et al., 2022) that conform to the surface by carefully cutting and folding two-dimensional sheets, providing a unique manufacturing method for soft electronics. This has great potential in soft robotics, biomedical devices, and wearable electronic devices. Kawano et al. presented a highly stretchable, deformable, and soft biological probe thin-film device designed based on the kirigami process (Morikawa et al., 2017). They utilized the kirigami process to fabricate a large number of elongated slits on a parylene film substrate, resulting in a high degree of stretchability (up to 470%). The structure of the device is shown in Figure 2.6a. The device can be adapted to the shape of the brain surface and record EEG signals from the visual cortex and occipital cortex of mice as shown in Figure 2.6b. Limited mechanical-type deformation (<2%) restricts the application of 2D materials to flexible devices. Hu et al. greatly improved the ability of 2D materials to be applied to flexible electronics by increasing the stretchability of MOS_2 deposited on PDMS from 0.75% to ~15% through the kirigami process (the preparation process is schematically shown in Figure 2.6c) (Zheng et al., 2018). Figure 2.6d shows the optical photographs of MoS_2/PDMS with different structures before and after stretching. The traditional rigid Si thin films can also be applied to kirigami designs to achieve folding structures (K. Zhang et al., 2017a). Figure 2.6e shows the schematic illustrations of pressing the Si thin films using the kirigami process into hemispherical protrusions and concave molds, respectively. Figure 2.6f shows a photograph of the convex hemispherical structure made of Si thin film.

2.6.2 Spray Coating Technology

Spraying techniques are commonly used in the field of soft electronics to prepare thin films and pictorial structures, usually using a spray gun to uniformly deposit a solution

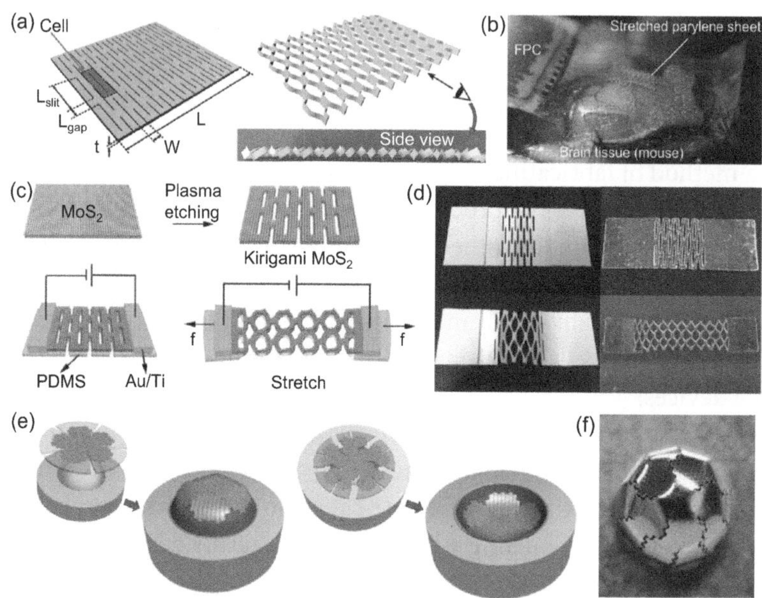

FIGURE 2.6 Applications of the kirigami process to soft electronics manufacturing. (a) Schematic of the structure fabricated by the kirigami process before and after stretching. The bottom right picture shows the side view. (b) Planar electrode (Pt) array devices placed on the surface of the cerebral cortex of living mice based on kirigami fabrication can be adjusted by stretching the film to adjust the position of the electrodes. (c) Schematic diagram of the process for manufacturing stretchable MoS_2/PDMS. (d) The photo of MoS_2/PDMS kirigami structures. (e) Schematic diagrams of a half-truncated icosahedral mesh based on silicon nanomembranes pressed into a hemispherical concave mold (right) and covered with a hemispherical convex mold (left), respectively. (f) Photographs of half-truncated icosahedra printed on a soft polyimide film. ([a] Adapted with permission (Morikawa et al., 2017). Copyright 2017, Wiley-VCH; [b] Adapted with permission (Morikawa et al., 2017). Copyright 2017, Wiley-VCH; [c] Adapted with permission (Zheng et al., 2018). Copyright 2018, American Chemical Society; [d] Adapted with permission (Zheng et al., 2018). Copyright 2018, American Chemical Society; [e] Adapted with permission (K. Zhang et al., 2017a). Copyright 2017, Springer Nature; [f] Adapted with permission (K. Zhang et al., 2017a). Copyright 2017, Springer Nature.)

or suspension onto a substrate to form the desired conductive film. Solutions or suspensions are formed from silver, MXene, copper, or carbon nanotube/graphene conductive particles suspended in an acrylic or polyurethane binder. The SEM images of Ag NWs, Ag NPs, and MXene deposited on the substrate surface are shown in Figure 2.7a (Jia et al., 2021; Li et al., 2021).

To fabricate conductive coatings on soft materials by spray coating, start by cleaning the material surface. Apply surface treatments if needed to improve adhesion. Load conductive paint into a spray gun, adjust viscosity, and spray multiple thin, overlapping coats allowing proper drying time between passes. Masks or grids can be used to define personalized patterns when spraying. Once fully cured, anneal the coated materials at 100–150°C to sinter the conductive particles, improving conductivity and durability. Test the sheet resistance, adhesion, and flexibility.

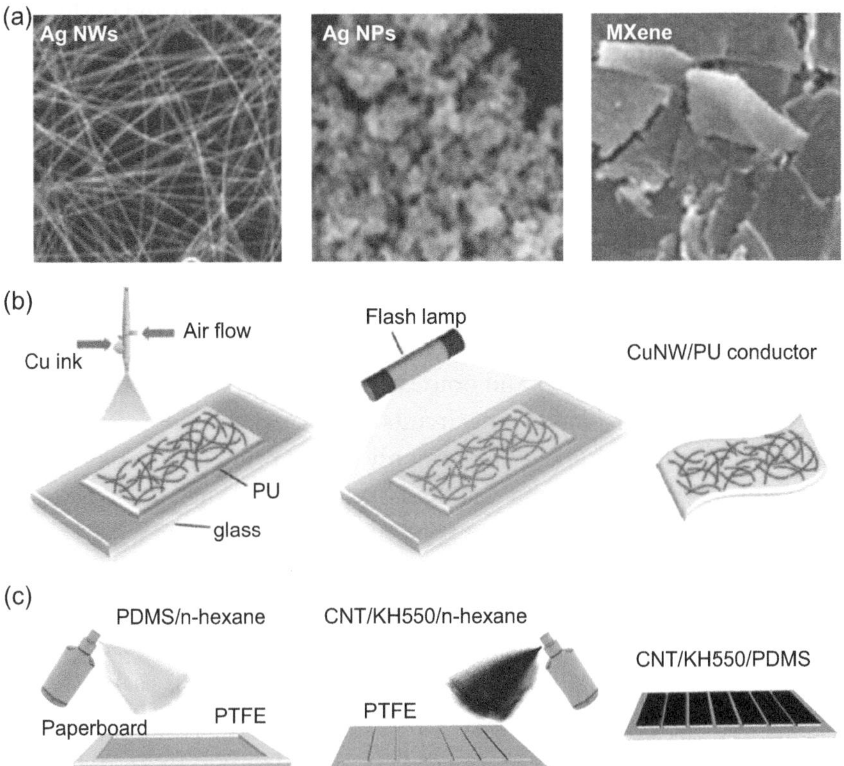

FIGURE 2.7   Applications of the spray coating process in soft electronic manufacturing. (a) SEM images of spray coating prepared Ag NWs, Ag NPs, and MXene, respectively. (b) Schematic diagram of Cu NW/PU conductors fabricated based on the spraying coating process. (c) Schematic diagram of CNT/KH550/PDMS sensor fabricated based on the spraying coating process. ([a] Adapted with permission (Li et al., 2021). Copyright 2021, Wiley-VCH. Adapted with permission (Jia et al., 2021). Copyright 2021, Spring Nature; [b] Adapted with permission (Ding et al., 2016). Copyright 2016, American Chemical Society; [c] Adapted with permission (Zhou et al., 2018). Copyright 2018, American Chemical Society.)

Utilizing the intrinsic properties of materials sprayed onto the substrate surface to design flexible electronic devices has made progress in flexible sensors. Using Cu ink sprayed onto the substrate to form Cu NWs as a replacement for expensive Ag NWs has been verified (Ding et al., 2016). The preparation process is shown in Figure 2.7b. Due to its good mechanical and conductive properties, this flexible device can be applied to wearable devices. Figure 2.7c verifies the process of preparing a CNT/KH550/PDMS strain sensor using a spray coating method (Zhou et al., 2018). The sensing of this sensor utilizes the brittle mechanical behavior of the conductive CNT/KH550 layer.

Spray coating technology allows versatile, scalable, and low-cost fabrication of conductive coatings on flexible substrates. Thickness and conductivity can be adjusted by multiple coats. Coatings are usually 10 to 100 µm thick. However, spray painting offers less control compared to technology like inkjet printing. It requires skill to achieve smooth, durable coatings and often needs protective overlaminates. Overall, spraying as a rapid prototyping method for simple conductive coatings lacks precision and performance compared to other advanced manufacturing methods.

2.6.3 Screen-Printing Technology

Screen printing, also known as silk screening or serigraphy, is a printing technique that uses a mesh screen to transfer ink onto a surface. It is a common technique for patterning conductive inks and pastes onto flexible substrates like textiles, plastic films, and paper. This allows the creation of flexible printed circuit boards and components.

The fabricating process is illustrated in Figure 2.8a (Gong et al., 2022). It involves using a mesh screen with the desired pattern and then using a squeegee to push ink deposited in unwanted areas through the mesh and onto the substrate below. With the right inks and substrates, both simple and complex soft circuits can be realized. For soft electronics, silver and carbon-based conductive inks are commonly screen printed. The inks need to cure or sinter after printing to achieve good conductivity. Polymers such as PI and PET are the most used flexible substrates, which have good mechanical properties.

Screen printing is a fast, scalable, and cost-effective process suitable for large-scale production of printed electronics. It allows the printing of complex circuit patterns and features down to around 100 µm resolution on a wide variety of flexible substrates like textiles, polymers, and paper. Screen printing uses simple equipment and is easy to set up at lower costs than cleanroom-based processes like photolithography. While screen printing has advantages in speed, cost, and flexibility compared to other processes, challenges include getting consistent prints on fabrics that absorb ink at different rates and registration issues when printing on flexible materials. Pre-treatments of fabrics are often needed. Overall, screen printing is suited for moderate-resolution circuits and components on flexible substrates for lower-performance printed electronics devices.

The concept of utilizing screen-printing techniques to combine different inks and different substrates to achieve different electronic functions has been validated. Figure 2.8b shows a flexible self-powered system for human pressure sensing, where the microbattery module and sensor module are based on MXene inks doped with different materials and prepared by screen printing on PET substrate (Zheng et al., 2021). Hiltunen et al. demonstrated a pressure sensor fabricated by screen-printing Ag/AgCl electrodes and interconnects on PDMS substrate (Figure 2.8c) (Huttunen et al., 2022) and successfully applied it to human physiological sensing. Figure 2.8d shows an exploded view of a human pressure sensor, where they successfully screen-printed Cu interdigitated electrodes on filter paper (Z. Wang et al., 2023a). The method of screen-printing Ag ink as electrodes on fabric has been validated (Seesaard & Wongchoosuk, 2023). Figure 2.8e shows four Ag electrodes screen printed on fabric. In addition to human physiological signals, flexible sensors in other fields such as sonar sensing have also been realized through screen-printing technology. Figure 2.8f shows a fully screen-printed sonar sensor, with all structures including the sensing layer printed layer-by-layer (Keller et al., 2023). In addition to sensor research, screen printing also plays an important role in the display field. Figure 2.8g shows a flexible mini LED panel prepared based on screen-printing technology, which finally achieved a size of 65 inches (X. Wang et al., 2023b).

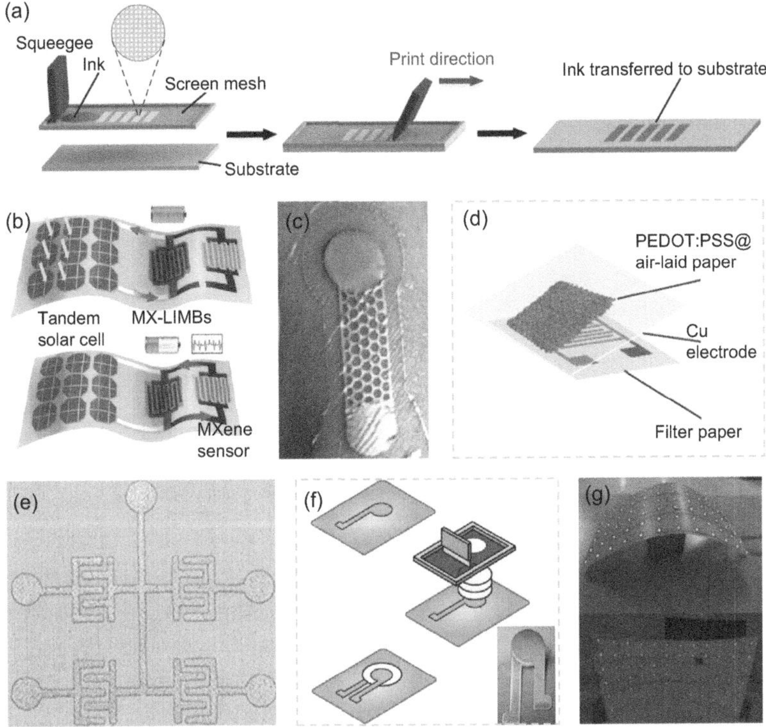

FIGURE 2.8 Screen-printing technology for soft electronics manufacturing. (a) The manufacturing process of screen-printing technology. Adapted with permission (Gong et al., 2022). Copyright 2022, Elsevier. (b) Schematic of the charging and discharging of a flexible self-powered pressure-sensing system based on MXene, which is fabricated by the screen-printing process. Adapted with permission (Zheng et al., 2021). Copyright 2021, Elsevier. (c) Optical images of screen-printing electronic tattoos on the epidermis. Adapted with permission (Huttunen et al., 2022). Copyright 2022, Wiley-VCH. (d) The schematic of the printable all-paper pressure sensor. Adapted with permission (Z. Wang et al., 2023a). Copyright 2023, American Chemical Society. (e) Four fabric-based electrode arrays by the screen-printing process. Adapted with permission (Seesaard & Wongchoosuk, 2023). Copyright 2023, Elsevier. (f) The manufacturing process for printed ultrasonic transducers. Adapted with permission (Keller et al., 2023). Copyright 2023, Wiley-VCH. The inset shows a photograph of ultrasonic transducers. (g) Flexible mini-LED panel manufactured by the screen-printing process. Adapted with permission (X. Wang et al., 2023b). Copyright 2023, Wiley-VCH.

2.7 SUMMARY AND OUTLOOK

This chapter provides a comprehensive summary of typical advanced fabrication technologies for soft electronics, as also depicted in Table 2.1. Soft electronics represents a cutting-edge interdisciplinary field that encompasses materials, devices, processes, and systems. It serves as a technical foundation for enhancing the functionality and performance of soft electronic devices while expanding their application scenarios. Advanced fabrication technologies, including soft lithography, soft transfer, 3D printing, and textile technology, play vital roles in shaping novel morphological devices in soft electronics.

TABLE 2.1   Advanced Fabrication Technologies for Soft Electronics and Their Application Potential

Technology	Classification	Resolution	Fabrication Efficiency	Applications	Ref.
Soft lithography	Replica molding (REM)	100 nm	High	Microstructures, nanowires, and lenses	Xia et al. (2004)
	Microtransfer molding (µTM)	0.5 µm	High	Thin films, nanomembranes, and LEDs	Sabahi-Kaviani and Luttge (2021)
	Microcontact printing (µCP)	1 µm	High	Self-assembled monolayers, biosensors, and microarrays	Jackman et al. (1995)
	Capillary microforming (MIMIC)	100 nm–5 µm	High	Microchannels, microlenses, and microcapsules	Wang et al. (2019)
	Solvent-assisted micromolding in capillaries (SAMIM)	1 µm	High	Microfluidic devices, porous structures, and scaffolds	Kim et al. (2004)
Soft transferring	Kinetically controlled transfer printing	<100 nm	High	Curved electronics, bioelectronics, and 3D integrated electronics	Meitl et al. (2006)
	Surface protrusions of adhesion-assisted transfer	100 µm	High	Flexible electronics, stretchable electronics, and wearable electronics	Huang et al. (2016)
	Inflatable stamp-assisted transfer	250 µm	High	Curved electronics, bioelectronics, and 3D integrated electronics	Carlson et al. (2012)
	Glue-assisted and surface chemical transfer	<20 nm	High	Flexible electronics, stretchable electronics, and wearable electronics	Jeong et al. (2014)
	Laser-based non-contact transfer	32 µm	High	Flexible electronics, stretchable electronics, and wearable electronics	Marinov (2018)
	Adhesion pad-assisted transfer	100 µm	High	Flexible electronics, stretchable electronics, and wearable electronics	Kim, Carlson, et al. (2012)
3D printing	Stereolithography (SLA)	0.1–50 µm	Moderate	Optical devices, microfluidics, and biomedical implants	Park et al. (2009); Wallin et al. (2017)
	Inkjet printing	0.2–50 µm	High	Flexible circuits, sensors, and displays	Yin et al. (2022)
	Selective laser sintering (SLS)	5–100 µm	Moderate	Functional parts, molds, and prototypes	Roy et al. (2019)
	Direct ink writing (DIW)	1–100 µm	Moderate	Conductive wires, antennas, and heaters	Truby and Lewis (2016)
	Shape deposition manufacturing (SDM)	–	Low	Soft actuators, robots, and artificial muscles	–
	Fused deposition modeling (FDM)	100 µm	High	Structural parts, housings, and enclosures	(Hong et al., (2016)

(Continued)

TABLE 2.1 (Continued)

Technology	Classification	Resolution	Fabrication Efficiency	Applications	Ref.
Textile technology	Coating	–	High	Conductive fabrics, sensors, and heaters	–
	Spinning	3 nm–5 μm	High	Functional fibers, yarns, and textiles	Carthew et al. (2022)
	Thermal drawing	50 μm–1 mm	High	Optical fibers, microstructured fibers, and devices	T. Zhang et al. (2017b)
Others	Screen printing	22–100 μm	High	Flexible circuits, sensors, and displays	Zavanelli and Yeo (2021)
	Spray coating	tens of μm	High	Thin films, nanomaterials, and devices	Hwang et al. (2016)
	Kirigami	a few mm	High	Stretchable electronics, actuators, and sensors	Uetani et al. (2021)

Soft lithography utilizes polymer elastomers as masks, stamps, or templates to fabricate micro/nanoscale structures. It enables the application of various materials to create intricate patterns on surfaces with different chemical properties and irregular curved surfaces. However, soft lithography demands high optical transparency, mechanical flexibility, and thermal stability of the flexible substrate. Addressing alignment precision during the process is also a challenge that needs high resolution.

Soft transfer involves transferring flexible electronics from rigid substrates to flexible ones, facilitating high-quality device transfer. Challenges persist in addressing issues such as peeling between the device and the rigid substrate, alignment accuracy, and maintaining device integrity. 3D printing offers a highly personalized and customizable approach for flexible electronics, boasting advantages such as design flexibility, rapid manufacturing, and scalability. However, challenges remain in material selection, print resolution, material compatibility, and interfacial adhesion.

Textile technology enables the integration of soft electronics into textiles, providing excellent flexibility, comfort, and adaptability. However, the structure and performance of fabrics are easily affected by environmental factors, and consideration must be given to solid fixation and reliable connections on textiles.

From a developing trend perspective, the critical focus of this field remains to enhance fabrication accuracy and preparation efficiency. Although different fabrication technologies encounter distinct challenges, they share common concerns such as material selection, process compatibility, cost control, reliability, and scalability. To address these challenges, effective strategies involve exploiting high-performance new materials and developing device fabrication processes with advancements in precision, efficiency, and reproducibility, which are driving the rapid iteration of soft electronics manufacturing. Remarkably, leveraging advanced fabrication technologies holds the potential for continuous evolution within the field of soft electronics. This progression paves the way for the development of novel intelligent sensory systems that exhibit enhanced performance, expanded functionality, and increased accessibility to a wider range of applications.

REFERENCES

Cadarso, V. J., Chidambaram, N., Jacot-Descombes, L., & Schift, H. (2017). High-aspect-ratio nanoimprint process chains. *Microsystems & Nanoengineering*, 3(1), 1–12.

Carlson, A., Wang, S., Elvikis, P., Ferreira, P. M., Huang, Y., & Rogers, J. A. (2012). Active, programmable elastomeric surfaces with tunable adhesion for deterministic assembly by transfer printing. *Advanced Functional Materials*, 22(21), 4476–4484.

Carthew, J., Taylor, J. B. J., Garcia-Cruz, M. R., Kiaie, N., Voelcker, N. H., Cadarso, V. J., & Frith, J. E. (2022). The bumpy road to stem cell therapies: Rational design of surface topographies to dictate stem cell mechanotransduction and fate. *ACS Applied Materials & Interfaces*, 14(20), 23066–23101.

Cavallo, F., & Lagally, M. G. (2010). Semiconductors turn soft: Inorganic nanomembranes. *Soft Matter*, 6(3), 439–455.

Choi, M. K., Yang, J., Kang, K., Kim, D. C., Choi, C., Park, C., Kim, S. J., Chae, S. I., Kim, T.-H., Kim, J. H., Hyeon, T., & Kim, D.-H. (2015). Wearable red–green–blue quantum dot light–emitting diode array using high-resolution intaglio transfer printing. *Nature Communications*, 6(1), 7149.

Ding, S., Jiu, J., Gao, Y., Tian, Y., Araki, T., Sugahara, T., Nagao, S., Nogi, M., Koga, H., Suganuma, K., & Uchida, H. (2016). One-step fabrication of stretchable copper nanowire conductors by a fast photonic sintering technique and its application in wearable devices. *ACS Applied Materials & Interfaces*, 8(9), 6190–6199.

Dong, Y., Wang, L., Xia, N., Yang, Z., Zhang, C., Pan, C., Jin, D., Zhang, J., Majidi, C., & Zhang, L. (2022). Untethered small-scale magnetic soft robot with programmable magnetization and integrated multifunctional modules. *Science Advances*, 8(25), eabn8932.

Gafford, J., Ding, Y., Harris, A., McKenna, T., Polygerinos, P., Holland, D., Walsh, C., & Moser, A. (2015). Shape deposition manufacturing of a soft, atraumatic, and deployable surgical grasper. *Journal of Mechanisms and Robotics*, 7(2), 021006.

Gao, W., Emaminejad, S., Nyein, H. Y. Y., Challa, S., Chen, K., Peck, A., Fahad, H. M., Ota, H., Shiraki, H., Kiriya, D., Lien, D.-H., Brooks, G. A., Davis, R. W., & Javey, A. (2016). Fully integrated wearable sensor arrays for multiplexed in situ perspiration analysis. *Nature*, 529(7587), 509–514.

Gong, X., Huang, K., Wu, Y.-H., & Zhang, X.-S. (2022). Recent progress on screen-printed flexible sensors for human health monitoring. *Sensors and Actuators A: Physical*, 345, 113821.

Gul, J. Z., Sajid, M., Rehman, M. M., Siddiqui, G. U., Shah, I., Kim, K.-H., Lee, J.-W., & Choi, K. H. (2018). 3D printing for soft robotics – A review. *Science and Technology of Advanced Materials*, 19(1), 243–262.

Hong, K. Y., Hui, Y. N., & Chen, H. Y. (2016). High-force soft printable pneumatics for soft robotic applications. *Soft Robotics*, 3(3), 144–158.

Huang, Y., Zheng, N., Cheng, Z., Chen, Y., Lu, B., Xie, T., & Feng, X. (2016). Direct laser writing-based programmable transfer printing via bioinspired shape memory reversible adhesive. *ACS Applied Materials & Interfaces*, 8(51), 35628–35633.

Huang, Y., Zhou, J., Ke, P., Guo, X., Yiu, C. K., Yao, K., Cai, S., Li, D., Zhou, Y., Li, J., Wong, T. H., Liu, Y., Li, L., Gao, Y., Huang, X., Li, H., Li, J., Zhang, B., Chen, Z., & Yu, X. (2023). A skin-integrated multimodal haptic interface for immersive tactile feedback. *Nature Electronics*, 6, 1020–1031.

Huttunen, O. H., Behfar, M. H., Hiitola-Keinänen, J., & Hiltunen, J. (2022). Electronic tattoo with transferable printed electrodes and interconnects for wireless electrophysiology monitoring. *Advanced Materials Technologies*, 7(8), 2101496.

Hwang, H., Kim, A., Zhong, Z., Kwon, H. C., Jeong, S., & Moon, J. (2016). Reducible-shell-derived pure-copper-nanowire network and its application to transparent conducting electrodes. *Advanced Functional Materials*, 26(36), 6545–6554.

Jackman, R. J., Wilbur, J. L., & Whitesides, G. M. (1995). Fabrication of submicrometer features on curved substrates by microcontact printing. *Science*, 269(5224), 664–666.

Jeong, J. W., Yang, S. R., Hur, Y. H., Kim, S. W., Baek, K. M., Yim, S., Jang, H.-I., Park, J. H., Lee, S. Y., Park, C.-O., & Jung, Y. S. (2014). High-resolution nanotransfer printing applicable to diverse surfaces via interface-targeted adhesion switching. *Nature Communications, 5*(1), 5387.

Jia, Y., Pan, Y., Wang, C., Liu, C., Shen, C., Pan, C., Guo, Z., & Liu, X. (2021). Flexible Ag microparticle/MXene-based film for energy harvesting. *Nano-Micro Letters, 13*(1), 201.

Keller, K., Leitner, C., Baumgartner, C., Benini, L., & Greco, F. (2023). Fully printed flexible ultrasound transducer for medical applications. *Advanced Materials Technologies, 8*(18), 2300577.

Kim, E., Xia, Y., & Whitesides, G. M. (2004). Two- and three-dimensional crystallization of polymeric microspheres by micromolding in capillaries. *Advanced Materials, 8*(3), 245–247.

Kim, K., Choi, J., Jeong, Y., Cho, I., Kim, M., Kim, S., Oh, Y., & Park, I. (2019a). Highly sensitive and wearable liquid metal-based pressure sensor for health monitoring applications: Integration of a 3D-printed microbump array with the microchannel. *Advanced Healthcare Materials, 8*(22), 1900978.

Kim, S., Carlson, A., Cheng, H., Lee, S., Park, J.-K., Huang, Y., & Rogers, J. A. (2012a). Enhanced adhesion with pedestal-shaped elastomeric stamps for transfer printing. *Applied Physics Letters, 100*(17).

Kim, S., Su, Y., Mihi, A., Lee, S., Liu, Z., Bhandakkar, T. K., Wu, J., Geddes III, J. B., Johnson, H. T., Zhang, Y., Park, J.-K., Braun, P. V., Huang, Y., & Rogers, J. A. (2012b). Imbricate scales as a design construct for microsystem technologies. *Small, 8*(6), 901–906.

Kim, S., Wu, J., Carlson, A., Jin, S. H., Kovalsky, A., Glass, P., Liu, Z., Ahmed, N., Elgan, S. L., Chen, W., Ferreira, P. M., Sitti, M., Huang, Y., & Rogers, J. A. (2010). Microstructured elastomeric surfaces with reversible adhesion and examples of their use in deterministic assembly by transfer printing. *Proceedings of the National Academy of Sciences, 107*(40), 17095–17100.

Kim, Y., Chortos, A., Xu, W., Liu, Y., Oh, J. Y., Son, D., Kang, J., Foudeh, A. M., Zhu, C., Lee, Y., Niu, S., Liu, J., Pfattner, R., Bao, Z., & Lee, T.-W. (2018). A bioinspired flexible organic artificial afferent nerve. *Science, 360*(6392), 998–1003.

Kim, Y. S., Mahmood, M., Lee, Y., Kim, N. K., Kwon, S., Herbert, R., Kim, D., Cho, H. C., & Yeo, W. H. (2019b). All-in-one, wireless, stretchable hybrid electronics for smart, connected, and ambulatory physiological monitoring. *Advanced Science, 6*(17), 1900939.

Kong, Y. L., Tamargo, I. A., Kim, H., Johnson, B. N., Gupta, M. K., Koh, T.-W., Chin, H.-A., Steingart, D. A., Rand, B. P., & McAlpine, M. C. (2014). 3D Printed quantum dot light-emitting diodes. *Nano Letters, 14*(12), 7017–7023.

Li, H., Wang, H., Chan, D., Xu, Z., Wang, K., Ge, M., Zhang, Y., Chen, S., & Tang, Y. (2022). Nature-inspired materials and designs for flexible lithium-ion batteries. *Carbon Energy, 4*(5), 878–900.

Li, J., Yuan, Z., Han, X., Wang, C., Huo, Z., Lu, Q., Xiong, M., Ma, X., Gao, W., & Pan, C. (2021). Biologically inspired stretchable, multifunctional, and 3D electronic skin by strain visualization and triboelectric pressure sensing. *Small Science, 2*(1), 2100083.

Li, S., Wang, H., Ma, W., Qiu, L., Xia, K., Zhang, Y., Lu, H., Zhu, M., Liang, X., Wu, X.-E., Liang, H., & Zhang, Y. (2023). Monitoring blood pressure and cardiac function without positioning via a deep learning–assisted strain sensor array. *Science Advances, 9*(32), eadh0615.

Libanori, A., Chen, G., Zhao, X., Zhou, Y., & Chen, J. (2022). Smart textiles for personalized healthcare. *Nature Electronics, 5*(3), 142–156.

Liu, J., Jiang, S., Xiong, W., Zhu, C., Li, K., & Huang, Y. (2022). Self-healing kirigami assembly strategy for conformal electronics. *Advanced Functional Materials, 32*(12), 2109214.

Loke, G., Khudiyev, T., Wang, B., Fu, S., Payra, S., Shaoul, Y., Fung, J., Chatziveroglou, I., Chou, P.-W., Chinn, I., Yan, W., Gitelson-Kahn, A., Joannopoulos, J., & Fink, Y. (2021). Digital electronics in fibres enable fabric-based machine-learning inference. *Nature Communications, 12*(1), 3317.

Luo, H., Wang, S., Wang, C., Linghu, C., & Song, J. (2021). Thermal controlled tunable adhesive for deterministic assembly by transfer printing. *Advanced Functional Materials, 31*(16), 2010297.

Marinov, V. R. (2018). 52-4: Laser-enabled extremely-high rate technology for μLED assembly. *SID Symposium Digest of Technical Papers, 49*(1), 692–695.

Mazzolai, B., & Mattoli, V. (2016). Generation soft. *Nature, 536*(7617), 400–401.

Meitl, M. A., Zhu, Z.-T., Kumar, V., Lee, K. J., Feng, X., Huang, Y. Y., Adesida, I., Nuzzo, R. G., & Rogers, J. A. (2006). Transfer printing by kinetic control of adhesion to an elastomeric stamp. *Nature Materials, 5*(1), 33–38.

Mikkonen, R., Puistola, P., Jönkkäri, I., & Mäntysalo, M. (2020). Inkjet printable polydimethylsiloxane for all-inkjet-printed multilayered soft electrical applications. *ACS Applied Materials & Interfaces, 12*(10), 11990–11997.

Mishra, A. K., Wallin, T. J., Pan, W., Xu, A., Wang, K., Giannelis, E. P., Mazzolai, B., & Shepherd, R. F. (2020). Autonomic perspiration in 3D-printed hydrogel actuators. *Science Robotics, 5*(38), eaaz3918.

Morikawa, Y., Yamagiwa, S., Sawahata, H., Numano, R., Koida, K., Ishida, M., & Kawano, T. (2017). Ultrastretchable Kirigami Bioprobes. *Advanced Healthcare Materials, 7*(3), 1701100.

Mukherjee, A. (2019). Organic field effect transistors fabricated using solution based aggregation and soft lithography. https://spiral.imperial.ac.uk/handle/10044/1/84850

Park, S.-H., Yang, D.-Y., & Lee, K.-S. (2009). Two-photon stereolithography for realizing ultraprecise three-dimensional nano/microdevices. *Laser & Photonics Reviews, 3*(1–2), 1–11.

Paul, M. T. Y., Kim, D., Saha, M. S., Stumper, J., & Gates, B. D. (2020). Patterning catalyst layers with microscale features by soft lithography techniques for proton exchange membrane fuel cells. *ACS Applied Energy Materials, 3*(1), 478–486.

Roy, N. K., Behera, D., Dibua, O. G., Foong, C. S., & Cullinan, M. A. (2019). A novel microscale selective laser sintering (µ-SLS) process for the fabrication of microelectronic parts. *Microsystems & Nanoengineering, 5*(1), 64.

Sabahi-Kaviani, R., & Luttge, R. (2021). Investigating the pattern transfer fidelity of Norland Optical Adhesive 81 for nanogrooves by microtransfer molding. *Journal of Vacuum Science & Technology B, Nanotechnology and Microelectronics: Materials, Processing, Measurement, and Phenomena, 39*(6), 062810.

Seesaard, T., & Wongchoosuk, C. (2023). Fabric-based piezoresistive Ti3AlC2/PEDOT:PSS force sensor for wearable E-textile applications. *Organic Electronics, 122*, 106894.

Sim, K., Chen, S., Li, Y., Kammoun, M., Peng, Y., Xu, M., Gao, Y., Song, J., Zhang, Y., Ardebili, H., & Yu, C. (2015). High fidelity tape transfer printing based on chemically induced adhesive strength modulation. *Scientific Reports, 5*(1), 16133.

Song, T. E., Yun, H., Kim, Y. J., Jeon, H. S., Ha, K., Jung, H. T., Han, H., Gogotsi, Y., Ahn, C. W., & Lee, Y. (2020). Vertically aligned nanopatterns of amine-functionalized Ti3C2 MXene via soft lithography. *Advanced Materials Interfaces, 7*(18), 2000424.

Sun, S., Fei, G., Wang, X., Xie, M., Guo, Q., Fu, D., Wang, Z., Wang, H., Luo, G., & Xia, H. (2021). Covalent adaptable networks of polydimethylsiloxane elastomer for selective laser sintering 3D printing. *Chemical Engineering Journal, 412*, 128675.

Truby, R. L., & Lewis, J. A. (2016). Printing soft matter in three dimensions. *Nature, 540*(7633), 371–378.

Uetani, K., Kasuya, K., Wang, J., Huang, Y., Watanabe, R., Tsuneyasu, S., Satoh, T., Koga, H., & Nogi, M. (2021). Kirigami-processed cellulose nanofiber films for smart heat dissipation by convection. *NPG Asia Materials, 13*(1), 62.

Wallin, T. J., Pikul, J. H., Bodkhe, S., Peele, B. N., Mac Murray, B. C., Therriault, D., McEnerney, B. W., Dillon, R. P., Giannelis, E. P., & Shepherd, R. F. (2017). Click chemistry stereolithography for soft robots that self-heal. *Journal of Materials Chemistry B, 5*(31), 6249–6255.

Wang, C., Linghu, C., Nie, S., Li, C., Lei, Q., Tao, X., Zeng, Y., Du, Y., Zhang, S., Yu, K., Jin, H., Chen, W., & Song, J. (2020b). Programmable and scalable transfer printing with high reliability and efficiency for flexible inorganic electronics. *Science Advances, 6*(25), eabb2393.

Wang, H., Li, X., Luan, K., & Bai, X. (2019). Capillary liquid bridge soft lithography for micropatterning preparation based on SU-8 photoresist templates with special wettability. *RSC Advances, 9*(41), 23986–23993.

Wang, S., Xu, J., Wang, W., Wang, G.-J. N., Rastak, R., Molina-Lopez, F., Chung, J. W., Niu, S., Feig, V. R., Lopez, J., Lei, T., Kwon, S.-K., Kim, Y., Foudeh, A. M., Ehrlich, A., Gasperini, A., Yun, Y., Murmann, B., Tok, J. B. H., & Bao, Z. (2018). Skin electronics from scalable fabrication of an intrinsically stretchable transistor array. *Nature, 555*(7694), 83–88.

Wang, X., Wang, D., Li, J., Zheng, H., Kano, R., Zou, Q., & Yue, C. (2023b). 13.1: The design and preparation of flexible MiniLED plate with nano-Ag paste. *SID Symposium Digest of Technical Papers, 54*(S1), 114–117.

Wang, X. Q., Chan, K. H., Cheng, Y., Ding, T., Li, T., Achavananthadith, S., Ahmet, S., Ho, J. S., & Ho, G. W. (2020a). Somatosensory, light-driven, thin-film robots capable of integrated perception and motility. *Advanced Materials, 32*(21), 2000351.

Wang, Z., Ding, J., & Guo, R. (2023a). Printable all-paper pressure sensors with high sensitivity and wide sensing range. *ACS Applied Materials & Interfaces, 15*(3), 4789–4798.

Xia, Y., McClelland, J. J., Gupta, R., Qin, D., Zhao, X. M., Sohn, L. L., Celotta, R. J., & Whitesides, G. M. (2004). Replica molding using polymeric materials: A practical step toward nanomanufacturing. *Advanced Materials, 9*(2), 147–149.

Xu, H., Tao, J., Liu, Y., Mo, Y., Bao, R., & Pan, C. (2022). Fully fibrous large-area tailorable triboelectric nanogenerator based on solution blow spinning technology for energy harvesting and self-powered sensing. *Small, 18*(37), 2202477.

Yan, J., Zhang, Y., Zhao, Y., Song, J., Xia, S., Liu, S., Yu, J., & Ding, B. (2020). Transformation of oxide ceramic textiles from insulation to conduction at room temperature. *Science Advances, 6*(6), eaay8538.

Yin, Z., Huang, Y., Yang, H., Chen, J., Duan, Y., & Chen, W. (2022). Flexible electronics manufacturing technology and equipment. *Science China Technological Sciences, 65*(9), 1940–1956.

Zavanelli, N., & Yeo, W.-H. (2021). Advances in screen printing of conductive nanomaterials for stretchable electronics. *ACS Omega, 6*(14), 9344–9351.

Zhang, K., Jung, Y. H., Mikael, S., Seo, J.-H., Kim, M., Mi, H., Zhou, H., Xia, Z., Zhou, W., Gong, S., & Ma, Z. (2017a). Origami silicon optoelectronics for hemispherical electronic eye systems. *Nature Communications, 8*(1), 1782.

Zhang, T., Li, K., Zhang, J., Chen, M., Wang, Z., Ma, S., Zhang, N., & Wei, L. (2017b). High-performance, flexible, and ultralong crystalline thermoelectric fibers. *Nano Energy, 41*, 35–42.

Zhao, H., Wie, J. J., Copic, D., Oliver, C. R., Orbaek White, A., Kim, S., & Hart, A. J. (2016). High-fidelity replica molding of glassy liquid crystalline polymer microstructures. *ACS Applied Materials & Interfaces, 8*(12), 8110–8117.

Zheng, S., Wang, H., Das, P., Zhang, Y., Cao, Y., Ma, J., Liu, S., & Wu, Z. S. (2021). Multitasking MXene inks enable high-performance printable microelectrochemical energy storage devices for all-flexible self-powered integrated systems. *Advanced Materials, 33*(10), 2005449.

Zheng, W., Huang, W., Gao, F., Yang, H., Dai, M., Liu, G., Yang, B., Zhang, J., Fu, Y. Q., Chen, X., Qiu, Y., Jia, D., Zhou, Y., & Hu, P. (2018). Kirigami-inspired highly stretchable nanoscale devices using multidimensional deformation of monolayer MoS2. *Chemistry of Materials, 30*(17), 6063–6070.

Zheng, Y., Chen, K., Yang, W., Wu, L., Qu, K., Zhao, J., Jiang, T., & Feng, Y. (2022). Kirigami reconfigurable gradient metasurface. *Advanced Functional Materials, 32*(5), 2107699.

Zhou, K., Zhao, Y., Sun, X., Yuan, Z., Zheng, G., Dai, K., Mi, L., Pan, C., Liu, C., & Shen, C. (2020). Ultra-stretchable triboelectric nanogenerator as high-sensitive and self-powered electronic skins for energy harvesting and tactile sensing. *Nano Energy, 70*, 104546.

Zhou, X., Zhu, L., Fan, L., Deng, H., & Fu, Q. (2018). Fabrication of highly stretchable, washable, wearable, water-repellent strain sensors with multi-stimuli sensing ability. *ACS Applied Materials & Interfaces, 10*(37), 31655–31663.

Zhuo, F., Zhou, J., Liu, Y., Xie, J., Chen, H., Wang, X., Luo, J., Fu, Y. (2023). Elmarakbi, A., & Duan, H. Kirigami–inspired 3D-printable MXene organohydrogels for soft electronics. *Advanced Functional Materials, 33*, 2308487.

CHAPTER 3

Soft Electronics for Monitoring and Diagnostics

Bojing Shi

3.1 MAIN PRINCIPLES AND TYPES OF SOFT SENSORS

3.1.1 Piezoresistive and Capacitive Devices

Resistance and capacitance are electrical parameters that are relatively easy to detect. Piezoresistive sensors are based on the characteristic that the resistance value of materials changes when subjected to force or deformation, providing flexibility and real-time monitoring capability for wearable technology, widely used in wearable devices to monitor and record physiological and motion data related to pressure, force, deformation, etc. The piezoresistive effect refers to the change in the resistance value inside an elastic material when it is subjected to external pressure or deformation. This change is due to the deformation of conductive particles or conductive networks inside the material under external pressure, which affects the flow of charges. These types of sensors are typically composed of two layers of material, one of which is conductive and the other is insulating. The conductive layer usually contains conductive particles or thin films, forming a resistance network. When this structure is subjected to external pressure, the resistance value inside the conductive layer will change. By measuring this change, information about external pressure or deformation can be obtained. In a piezoresistive sensor, there is usually a gap between the two layers of material, which allows the sensor to maintain high resistance when not subjected to force. When external pressure is applied, the particles or structures of the conductive layer undergo compression or stretching and the resistance value changes accordingly. This change is usually nonlinear, but after calibration and calculation, the resistance change can correspond to the strength of the force (Figure 3.1).

Capacitive sensors are based on the capacitance changes between materials, providing highly sensitive and real-time feedback capabilities for wearable devices, widely used in wearable devices to monitor and record physiological and motion data related to contact, touch, gesture, etc. The working principle of capacitive sensors is based on the capacitance effect, which means that the capacitance value between two conductive bodies changes with the distance and relative position between them. These conductive materials typically

DOI: 10.1201/9781003493631-3

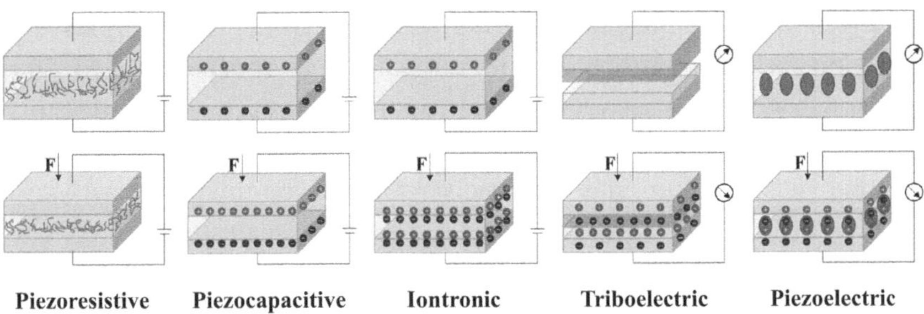

FIGURE 3.1 Structural diagrams of four types of soft sensors. Adapted with permission (Wang et al., 2023). Copyright 2023, Springer Nature.

exist in the form of electrodes, which can be metals, conductive coatings, or conductive fibres. Capacitive sensors typically consist of two electrodes, when the user touches or approaches these two electrodes, the conductivity of the body tissue will cause a change in capacitance. This change can be detected and recorded by measuring changes in capacitance values, including contact, touch, gestures, and other information. The capacitance value of the sensor is inversely proportional to the distance between electrodes and is related to factors such as the shape and size of the conductive body, as well as the electrical properties of nearby objects. When the user approaches or touches the electrode, the electric field between the conductors changes, resulting in a change in capacitance value. This change can be detected and analysed through relevant sensors and processing units in the circuit.

3.1.2 Piezoelectric and Triboelectric Devices

Both piezoelectric and triboelectric devices can directly convert mechanical changes into electrical signals. The advantage is no need for a complex driving system, and the sensors themselves can convert the target parameters into electrical signals, facilitating information collection and processing. It is worth mentioning that in addition to using piezoelectric devices to detect a pulse, researchers have also prepared wearable ultrasound devices using piezoelectric materials for detecting blood flow and heart activity. Piezoelectric sensors detect pressure or force by utilising the charge generation and potential changes of piezoelectric materials. This technology is used in monitoring physiological parameters, gesture recognition, motion analysis, and other aspects. The piezoelectric effect refers to the phenomenon of charge separation and potential changes in certain specific crystal or ceramic materials when subjected to mechanical pressure or deformation, which leads to the uneven distribution of positive and negative charges inside, resulting in the formation of charge dipoles. Piezoelectric sensors typically utilise this effect to measure external pressure or force.

In piezoelectric sensors, piezoelectric materials are typically made into thin films, flakes, or other shapes and integrated into the structure of wearable devices. When the sensor is subjected to external pressure or deformation, the piezoelectric material undergoes slight deformation, resulting in uneven distribution of internal charges and ultimately generating charges. The generated charge can be measured to determine external pressure or force. For example, piezoelectric sensors can be integrated into sports gloves to capture hand movements and gestures. This is very useful in applications such as virtual reality and gesture control, where users can complete operations through gestures without touching the screen or other devices. Then, piezoelectric sensors can be integrated into the insole to monitor pressure distribution and gait of the feet and realise posture correction. This is of great significance for athlete training, gait analysis of the elderly, and monitoring during the rehabilitation process. Intelligent insoles can provide real-time walking data to help users adjust their gait and reduce joint pressure. In addition, by embedding sensors into clothing, it is possible to monitor the user's body posture. Piezoelectric sensors are also used in smart mattresses to monitor sleep quality. The sensors on the mattress can detect changes in the user's sleeping posture, turning frequency, and movement during sleep, providing personalised sleep analysis and improvement suggestions.

Triboelectric sensors are based on the triboelectric effect, which detects motion, touch, or deformation through potential changes caused by friction or contact between materials. The triboelectric effect is a phenomenon of converting frictional force into electrical energy. Triboelectric sensors are typically composed of two layers of materials: One is frictional material and the other is conductive material. When these two layers of materials move relative to each other or experience friction, the charges generated by friction will cause potential changes in the conductive material. This change can be detected and recorded by measuring the changes in potential values to detect and record the effects of friction, thereby achieving perception of motion, touch, or deformation. Triboelectric sensors can be used in gesture recognition and monitoring human motion. For example, by integrating sensors into gloves, the potential changes generated by friction when users make gestures in the air can be used to recognise gestures. This application scenario plays an important role in fields such as virtual reality and game control. Meanwhile, by integrating triboelectric sensors in sports equipment, such as sports shoes, sportswear, etc., we can detect the potential changes generated by friction and record real-time information such as the user's gait and movement trajectory. This is very helpful for athlete training and sports health monitoring. Triboelectric sensors can be used for touch interaction. By embedding sensors into devices such as wristbands and watches, users can convert the frictional potential changes generated by sliding or tapping their fingers on the surface of the device into corresponding instructions or operations.

3.1.3 Photoelectric Devices

Infrared light can penetrate biological tissues such as skin and muscles well. So, infrared sensing can be used for detecting blood vessels. Optoelectronic sensors are based on the photoelectric effect, which can monitor the surrounding environment, physiological parameters, or user behaviour by sensing changes in light. This technology has been widely applied in the field of wearable devices, covering multiple aspects such as physiological monitoring, gesture recognition, and environmental perception.

Photoelectric sensors typically include photosensitive components (such as photoresistors, photodiodes, phototransistors, etc.) and related circuits. When light reaches the

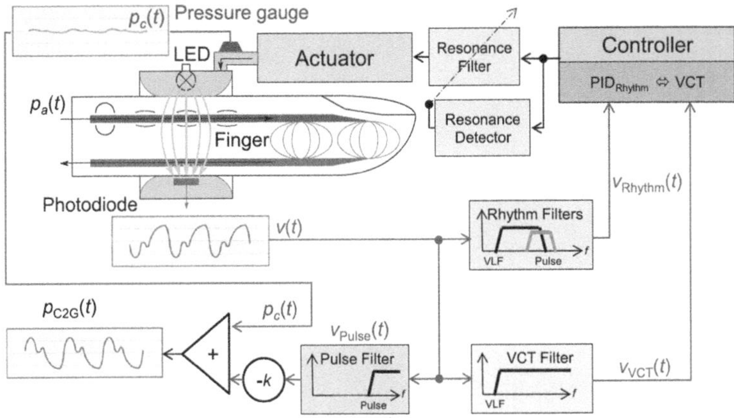

FIGURE 3.2   Schematic diagram of a photoelectric sensor for detecting fingertip pulse. Adapted with permission (Fortin et al., 2021). Copyright 2021, Springer Nature.

photosensitive element, the energy of photons excites electrons inside the material, thereby changing electrical properties such as resistance and current (Figure 3.2). By measuring these changes, information about light intensity, spectral distribution, and other factors can be obtained. Photoelectric sensors are widely used for monitoring heart rate, blood oxygen, and pulse waves. Usually, these types of sensors are embedded in devices such as wristbands and smartwatches, and calculate heart rate by shining on the skin and measuring the reflected light, analysing blood pulsation. Such applications are very useful for health tracking and exercise monitoring. Then, by irradiating the skin with different wavelengths of light and measuring the absorption characteristics of haemoglobin, the oxygen content in the blood can be calculated. This plays an important role in monitoring the respiratory function and sleep quality of patients. Photoelectric sensors can also be used for posture monitoring. By placing sensors in different parts of the body, it is possible to perceive changes in posture. This has practical applications for athlete training, posture correction, and other aspects.

3.1.4 Electrochemical Devices

A wearable electrochemical device integrates micro-electrochemical sensors to monitor and analyse various physiological and environmental parameters in real time. The technology uses the principles of electrochemistry, the chemical discipline that studies the interaction between electric currents and chemical reactions for the detection and quantification of specific analytes. The core components of a wearable electrochemical sensor usually include electrodes, electrolytes, and sensing elements. The electrode causes the electrochemical reaction, while the electrolyte provides the medium for ion transport. The sensing element is designed to selectively interact with the target analyte to produce a measurable electrochemical signal (Figure 3.3).

These sensors are often designed to monitor biomarkers such as glucose, lactic acid, and various ions. Integrating these sensors into wearables enables continuous, non-invasive

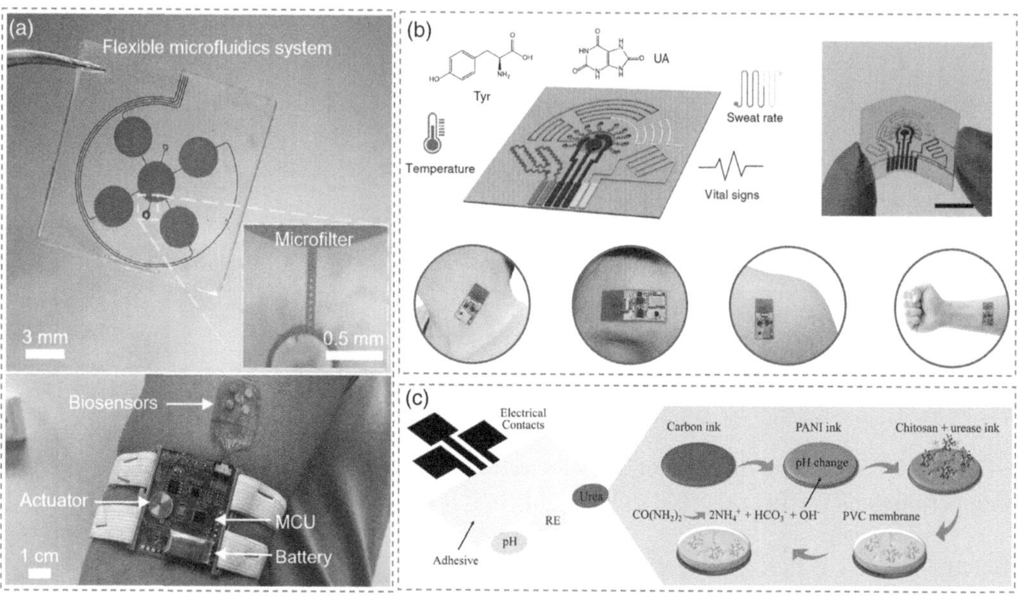

FIGURE 3.3 Electrochemical sensors. (a) Wearable sweat sensor. (b) Wearable sensor for detecting uric acid and tyrosine in sweat. (c) Wearable sensor for analysing urea in sweat. ([a] Adapted with permission (Huang et al., 2023). Copyright 2023, Wiley-VCH; [b] Adapted with permission (Yang et al., 2020). Copyright 2020, Springer Nature; [c] Adapted with permission (Ibáñez-Redín et al., 2023). Copyright 2023, Elsevier.)

monitoring, providing valuable insights into the user's health and environmental exposure. Selective binding of sensing elements to target analytes in biological or environmental samples. This interaction is specific, allowing the sensor to target a specific substance. Combined with the event to trigger the electrochemical reaction of the electrode-sensing element interface, this reaction results in the production or consumption of electrons, which changes the electrical signal. Changes in electrochemical signals are transduced into measurable outputs, such as voltage or current. The electronics of the wearable device then process this signal. The processed data can be transferred to connected devices, such as smartphones or cloud platforms, for further analysis and interpretation. Wearable electrochemical sensors often integrate wireless communication technology for seamless data transmission. The benefits of wearable electrochemical sensing include real-time monitoring, portability, and the potential for personalised medicine. These devices have a wide range of application prospects in fitness tracking, disease management, and environmental monitoring, providing hope for a more connected and information-based personal health management.

3.1.5 Hydrogel Devices

Hydrogel sensors aim to achieve highly sensitive detection of physiological parameters, environmental pollution, etc. by monitoring the change of ion concentration in the hydrogel (Figure 3.4). This technology makes use of the special structure of the hydrogel material

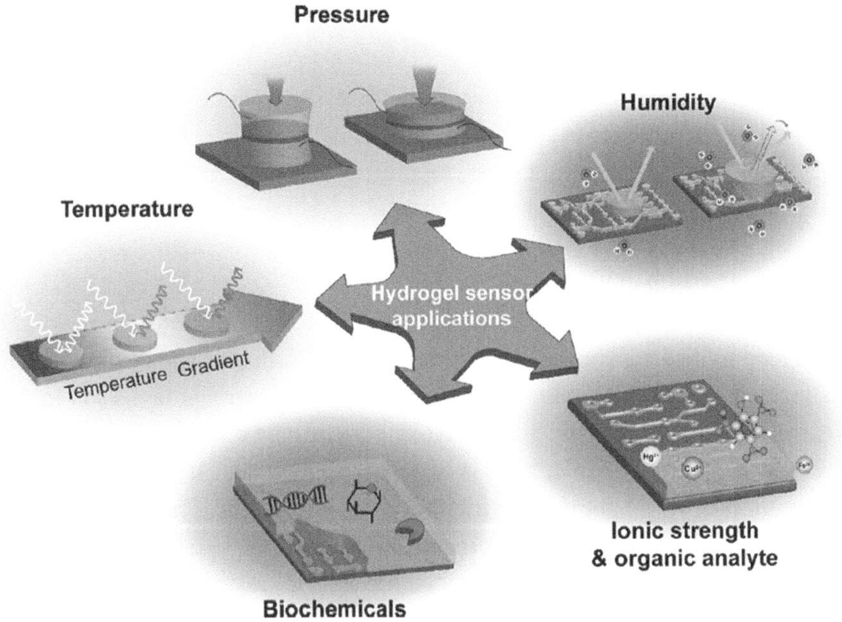

FIGURE 3.4 Main applications of hydrogel sensors. Adapted with permission (Sun et al., 2021). Copyright 2021, American Chemical Society.

and its sensitivity to the change of ion concentration, providing a new way of soft, comfortable, and real-time monitoring for wearable devices. The working principle of ionic hydrogel involves the structure of the hydrogel and the diffusion process of ions in water. Hydrogel is a kind of polymer material, whose structure is porous and can absorb and store a large amount of water. Ions dissolved in water, such as Na^+, K^+, Cl^-, etc., can penetrate the structure of the hydrogel. When the hydrogel comes in contact with a physiological liquid or water in the environment, the hydrogel begins to absorb water. Due to its porous structure, water rapidly permeates into the hydrogel, leading to the expansion of the hydrogel. This water absorption process not only makes the hydrogel softer but also creates conditions for ion diffusion. As the hydrogel absorbs water, the ions in the water begin to diffuse in the hydrogel. The diffusion rate of ions is related to the properties of ions and the structure of hydrogels. The diffusion degree of different ions in the hydrogel is different, which makes it possible to selectively detect specific ions. The diffusion of ions directly affects the conductivity of the hydrogel. In the presence of ions, the conductivity of hydrogels is enhanced because ions can conduct electricity. By measuring the change in the conductivity of the hydrogel, the change in ion concentration in the effluent gel can be indirectly reflected. The hydrogel sensor usually includes a measuring circuit to measure the conductivity of the hydrogel. These sensors measure changes in resistance or conductivity by connecting the hydrogel to a conductive element. Sensor readings can be interpreted and recorded through connected electronic devices.

3.2 MONITORING AND DIAGNOSIS OF CARDIAC AND VASCULAR DISEASES

Common cardiovascular and cerebrovascular diseases include vascular sclerosis, hypertension, plaques, and moderate stroke. To scientifically evaluate the state of blood vessels, it is necessary to detect many indicators, including heart rate and rhythm, blood pressure, blood oxygen, blood flow, and so on (Figure 3.5).

3.2.1 Heart Rate and Rhythm

Arrhythmias, including atrial fibrillation, ventricular fibrillation, tachycardia, or bradycardia, can lead to serious consequences such as heart failure. One of the commonly used methods for detecting heart rate and rhythm through wearable devices is to use electrocardiogram (ECG) for analysis. Soft electronic technology is an emerging field of electronic devices based on flexible, thin, and flexible materials. Its progress in monitoring heart rhythm has brought significant innovation to the medical field. With the increasing concern for health, monitoring and prevention of heart diseases have become particularly important. The application of soft electronic technology provides new possibilities for heart rate monitoring, providing patients with more convenient, accurate, and comfortable means of heart health monitoring. In the treatment of heart diseases, researchers have utilised flexible implantable triboelectric generators to achieve self-powered pacemakers, which use the energy of the heartbeat to drive electric pulse devices to regulate heart rhythm (Ouyang et al., 2019). In addition, scientists have also used biodegradable materials to make electronic blood vessels, which can improve endothelialisation through electrical stimulation (Cheng et al., 2020).

The flexibility and adaptability of soft electronic technology make traditional rigid electronic devices unmatched. Traditional heart rate monitoring devices are usually made of hard materials and are not suitable for fitting to the surface of the human body, which can easily cause discomfort when used. Soft electronic technology utilises flexible substrates and materials to manufacture sensors that are as thin as paper, lightweight, and soft and can tightly adhere to the surface of the skin without affecting the normal life and activities of patients. This flexible design effectively improves the comfort of monitoring equipment, making long-term monitoring possible. Soft electronic technology is beneficial for long-term disease monitoring. Traditional ECG monitoring devices typically require patients to undergo regular testing at hospitals or clinics, while soft electronic technology can achieve monitoring anytime, anywhere. Patients can attach flexible heart rate monitoring devices to their bodies and transmit real-time data to doctors or cloud databases through technologies such as Bluetooth. Doctors can access the patient's heart rate data for analysis at any time. This real-time monitoring method helps to detect arrhythmia earlier and improves the level of patient monitoring. In addition, the progress of soft electronic technology in heart rate monitoring has also driven the development of telemedicine. By combining monitoring devices with the internet, doctors can remotely monitor the heart health status of patients. This is particularly important for patients who cannot frequently go to the hospital for examination, especially during special periods such as epidemics. Remote

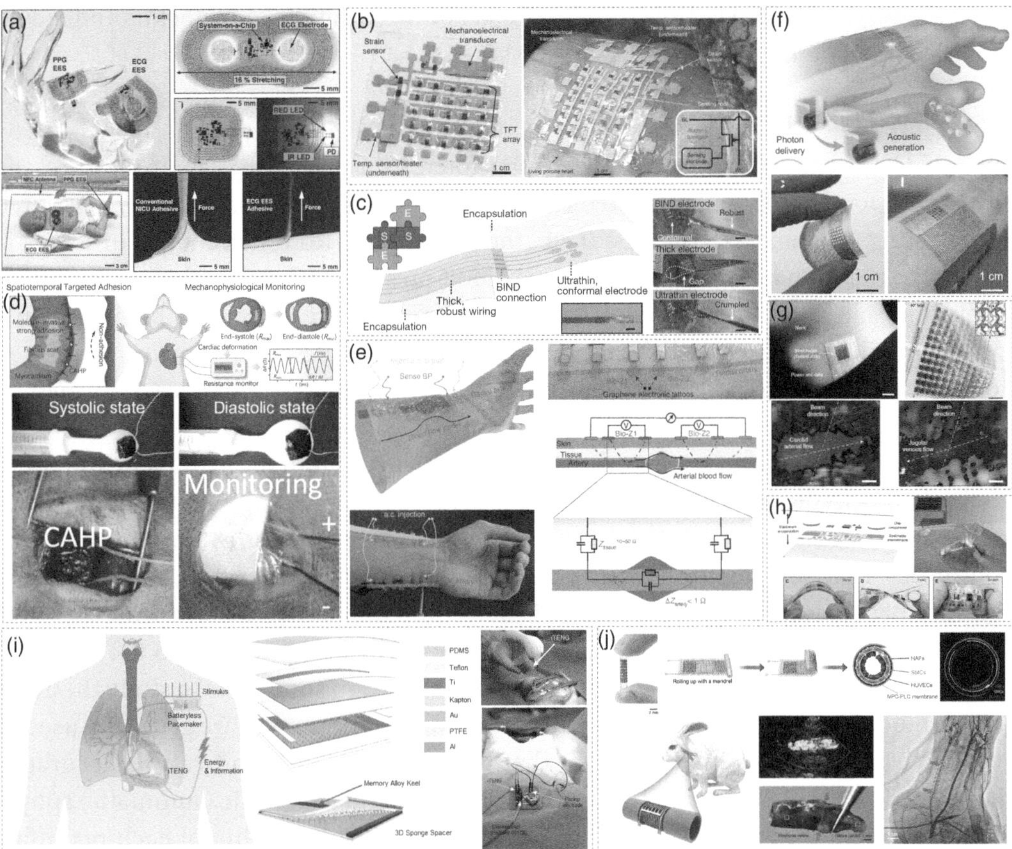

FIGURE 3.5 Soft electric devices for cardiac and vascular detection. (a) Soft wireless wearable electronic devices for neonatal critical care monitoring. (b) Soft rubbery epicardial bioelectronic patch. (c) Plug-and-play soft electrodes. (d) A hydrogel patch conformably integrated with the heart surface can be used to monitor heart activity. (e) Electronic tattoos for blood pressure monitoring. (f) Flexible optoacoustic sensor for vascular monitoring. (g) Wearable soft ultrasound device for deep tissue haemodynamic monitoring. (h) Soft ultrasound system. (i) A self-powered pacemaker based on an implanted triboelectric generator. (j) Cyborg vessel. ([a] Adapted with permission (Chung et al., 2019). Copyright 2019, AAAS; [b] Adapted with permission (Sim et al., 2020). Copyright 2020, Springer Nature; [c] Adapted with permission (Jiang et al., 2023). Copyright 2023, Springer Nature; [d] Adapted with permission (Yu et al., 2023). Copyright 2023, Springer Nature; [e] Adapted with permission (Kireev et al., 2022). Copyright 2022, Springer Nature; [f] Adapted with permission (Jin et al., 2023). Copyright 2023, Springer Nature; [g] Adapted with permission (Wang et al., 2021). Copyright 2021, Springer Nature; [h] Adapted with permission (Jin et al., 2021). Copyright 2021, AAAS; [i] Adapted with permission (Ouyang et al., 2019). Copyright 2019, Springer Nature; [j] Adapted with permission (Cheng et al., 2020; Zhang et al., 2020). Copyright 2020, Elsevier.)

medical care can effectively reduce direct contact between patients and doctors and reduce the risk of infection.

3.2.2 Blood Pressure

Since 1733, humans have developed a strong interest in measuring blood pressure and have continuously proposed measurement principles and methods, as well as prepared relevant testing instruments. Amongst them, the discovery of Korotkoff sounds in 1905 laid the theoretical foundation for non-invasive blood pressure today. To achieve continuous ambulatory blood pressure monitoring, researchers continue to develop blood pressure monitoring devices that can be worn for a long time. At present, the main methods of non-invasive blood pressure measurement are the cuff method and the sleeveless method (Figure 3.6).

Cuff measurement can be roughly divided into auscultation measurement and oscilloscope measurement according to measurement methods. Manual auscultation is the gold standard of non-invasive blood pressure measurement and is the most accurate non-invasive blood pressure measurement method. In the process of blood pressure measurement, the blood pressure value is determined by using a stethoscope to listen to the sound caused by poor blood pressure flow in the blood vessels, so the ability to hear accurately is the premise of accurate measurement. In some tests to study the accuracy of blood pressure measurement, two measurement personnel are generally used to auscultate at the same time to ensure that the auscultating sound can be accurately captured. The oscilloscope method is used by the general electronic (automatic) sphygmomanometer. Each manufacturer uses the oscilloscope algorithm of each manufacturer to infer the blood pressure value, and the accuracy is related to the tested person. The accuracy of oscillography is generally judged by comparison with auscultation, and the smaller the difference between the two, the more accurate it is generally considered.

There are currently two main theories for deriving blood pressure based on pulse waves: Pulse transit time (PTT) and pulse wave analysis (PWA). According to the theory of PTT, there is a certain correlation between blood pressure (P), vascular stiffness, and PTT (τ), which can be described by the following formula:

$$v = \frac{l}{\tau} = \sqrt{\frac{A}{\rho}\frac{dP}{dA}} \tag{3.1}$$

Where, A is the cross-sectional area of the artery, l is the wave travel length, v is the pulse wave velocity, and ρ is blood density. dA/dP is the arterial compliance, which is related to arterial stiffness. Therefore, researchers usually use multiple sensor devices to obtain multiple pulse waves, thereby calculating the propagation speed of pulse waves and obtaining blood pressure data.

The main method of PWA is to extract feature values from pulse waveforms, to calculate blood pressure data. The relationship between pulse waves $\Delta V(\omega)$ and blood pressure $\Delta P(\omega)$ can be described by the following formula:

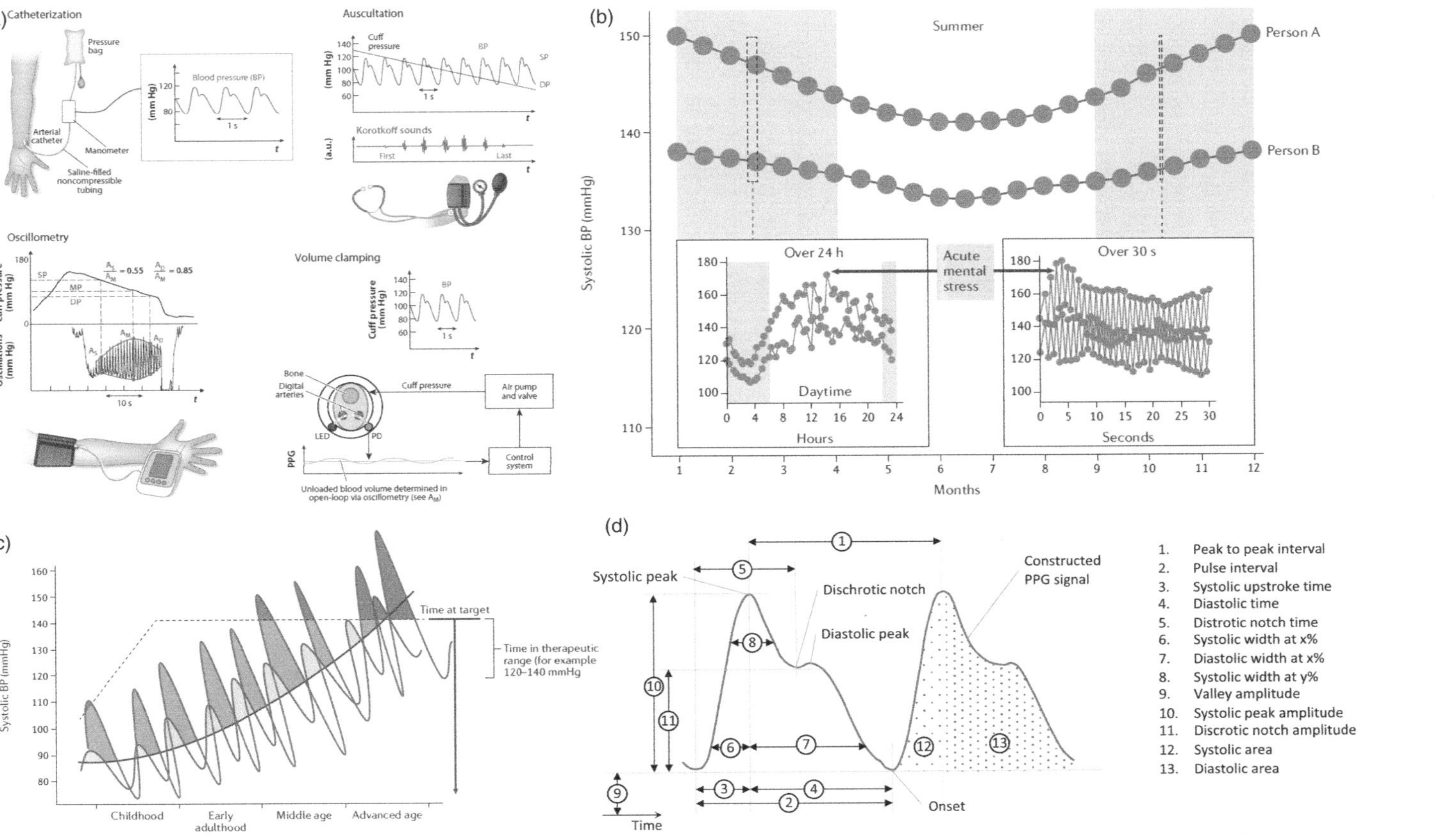

FIGURE 3.6 Non-invasive blood pressure detection. (a) Common blood pressure detection methods. (b) Blood pressure variability. (c) Time at target blood pressure levels. (d) Extracting blood pressure from PPG signals. ([a] Adapted with permission (Mukkamala et al., 2022). Copyright 2022, Annual Reviews Inc.; [b] Adapted with permission (Schutte et al., 2022). Copyright 2022, Springer Nature; [c] Adapted with permission (Schutte et al., 2022). Copyright 2022, Springer Nature; [d] Adapted with permission (Frey et al., 2022). Copyright 2022, Springer Nature.)

$$\Delta V(\omega) = \frac{1}{j\omega\eta + E}\Delta P(\omega) \tag{3.2}$$

Where, η is the coefficient of viscosity of the arterial wall and E is the elastic modulus of viscosity of the arterial wall. The advantage of the PWA method is that it only requires pulse wave data from one sensor to deduce blood pressure. The progress of soft electronic technology in monitoring blood pressure has brought a series of innovations to the medical field, providing patients with more convenient and comfortable blood pressure monitoring solutions. Traditional blood pressure monitoring devices typically use inflatable cuffs and rigid instruments, which limit the patient's freedom of movement. However, the introduction of soft electronic technology breaks this limitation, making blood pressure monitoring more intelligent, portable, and continuous.

The flexibility of soft electronic technology makes it possible to replace traditional blood pressure cuffs. Traditional cuffs are made of hard materials and need to be tightly wrapped around the upper arm to ensure accurate measurement. The soft electronic technology utilises soft and thin materials to prepare blood pressure sensors, which can better fit the skin curve and reduce discomfort during use. This flexible design allows patients to have more freedom in daily activities and no longer be constrained by monitoring equipment. Second, the application of soft electronic technology has promoted the implementation of continuous blood pressure monitoring. Traditional blood pressure measurement is usually point measurement, which requires patients to use instruments to measure at specific times, which often cannot obtain comprehensive information on blood pressure changes. The soft electronic technology of blood pressure sensors can achieve continuous monitoring, seamlessly integrate into wearable devices or close-fitting patches, and record real-time changes in the patient's blood pressure. This continuous monitoring method provides doctors with more detailed blood pressure data, which helps to better understand the patient's blood pressure status and improve the management level of cardiovascular diseases such as hypertension.

Soft electronic technology also has the characteristics of portability and intelligence. Traditional blood pressure monitoring devices are bulky and not portable, while the application of soft electronic technology makes blood pressure monitoring devices more lightweight and can be integrated into wearable devices, mobile phones, or other portable devices, allowing patients to monitor blood pressure anytime, anywhere. In addition, soft electronic technology can provide personalised health advice and warnings through intelligent analysis of sensor data, providing patients with more comprehensive health management services. The progress of soft electronic technology in monitoring blood pressure has provided patients with more convenient, comfortable, and accurate blood pressure monitoring methods. Its flexibility, continuous monitoring ability, portability, and intelligence make blood pressure monitoring no longer limited by time and location, providing a more comprehensive solution for the prevention and management of cardiovascular diseases. With the continuous innovation of technology, it is believed that flexible electronic technology will continue to make greater progress in the field of blood pressure monitoring.

3.2.3 Blood Oxygen

The measurement of non-invasive blood oxygen saturation (SaO_2) is based on Lambert–Beer law, and the light absorption characteristics of near-infrared spectroscopy are used to determine the measurement. Since the absorption rates of oxyhaemoglobin (HbO_2) and reduced haemoglobin (HbR) in the blood are different in the near-infrared light band for the same wavelength, the content of oxygen and haemoglobin in the blood can be calculated by measuring the attenuation degree of different light rays passing through the blood. The sensor is mainly composed of two light-emitting diodes and one photosensitive diode, which emit red light of 660 nm and infrared light of 940 nm, respectively, and can pass through the skin of the tested object. Usually parallel to the same side of the sensor, the opposite side is placed a photodiode.

$$SaO_2 = \frac{HbO_2}{HbO_2 + HbR} \times 100\% \tag{3.3}$$

Continuous wave spectroscopy, also known as steady-state spectroscopy, uses near-infrared light sources with constant intensity to calculate the change in the optical parameters of brain tissue according to the attenuation of light intensity transmitted or scattered through brain tissue. Time-resolved spectroscopy shoots an ultra-short pulsed light into a certain place on the surface of human tissue and detects the response after the propagation of incident light at another place a certain distance away. The distribution of light propagation path length and outgoing light intensity over time can be obtained, and then the absorption coefficient and scattering coefficient of the tissue can be obtained, and finally, the HbO_2 concentration can be obtained. Absolute values of HbR concentration and cerebral oxygen saturation can also be obtained. Based on FDPM technology, the propagation path length and migration time of photons are obtained, to obtain the optical parameters of brain tissue, and then the absolute value of cerebral blood oxygen saturation can be calculated by using appropriate algorithms.

3.2.4 Blood Flow

Blood flow sensors typically use various technologies, such as laser Doppler, electromagnetic induction, or pressure sensing, to measure parameters such as blood flow velocity, flow rate, and pressure on the blood vessel wall. These sensors can be placed directly on the surface of the skin or penetrate the skin to achieve real-time monitoring of haemodynamics. Through these sensing technologies, doctors can obtain detailed information about the patient's blood flow status, helping to diagnose and treat cardiovascular diseases, hypertension, and other conditions. Wearable devices combine advanced data processing technology to provide more in-depth blood flow analysis. Through built-in algorithms and data processing units, these devices can analyse and interpret blood flow data in real time, detecting any abnormal patterns or trends. This provides doctors with more comprehensive and quantitative information, which helps to develop personalised treatment plans and preventive measures. The technological advancement of wearable electronic devices in monitoring blood flow has brought tremendous changes to clinical medicine. These devices integrate highly sensitive sensing technology, advanced data processing, and wireless communication to achieve real-time monitoring and comprehensive evaluation of haemodynamics. In the future, with the continuous innovation of technology, wearable devices are expected to play an increasingly important role in cardiovascular health management, disease prevention, and rehabilitation processes, providing patients with more comprehensive and personalised medical services.

3.3 MONITORING AND DIAGNOSIS OF RESPIRATORY DISEASES

Parameters related to respiration, such as respiratory rhythm, intensity, volume, etc., are closely related to the health of the respiratory system. It is of great significance to use the sensor to accurately monitor the above respiratory parameters for a long time. In general, the monitoring of breath mainly monitors the breathing air stream and exhaled gas molecules (Figure 3.7).

Monitoring respiratory rhythm requires real-time detection of changes in respiratory airflow or chest undulations, using sensors such as piezoresistive, capacitive, piezoelectric, triboelectric, and so on. Accelerometers can be used for real-time detection of changes in chest undulations during breathing, but solving the problems of artefacts and low signal-to-noise ratio has become one of the bottlenecks restricting their widespread application. Based on the idea of bionics, researchers have proposed a variety of sensors that can detect changes in the thorax, including micro-airways that mimic fish lateral lines and shark gills. Wearable devices are equipped with highly sensitive respiratory sensors that can measure respiratory parameters in real time. These types of sensors include expiratory flow sensors, chest motion sensors, and pressure sensors. Through these sensors, the device can monitor key respiratory indicators such as respiratory rate, tidal volume, and end-of-breath carbon dioxide concentration. These data provide a comprehensive understanding of respiratory system function, which helps to detect respiratory diseases early, evaluate treatment effectiveness, and guide exercise and rehabilitation training.

The sensing technology of wearable respiratory monitoring devices is constantly evolving to provide more accurate measurements of respiratory capacity. The built-in sensors typically use technologies such as pressure, motion, or sound to monitor respiratory movement and expiratory flow rate. The application of flexible materials and microsensors enables these devices to comfortably fit the user's body and achieve long-term continuous monitoring. The development of these sensing technologies provides reliable means for real-time monitoring of key indicators such as respiratory rate, tidal volume, and lung capacity.

The technological progress of wearable electronic devices in monitoring breath molecules represents innovation in the field of medical technology, providing new possibilities for real-time and non-invasive breath analysis. These devices combine microsensor technology, data processing, and communication functions, allowing medical professionals to

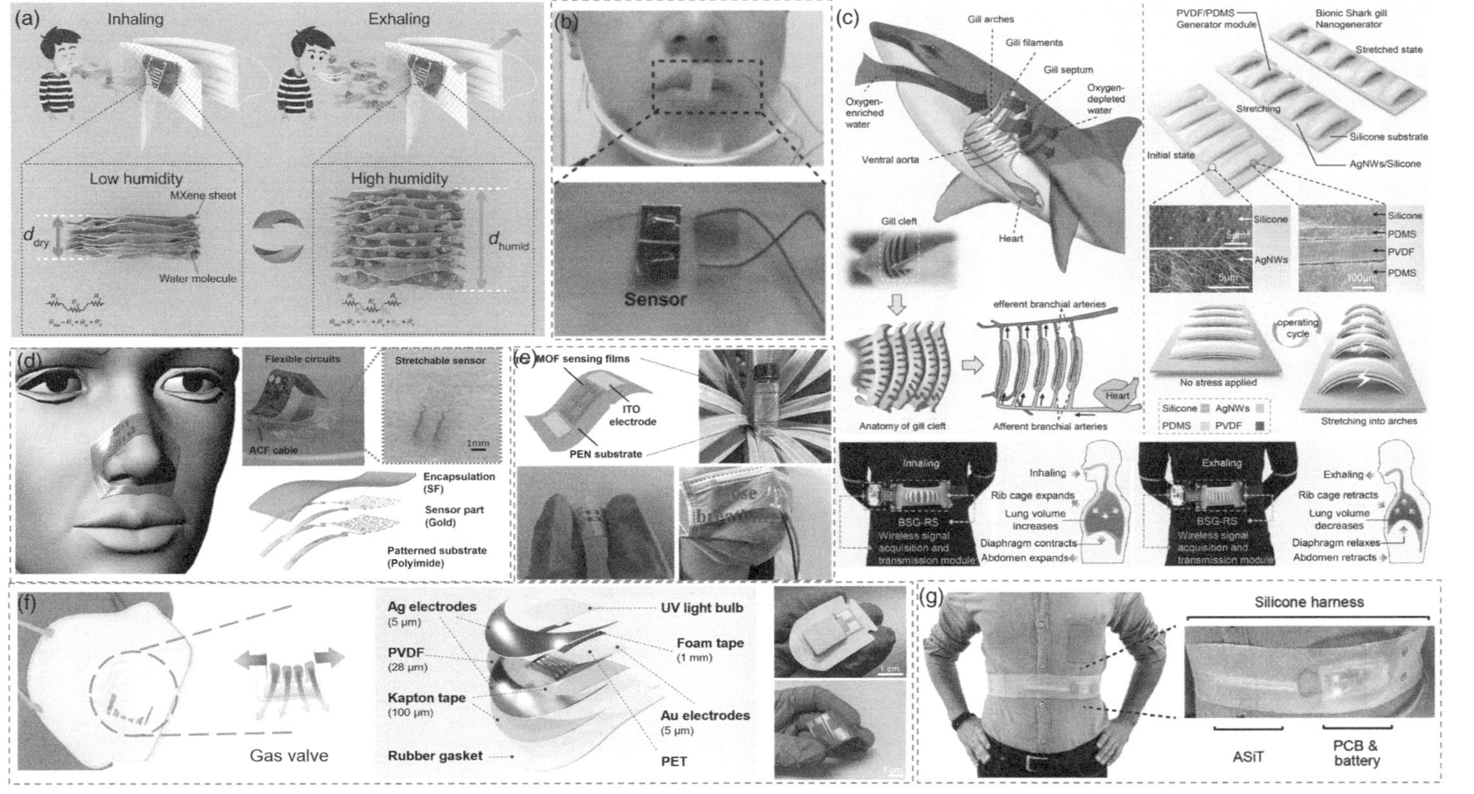

FIGURE 3.7   Soft sensors for respiratory detection. (a) Humidity sensor integrated into the mask. (b) Primary battery structured humidity sensor. (c) Biomimetic soft respiratory sensor. (d) Soft respiratory sensor. (e) Soft humidity sensor. (f) Wearable sensors capable of detecting respiratory mechanics and expiratory molecular signals. (g) Bioinspired soft respiratory sensor. ([a] Adapted with permission (Liu et al. n.d.). Copyright 2023, Wiley-VCH; [b] Adapted with permission (Duan et al., 2022). Copyright 2022, Elsevier; [c] Adapted with permission (Zou et al., 2022). Copyright 2022, Elsevier; [d] Adapted with permission (Chen et al., 2020). Copyright 2020, Wiley-VCH; [e] Adapted with permission (Zhang et al., 2022). Copyright 2022, Elsevier; [f] Adapted with permission (Dai et al., 2023). Copyright 2023, Wiley-VCH; [g] Adapted with permission (Cotur et al., 2022). Copyright 2022, Wiley-VCH.)

have a more detailed understanding of the patient's exhaled breath composition, providing important information for early diagnosis and treatment of diseases. Sensors typically use advanced technologies such as chemical sensing, nanotechnology, or optical sensing to identify and quantify specific molecules in exhaled breath, such as gases, volatile organic compounds (VOCs), etc. This enables these devices to monitor a range of exhaled components, including but not limited to metabolites, airway inflammation markers, and drug metabolites. These devices integrate highly sensitive sensing technology, intelligent data processing, and remote communication to provide medical professionals with more comprehensive exhalation data. In the future, these technologies are expected to play a more important role in the early diagnosis, treatment effectiveness evaluation, and personalised treatment plan formulation of respiratory system diseases, providing patients with more comprehensive and personalised medical services.

3.4 MONITORING AND DIAGNOSIS OF SKIN DISEASE

For skin monitoring, the main indicators include epidermal temperature, sweat composition, skin water, skin modulus, etc. The technological progress of wearable electronic devices in detecting skin diseases marks the intersection of medicine and technology, providing more convenient and real-time solutions for monitoring skin health. These devices combine advanced sensing technology, data processing, and communication functions, allowing medical professionals to have a more detailed understanding of the patient's skin condition, and providing new means for early detection and treatment of skin problems (Figure 3.8).

The sensing technology of wearable skin monitoring devices has been significantly improved, enabling highly sensitive detection of skin physiological and biochemical indicators. These devices are usually equipped with optical sensors, resistive sensors, or chemical sensors to detect various physiological parameters of the skin, such as humidity, temperature, conductivity, and light reflectivity. Through these sensing technologies, doctors can obtain detailed information about the skin layer, helping to diagnose and monitor various skin conditions such as eczema, psoriasis, etc. In terms of wound healing, scientists use flexible electrical stimulators to stimulate skin wounds, achieving the goal of anti-inflammatory and promoting wound healing. Some wearable skin monitoring devices also combine imaging technology, such as dermoscopy or infrared spectrometer, to achieve more detailed observations of the fine structures and blood flow on the skin surface. This comprehensive monitoring method helps doctors evaluate the condition of skin lesions more comprehensively.

3.5 MONITORING AND DIAGNOSIS OF ACTIONS AND POSTURES

Soft electronic devices in monitoring human muscle movement and posture provide convenient and efficient solutions for rehabilitation and sports. These devices integrate advanced sensing technology, data processing, and communication functions, enabling medical professionals and sports and health enthusiasts to have a more comprehensive understanding of muscle activity and body posture, promoting rehabilitation and improving exercise performance (Figure 3.9).

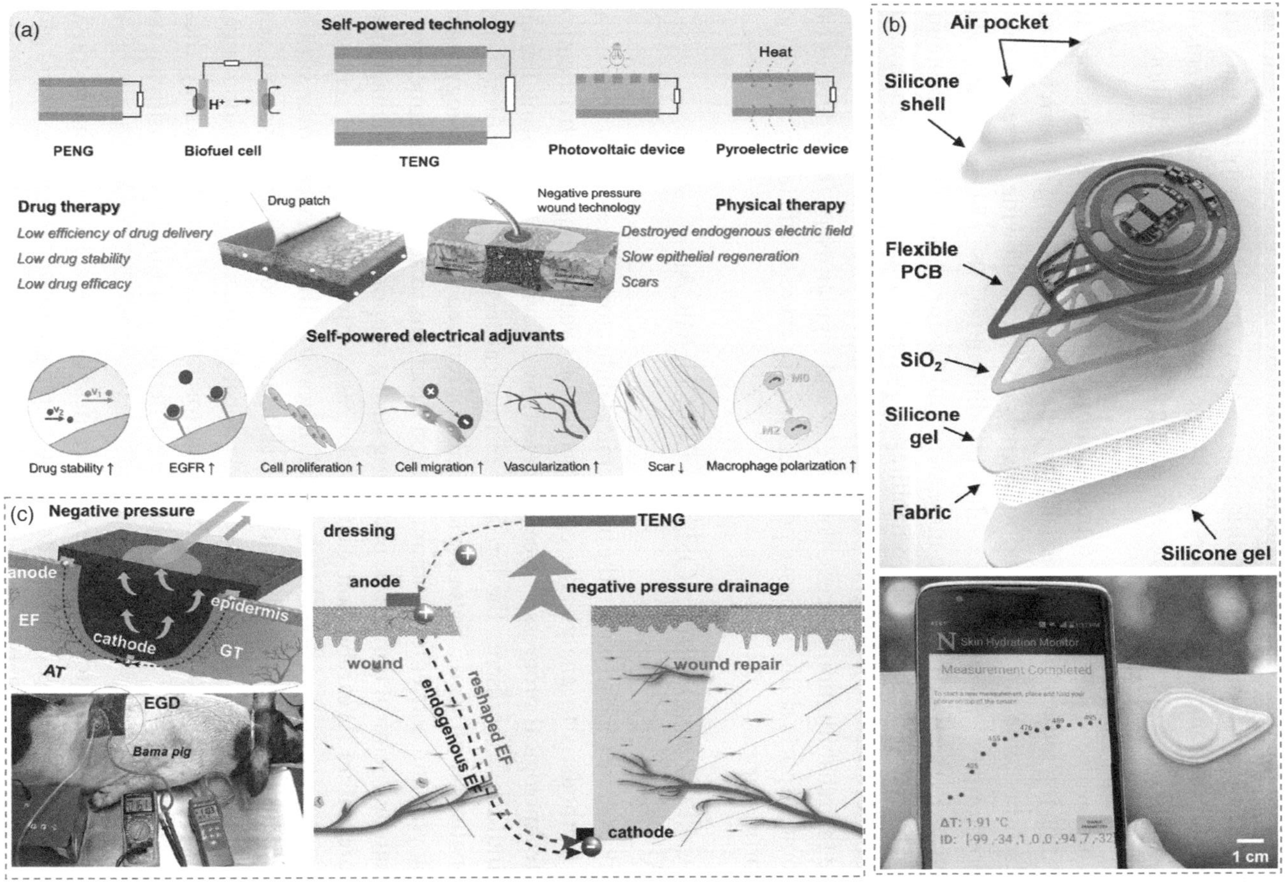

FIGURE 3.8 Soft electronic devices for wound healing and skin detection. (a) Wound healing method based on self-powered technology. (b) Soft sensor for monitoring and diagnosis of inflammatory skin diseases. (c) Boost wound repair via electrogenerative dressing. [a] Adapted with permission (Luo, Shi, et al., 2023b). Copyright 2023, Elsevier; [b] Adapted with permission (Madhvapathy et al., 2020). Copyright 2020, AAAS; [c] Adapted with permission (Luo, Liang, et al., 2023a). Copyright 2023, Wiley-VCH.)

Significant progress has been made in the sensing technology of wearable muscle movement and posture monitoring devices. These devices are typically equipped with various sensors such as accelerometers, gyroscopes, electromyography (EMG) sensors, etc., to detect and record body movements and muscle activity. Accelerometers and gyroscopes can measure the direction and velocity of the body, while EMG sensors can capture muscle electrical signals, providing information about muscle activity intensity and patterns. The combination of these sensors enables the device to track muscle movements and changes in body posture in real time, providing detailed data for rehabilitation and exercise training.

For individuals with swallowing difficulties, obtaining information on jaw muscle activity during swallowing movements is beneficial for rehabilitation training. Researchers use wearable soft sensors to obtain muscle motion signals during swallowing, thereby achieving remote monitoring of patients with swallowing difficulties. The progress of wearable electronic devices in monitoring muscle movement and posture has also had a profound impact on rehabilitation medicine. For rehabilitation patients, these devices can provide real-time motion feedback, help patients perform rehabilitation exercises more accurately, and accelerate the rehabilitation process. For athletes and regular users, these devices can be used to monitor sports skills, improve posture, increase exercise efficiency, and reduce the risk of sports injuries.

3.6 MONITORING AND DIAGNOSIS OF BIOCHEMICAL INDICATORS

The commonly used method to obtain the biochemical indicators of the human body using non-invasive methods is to analyse the composition of sweat through electrochemical devices. The technological progress of wearable electronic devices in monitoring human biochemical indicators represents the forefront of medical technology, providing a new way for personalised healthcare. These devices utilise advanced sensing technology, intelligent data analysis, and convenient communication functions to achieve real-time monitoring of human biochemical indicators, providing strong support for health management and disease prevention. Wearable soft electric devices continue to innovate, achieving highly sensitive detection of various biochemical indicators. These devices cover various sampling methods such as blood, body fluids, and skin, and are equipped with various sensors to achieve real-time monitoring of key biochemical parameters such as blood sugar, lactate, urea, protein, and electrolytes. By using microsensors and nanotechnology, these devices can achieve a smaller and lighter design while maintaining high sensitivity and improving wearing comfort.

Taking blood glucose monitoring as an example, these devices can provide more convenient and continuous blood glucose monitoring to help patients better manage blood glucose levels. The main manifestation of diabetes is the fluctuation of blood glucose beyond the normal range, so the detection of blood glucose concentration is of great significance. According to the trauma caused by blood glucose detection to the human body, the current blood glucose detection methods can be divided into invasive detection, minimally invasive detection, and non-invasive detection. Invasive testing can cause

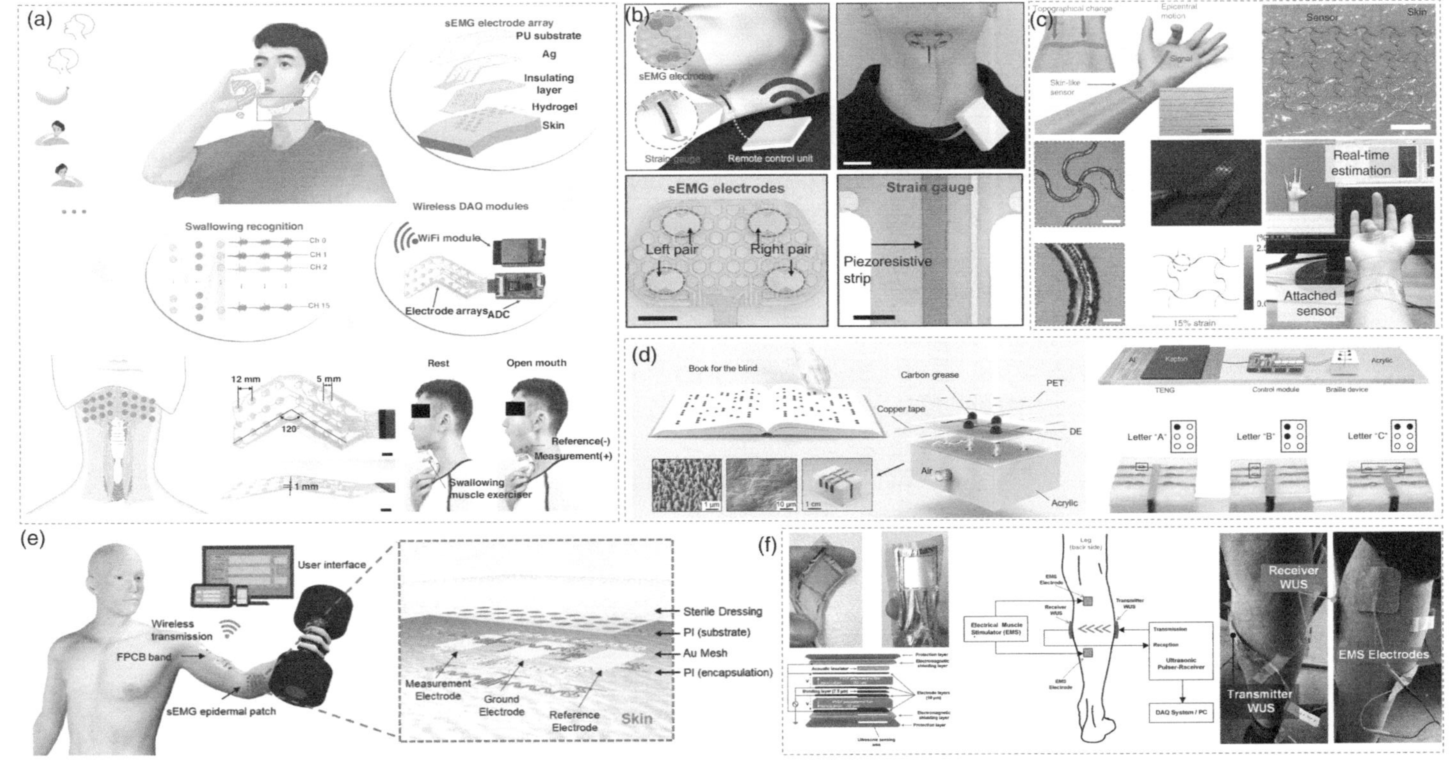

FIGURE 3.9 Soft electronic devices for muscle activity and posture recognition. (a) Soft electromyographic sensor for swallowing monitoring. (b) Soft sensors for monitoring oral swallowing. (c) Skin sensors that can recognise human movements. (d) Flexible and refreshable dynamic Braille display based on dielectric elastomer. (e) Wearable sensors for muscle strength monitoring. (f) Wearable soft ultrasound device for monitoring calf muscles. ([a] Adapted with permission (Zhang et al., 2023). Copyright 2023, Springer Nature; [b] Adapted with permission (Kim et al., 2019). Copyright 2019, AAAS; [c] Adapted with permission (Kim et al., 2020). Copyright 2020, Springer Nature; [d] Adapted with permission (Qu et al., 2021). Copyright 2021, Wiley-VCH; [e] Adapted with permission (Gong et al., 2023). Copyright 2023, Wiley-VCH; [f] Adapted with permission (AlMohimeed & Ono, 2020). Copyright 2020, MDPI.)

direct harm to patients. Although minimally invasive detection will not cause direct harm to patients, this method has high requirements for materials, the cost problem cannot be ignored, and it is difficult to obtain blood glucose values directly. Non-invasive testing means that testing is carried out under conditions that do not cause harm to the human body at all. Due to many problems in invasive and minimally invasive testing, non-invasive testing has become a research hotspot for many research institutions and companies.

The parts of non-invasive detection and measurement include fingers, arms, eyeballs, earlobes, etc. Alternative media include tissue fluid, tears, sweat, blood, etc. There are a variety of non-invasive detection methods, which can usually be divided into two categories: Optical detection and non-optical detection. Light is an ideal information carrier for non-invasive detection, which can realise non-invasive and non-contact detection. The optical detection method has the characteristics of simple operation and fast speed and has been widely concerned. In recent years, many domestic and foreign scholars have carried out research on optical detection methods and made certain progress. Optical detection methods mainly include photoacoustic spectroscopy, Raman spectroscopy, fluorescence method, polarised optical rotation method, optical coherence tomography and spectroscopy. The non-optical detection method refers to the method of blood glucose detection without the aid of light. The non-optical detection methods are based on different theories, including the reverse ion electroosmosis method, metabolic thermal conditioning method and bioimpedance method.

3.7 WEARABLE DISEASE MONITORING AND DIAGNOSIS BASED ON ARTIFICIAL INTELLIGENCE

Regardless of the type of sensors, ultimately it is necessary to evaluate human health and disease status based on the data obtained. Therefore, how to extract effective information from complex sensing signals is one of the important research topics in the field of flexible sensing. With the continuous development of artificial intelligence (AI), utilising AI for sensor signal analysis has become one of the increasingly popular methods.

The combination of soft electronic devices and AI provides users with a more intelligent and personalised experience. This combination has promoted the development of portable electronic technology, making it more intelligent and comprehensive, with a wider range of application prospects. First, the addition of artificial intelligence endows wearable devices with more advanced data processing and intelligent analysis capabilities. The large amount of data collected by sensors can be used for deep learning and pattern recognition through artificial intelligence algorithms, thereby more accurately understanding user behaviour, health status, and needs. This enables wearable devices to provide more personalised services, adjusting reminders, suggestions, and monitoring methods based on user habits and physical conditions.

Soft electronic devices combined with AI have achieved a higher degree of automation and intelligence. For example, in terms of health monitoring, wearable devices can automatically recognise the user's movement type, sleep stage, heart rate changes, etc. and generate corresponding reports and suggestions through artificial intelligence algorithms. In daily life, combining artificial intelligence with voice assistants allows users to easily control devices, query information, and even engage in voice interaction through voice commands. In addition, the integration of soft electric devices and AI makes real-time monitoring and immediate feedback possible. By analysing the data collected by sensors in real time, AI can quickly identify abnormal situations and issue alerts or reminders promptly. In terms of exercise and medical monitoring, for example, when the device detects a user's abnormal heart rate or excessive exercise, it can immediately remind the user to appropriately slow down the exercise intensity to prevent excessive fatigue. Medical monitoring equipment can analyse patients' physiological data through AI for early disease prediction and risk assessment. In the rehabilitation process, combining virtual reality and augmented reality technology of artificial intelligence, wearable devices can provide more personalised and vivid rehabilitation plans, improving the rehabilitation effect of patients (Figure 3.10).

In the future, the combination of soft electronic devices and AI will achieve more breakthroughs in multiple fields. In the field of smart homes, wearable devices will be part of smart home systems, enabling more intelligent home management and life services through artificial intelligence. In the industrial field, wearable devices combined with AI can improve work efficiency, ensure employee safety, and achieve more intelligent production and management.

3.8 SUMMARY AND PROSPECT

The rapid progress of flexible electronic technology in disease monitoring and diagnosis has injected new vitality into the medical field, providing patients with more convenient, accurate, and continuous monitoring and diagnostic methods. The innovation of this technology is mainly reflected in the flexibility, wearability, high sensitivity, and remote monitoring of sensors, providing strong support for the early detection and treatment of various diseases. The flexibility of soft electronic sensors makes medical devices closer to the patient's body curve, thus improving monitoring comfort. Traditional rigid medical devices are often limited by shape and material, while flexible electronic technology uses soft and thin materials to make sensors that fit the skin. The lightweight and soft characteristics allow patients to wear them more naturally without feeling uncomfortable with hard objects, thereby improving patient cooperation. Second, soft electronic technology has diverse and extensive applications in disease monitoring. By integrating various sensors, it is possible to monitor multiple physiological indicators, such as ECG, blood pressure, blood sugar, blood flow velocity, etc. The high sensitivity and resolution of flexible electronic sensors make monitoring data more accurate, providing doctors with more comprehensive patient information and helping to detect potential disease risks and abnormal changes early.

Soft electronic technology has shown outstanding performance in disease monitoring, especially in the management of chronic diseases. For example, for patients with diabetes, flexible electronic sensors can monitor blood glucose levels in real time, eliminating the need for patients to take blood frequently, improving the convenience of monitoring. For patients with cardiovascular diseases, flexible electronic sensors can continuously monitor ECG and blood pressure, providing doctors with more detailed cardiovascular function

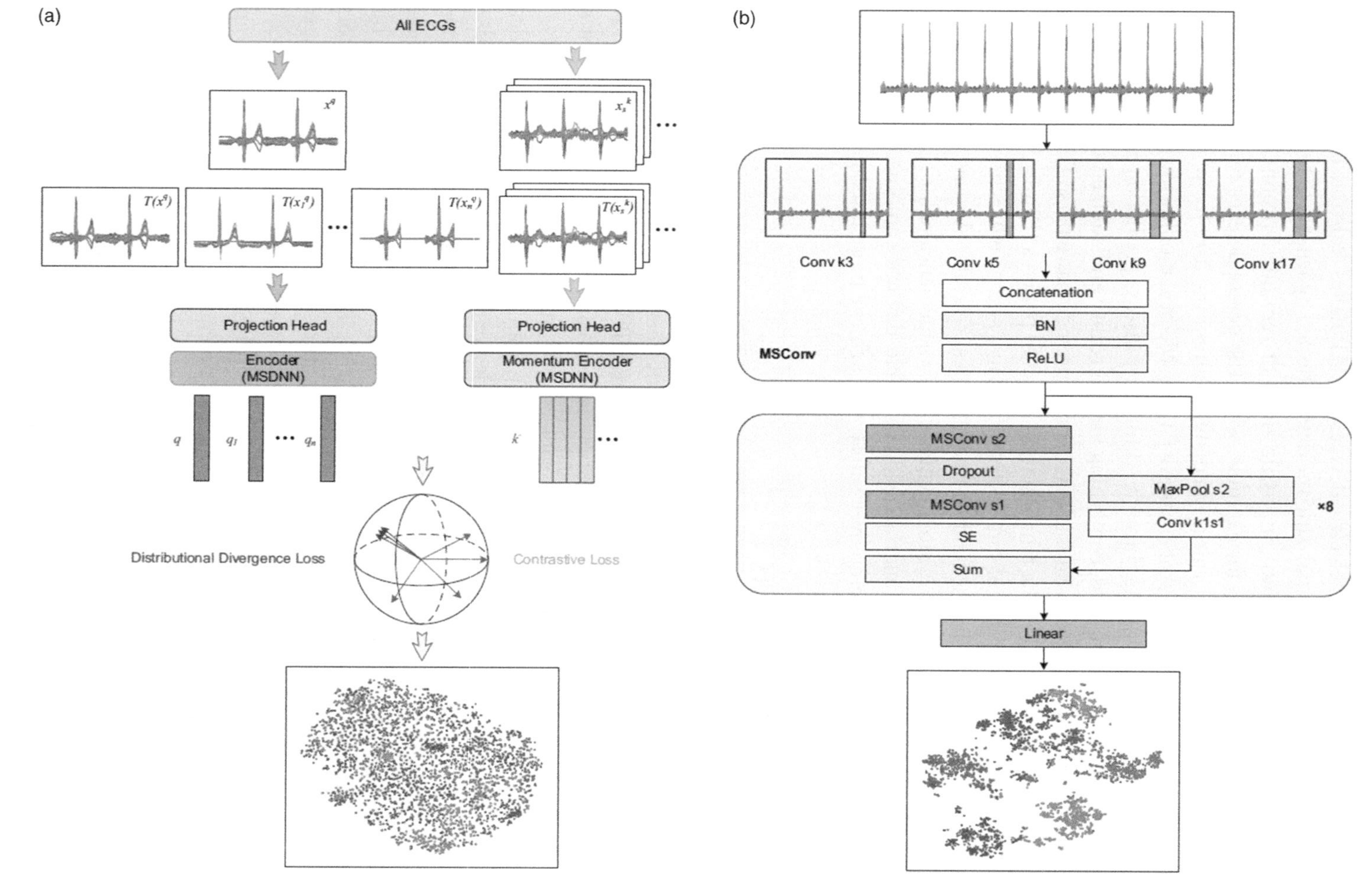

FIGURE 3.10   Using artificial intelligence to process sensing signals. Adapted with permission (Lai et al., 2023). Copyright 2023, Springer Nature.

information and achieving more personalised treatment plans. In addition, the development of flexible electronic technology has also promoted the implementation of telemedicine. Through wireless communication technology, patients can transmit real-time monitoring data generated by flexible electronic devices to the cloud or doctor's end, and doctors can monitor and analyse the health status of patients anytime and anywhere. This remote monitoring method can not only improve the work efficiency of doctors but also reduce the medical costs of patients, especially for some patients who require long-term monitoring, which has significant advantages.

The advancement of soft electronic technology in disease diagnosis has also brought breakthroughs to the field of medical imaging. Flexible electronic sensors can be flexibly applied inside or outside the body to achieve high-resolution imaging of tissue structure and function. For example, the application of flexible electronic sensors in medical imaging devices such as endoscopes and ultrasound imaging provides doctors with clearer and more accurate imaging information, which helps to detect lesions early and provide more accurate diagnoses. The progress of flexible electronic technology in disease monitoring and diagnosis has injected new vitality into the medical field, providing patients with more intelligent, convenient, and continuous medical services. With the continuous innovation of technology, flexible electronic technology is expected to provide more comprehensive and effective solutions for the early prevention, diagnosis, and treatment of more diseases in the future. Another innovative aspect of soft electronic technology is its versatility. The soft electronic devices can integrate multiple sensors, which can not only monitor ECG signals but also other physiological parameters such as skin temperature, humidity, and exercise status. This multifunctional monitoring device can provide doctors with more comprehensive patient health information, help to comprehensively understand the patient's physical condition, and develop more personalised treatment plans.

REFERENCES

AlMohimeed, I., & Ono, Y. (2020). Ultrasound measurement of skeletal muscle contractile parameters using flexible and wearable single-element ultrasonic sensor. *Sensors*, *20*(13), 3616.

Chen, Y., Liu, F., Lu, B., Zhang, Y., & Feng, X. (2020). Skin-like hybrid integrated circuits conformal to face for continuous respiratory monitoring. *Advanced Electronic Materials*, *6*(7), 2000145.

Cheng, S., Hang, C., Ding, L., Jia, L., Tang, L., Mou, L., Qi, J., Dong, R., Zheng, W., Zhang, Y., & Jiang, X. (2020). Electronic blood vessel. *Matter*, *3*(5), 1664–1684.

Chung, H. U., Kim, B. H., Lee, J. Y., Lee, J., Xie, Z., Ibler, E. M., Lee, K., Banks, A., Jeong, J. Y., Kim, J., Ogle, C., Grande, D., Yu, Y., Jang, H., Assem, P., Ryu, D., Kwak, J. W., Namkoong, M., Park, J. B., … Rogers, J. A. (2019). Binodal, wireless epidermal electronic systems with in-sensor analytics for neonatal intensive care. *Science*, *363*(6430), eaau0780.

Cotur, Y., Olenik, S., Asfour, T., Bruyns-Haylett, M., Kasimatis, M., Tanriverdi, U., Gonzalez-Macia, L., Lee, H. S., Kozlov, A. S., & Güder, F. (2022). Bioinspired stretchable transducer for wearable continuous monitoring of respiratory patterns in humans and animals. *Advanced Materials*, *34*(33), 2203310.

Dai, J., Meng, J., Zhao, X., Zhang, W., Fan, Y., Shi, B., & Li, Z. (2023). A wearable self-powered multiparameter respiration sensor. *Advanced Materials Technologies*, *8*(7), 2201535.

Duan, Z., Yuan, Z., Jiang, Y., Zhao, Q., Huang, Q., Zhang, Y., Liu, B., & Tai, H. (2022). Power generation humidity sensor based on primary battery structure. *Chemical Engineering Journal, 446*, 136910.

Fortin, J., Rogge, D. E., Fellner, C., Flotzinger, D., Grond, J., Lerche, K., & Saugel, B. (2021). A novel art of continuous noninvasive blood pressure measurement. *Nature Communications, 12*(1), 1387.

Frey, L., Menon, C., & Elgendi, M. (2022). Blood pressure measurement using only a smartphone. *npj Digital Medicine, 5*(1), 86.

Gong, Q., Jiang, X., Liu, Y., Yu, M., & Hu, Y. (2023). A flexible wireless sEMG system for wearable muscle strength and fatigue monitoring in real time. *Advanced Electronic Materials, 9*(9), 2200916.

Huang, X., Liu, Y., Park, W., Li, J., Ma, J., Yiu, C. K., Zhang, Q., Li, J., Wu, P., Zhou, J., Zeng, Y., He, X., Li, J., Wong, T. H., Yao, K., Zhao, L., Gao, Y., Shi, R., Li, H., Yu, X. (2023). Intelligent soft sweat sensors for the simultaneous healthcare monitoring and safety warning. *Advanced Healthcare Materials, 12*(15), 2202846.

Ibáñez-Redín, G., Rosso Cagnani, G.O., Gomes, N., Raymundo-Pereira, P. A. S., Machado, S. A., Gutierrez, M. A., Krieger, J. E., & Oliveira, O. N. (2023). Wearable potentiometric biosensor for analysis of urea in sweat. *Biosensors and Bioelectronics, 223*, 114994.

Jiang, Y., Ji, S., Sun, J., Huang, J., Li, Y., Zou, G., Salim, T., Wang, C., Li, W., Jin, H., Xu, J., Wang, S., Lei, T., Yan, X., Peh, W. Y. X., Yen, S.-C., Liu, Z., Yu, M., Zhao, H., Chen, X. (2023). A universal interface for plug-and-play assembly of stretchable devices. *Nature, 614*(7948), 456–462.

Jin, H., Zheng, Z., Cui, Z., Jiang, Y., Chen, G., Li, W., Wang, Z., Wang, J., Yang, C., Song, W., Chen, X., & Zheng, Y. (2023). A flexible optoacoustic blood 'stethoscope' for noninvasive multiparametric cardiovascular monitoring. *Nature Communications, 14*(1), 4692.

Jin, P., Fu, J., Wang, F., Zhang, Y., Wang, P., Liu, X., Jiao, Y., Li, H., Chen, Y., Ma, Y., & Feng, X. (2021). A flexible, stretchable system for simultaneous acoustic energy transfer and communication. *Science Advances, 7*(40), eabg2507.

Kim, K. K., Ha, I., Kim, M., Choi, J., Won, P., Jo, S., & Ko, S. H. (2020). A deep-learned skin sensor decoding the epicentral human motions. *Nature Communications, 11*(1), 2149.

Kim, M. K., Kantarcigil, C., Kim, B., Baruah, R. K., Maity, S., Park, Y., Kim, K., Lee, S., Malandraki, J. B., Avlani, S., Smith, A., Sen, S., Alam, M. A., Malandraki, G., & Lee, C. H. (2019). Flexible submental sensor patch with remote monitoring controls for management of oropharyngeal swallowing disorders. *Science Advances, 5*(12), eaay3210.

Kireev, D., Sel, K., Ibrahim, B., Kumar, N., Akbari, A., Jafari, R., & Akinwande, D. (2022). Continuous cuffless monitoring of arterial blood pressure via graphene bioimpedance tattoos. *Nature Nanotechnology, 17*(8), 864–870.

Lai, J., Tan, H., Wang, J., Ji, L., Guo, J., Han, B., Shi, Y., Feng, Q., & Yang, W. (2023). Practical intelligent diagnostic algorithm for wearable 12-lead ECG via self-supervised learning on large-scale dataset. *Nature Communications, 14*(1), 3741.

Liu, T., Qu, D., Guo, L., Zhou, G., Zhang, G., Du, T., & Wu, W. (n.d.). MXene/TPU composite film for humidity sensing and human respiration monitoring. *Advanced Sensor Research, 3*, 2300014.

Luo, R., Liang, Y., Yang, J., Feng, H., Chen, Y., Jiang, X., Zhang, Z., Liu, J., Bai, Y., Xue, J., Chao, S., Xi, Y., Liu, X., Wang, E., Luo, D., Li, Z., & Zhang, J. (2023a). Reshaping the endogenous electric field to boost wound repair via electrogenerative dressing. *Advanced Materials, 35*(16), 2208395.

Luo, R., Shi, B., Luo, D., & Li, Z. (2023b). Self-powered electrical stimulation assisted skin wound therapy. *Science Bulletin, 68*(16), 1740–1743.

Madhvapathy, S. R., Wang, H., Kong, J., Zhang, M., Lee, J. Y., Park, J. B., Jang, H., Xie, Z., Cao, J., Avila, R., Wei, C., D'Angelo, V., Zhu, J., Chung, H. U., Coughlin, S., Patel, M., Winograd, J., Lim, J., Banks, A., … Rogers, J. A. (2020). Reliable, low-cost, fully integrated hydration sensors for monitoring and diagnosis of inflammatory skin diseases in any environment. *Science Advances, 6*(49), eabd7146.

Mukkamala, R., Stergiou, G. S., & Avolio, A. P. (2022). Cuffless blood pressure measurement. *Annual Review of Biomedical Engineering, 24*(1), 203–230.

Ouyang, H., Liu, Z., Li, N., Shi, B., Zou, Y., Xie, F., Ma, Y., Li, Z., Li, H., Zheng, Q., Qu, X., Fan, Y., Wang, Z. L., Zhang, H., & Li, Z. (2019). Symbiotic cardiac pacemaker. *Nature Communications, 10*(1), 1821.

Qu, X., Ma, X., Shi, B., Li, H., Zheng, L., Wang, C., Liu, Z., Fan, Y., Chen, X., Li, Z., & Wang, Z. L. (2021). Refreshable braille display system based on triboelectric nanogenerator and dielectric elastomer. *Advanced Functional Materials, 31*(5), 2006612.

Schutte, A. E., Kollias, A., & Stergiou, G. S. (2022). Blood pressure and its variability: Classic and novel measurement techniques. *Nature Reviews Cardiology, 19*(10), 643–654.

Sim, K., Ershad, F., Zhang, Y., Yang, P., Shim, H., Rao, Z., Lu, Y., Thukral, A., Elgalad, A., Xi, Y., Tian, B., Taylor, D. A., & Yu, C. (2020). An epicardial bioelectronic patch made from soft rubbery materials and capable of spatiotemporal mapping of electrophysiological activity. *Nature Electronics, 3*(12), 775–784.

Sun, X., Agate, S., Salem, K. S., Lucia, L., & Pal, L. (2021). Hydrogel-based sensor networks: Compositions, properties, and applications—A review. *ACS Applied Bio Materials, 4*(1), 140–162.

Wang, C., Qi, B., Lin, M., Zhang, Z., Makihata, M., Liu, B., Zhou, S., Huang, Y.-H., Hu, H., Gu, Y., Chen, Y., Lei, Y., Lee, T., Chien, S., Jang, K.-I., Kistler, E. B., & Xu, S. (2021). Continuous monitoring of deep-tissue haemodynamics with stretchable ultrasonic phased arrays. *Nature Biomedical Engineering, 5*(7), 749–758.

Wang, Y., Adam, M. L., Zhao, Y., Zheng, W., Gao, L., Yin, Z., & Zhao, H. (2023). Machine learning-enhanced flexible mechanical sensing. *Nano-Micro Letters, 15*(1), 55.

Yang, Y., Song, Y., Bo, X., Min, J., Pak, O. S., Zhu, L., Wang, M., Tu, J., Kogan, A., Zhang, H., Hsiai, T. K., Li, Z., & Gao, W. (2020). A laser-engraved wearable sensor for sensitive detection of uric acid and tyrosine in sweat. *Nature Biotechnology, 38*(2), 217–224.

Yu, C., Shi, M., He, S., Yao, M., Sun, H., Yue, Z., Qiu, Y., Liu, B., Liang, L., Zhao, Z., Yao, F., Zhang, H., & Li, J. (2023). Chronological adhesive cardiac patch for synchronous mechanophysiological monitoring and electrocoupling therapy. *Nature Communications, 14*(1), 6226.

Zhang, D., Chen, Z., Xiao, L., Zhu, B., Wu, R., Ou, C., Ma, Y., Xie, L., & Jiang, H. (2023). Stretchable and durable HD-sEMG electrodes for accurate recognition of swallowing activities on complex epidermal surfaces. *Microsystems & Nanoengineering, 9*(1), 115.

Zhang, S., Li, L., Lu, Y., Liu, D., Zhang, J., Hao, D., Zhang, X., Xiong, L., & Huang, J. (2022). Sensitive humidity sensors based on ionically conductive metal-organic frameworks for breath monitoring and non-contact sensing. *Applied Materials Today, 26*, 101391.

Zhang, Y., Yu, J., & Gu, Z. (2020). Cyborg Vessel. *Matter, 3*(5), 1393–1395.

Zou, Y., Gai, Y., Tan, P., Jiang, D., Qu, X., Xue, J., Ouyang, H., Shi, B., Li, L., Luo, D., Deng, Y., Li, Z., & Wang, Z. L. (2022). Stretchable graded multichannel self-powered respiratory sensor inspired by shark gill. *Fundamental Research, 2*(4), 619–628.

CHAPTER 4

Soft Electronics for Medical Treatment

Meng Wang

4.1 INTRODUCTION

Medical treatment is the most important and promising application field of soft electronics and it is also an emerging research direction (Zhang et al., 2023c). Compared with traditional rigid medical devices, medical devices made with soft electronic technology have the advantages of being flexible, lightweight, and deformable (Luo et al., 2020). Therefore, soft medical electronic devices can fit well to the arbitrary surfaces of the human body and can adapt to the shape and movement deformation of different joint parts (Ma et al., 2020). These features not only ensure the accuracy and reliability of soft electronic devices during diagnosis and treatment but also ensure the patient's wearing comfort (Vaghasiya et al., 2023; T. Zhang et al., 2023b). In addition, the power efficiency of soft electronic devices is usually low and many self-powered and wireless power supply solutions have been proposed to replace batteries, which makes them suitable for long-term diagnostic and therapeutic work needs (Guo et al., 2021).

Currently, soft bioelectronic devices have been widely developed and used in precision medicine. Combining the sensing and therapeutic capabilities of soft bioelectronics is a core goal to enable personalized, decentralized healthcare (Zhang et al., 2023c). So far, many studies have successfully used soft bioelectronic devices for continuous health monitoring of the human body, such as common human physiological indicators: body temperature, ECG, pulse, and blood pressure (Cheng et al., 2020; Kang et al., 2022; Meng et al., 2019; Yamamoto et al., 2017). Furthermore, through complex and advanced biochemical sensor systems, these soft bioelectronic devices can further detect and analyze biomolecules and chemical substances inside the human body, such as electrolytes, glucose, lactic acid, and uric acid (Emaminejad et al., 2017; Gao et al., 2016; Yang et al., 2020b). Not only that, soft bioelectronic devices can provide patients with real-time, continuous on-demand treatment services in a convenient, controllable, and precise manner. This makes them particularly advantageous in the diagnosis and treatment of complex diseases and chronic diseases (Qiao et al., 2023). Integrating various responsive soft actuators and controllable stimulators, soft bioelectronic devices can also achieve highly controllable drug delivery

DOI: 10.1201/9781003493631-4

and release operations, providing personalized and precise medical services to patients (Kar et al., 2022; Zheng et al., 2023). In addition, with the characteristics of ultra-thin, soft, conformable, and low elastic modulus, soft electronic devices have stronger in vivo compatibility than traditional rigid flat implantable devices (Kim et al., 2017; Koo et al., 2021). This has led to high hopes for its application in implantable medicine and has received widespread attention and research.

This chapter will focus on the application of soft bioelectronic devices in the medical field, review significant research progress and results achieved in recent years, and provide detailed insights into the progress and role of soft bioelectronic devices in treating various diseases. Additionally, it will propose exciting development possibilities for soft bioelectronics in future medical treatments. The main content includes the following four parts: smart wound dressings, bioelectronic patches for transdermal and epidermal treatments, soft actuators for drug delivery, and other soft electronics for medical treatment.

4.2 SMART WOUND DRESSINGS

Wound management has always been an important topic in the medical field and is one of the common ailments in people's daily lives (Singer & Clark, 1999). Each year, billions of dollars are invested in wound management around the world (Sen, 2021). In particular, chronic difficult-to-heal wounds will bring a heavy burden to patients' economy and life (Falanga et al., 2022; Sun et al., 2022). Therefore, nations worldwide prioritize medical research in wound treatment. Wound healing is a dynamic and complex process. A typical wound-healing process includes four stages: hemostasis, inflammation, proliferation, and remodeling (Figure 4.1) (Li et al., 2023). The healing cycle of chronic wounds usually lasts for more than 12 weeks (Trinh et al., 2022). Among the tools utilized in wound treatment, wound dressing stands as the most commonly employed method. It can cover the wound, protect it from damage, and promote wound healing (Derakhshandeh et al., 2018). To date, thousands of different wound dressings have been developed to treat different types of wounds, including gauze, bandages, foams, and hydrogels (Brumberg et al., 2021; Ghomi et al., 2019; Kus & Ruiz, 2020). While traditional wound dressings boast a rich history of

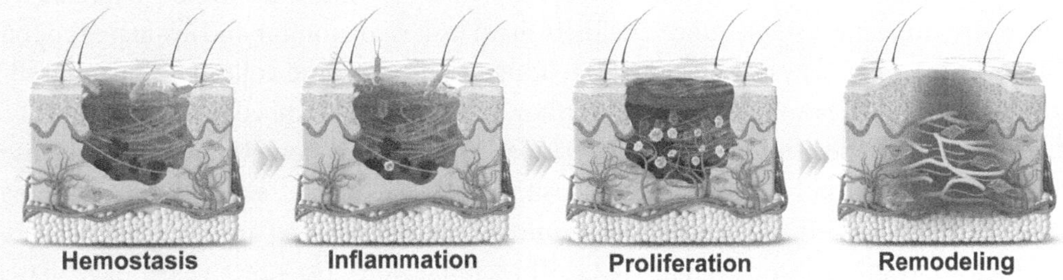

FIGURE 4.1   Schematic of the wound healing process from left to right: hemostasis, inflammation, proliferation, and remodeling. Adapted with permission (Li et al., 2023). Copyright 2023, Springer Nature.

development and clinical practice, they still fall short of meeting certain treatment needs. For example, they cannot obtain real-time status information of the wound during the healing process nor can they dynamically respond and provide on-demand treatment based on the actual condition of the wound, which makes traditional wound dressings play a limited and passive role in wound management (Dong & Guo, 2021). Fortunately, the rapid development of soft electronic technology in recent years and its monitoring and treatment capabilities in biomedicine have brought new strategies to the construction of intelligent wound dressings.

In wound treatment, monitoring of the wound environment is of great significance. There are many types of wounds such as acute wounds, burns, and chronic ulcers. The environment of these wounds varies, and changes in the wound-healing process are reflected in the wound environment (Castaño et al., 2018; Kruse et al., 2015). Clinical studies have found that wound status is closely related to temperature, pH, humidity, uric acid, and oxygen levels in the wound environment (Brett, 2006; Castilla & Velazquez, 2012; Haller et al., 2021; Maliyar et al., 2020). For example, when a wound becomes infected, the wound is often accompanied by an increase in temperature and a change in pH (Chanmugam et al., 2017; Derwin et al., 2023; Metcalf et al., 2019); the concentration of uric acid in the wound exudate is related to the colonization of *Staphylococcus aureus* and the severity of the wound injury (Fernandez et al., 2012). Therefore, obtaining physiological parameters of the wound environment can help medical staff understand the wound status more intuitively (McLister et al., 2016). Compared with traditional wound dressings, smart wound dressings based on soft bioelectronics technology carry numerous biochemical sensing and stimulation modules, which can monitor the biochemical information in the wound environment in real time and convert it into readable data. This helps medical staff understand the status and healing process of the wound and propose precise treatment plans. Furthermore, they can also treat wounds according to the instructions of medical staff, such as on-demand controlled release of drugs and programmed electrical stimulation therapy (Jiang et al., 2023b; Sani et al., 2023; Xu et al., 2021).

Although the research history of smart wound dressings based on soft electronic devices is not long, their development is amazing and inspiring. In the past decade or so, soft electronic smart wound dressings have undergone many advancements and updates (Farahani & Shafiee, 2021). In the initial stage of research, smart wound dressings have a relatively simple structure and a single function. Their main task is to monitor and evaluate the condition of the wound. For example, in 2014, Tomàs Guinovart and colleagues introduced a wearable wound dressing that could monitor wound pH by embedding screen-printed potentiometric sensors into an adhesive bandage (2014). This potentiometric sensor uses electropolymerized polyaniline as the sensitive material for pH sensing and combines screen printing and all-solid-state potentiometric methods to prepare the reference electrode and working electrode (Figure 4.2a). This simple, low-cost adhesive bandage–based pH sensor exhibits Nernstian sensitivity over a pH range of 4.35–8.00. They verified the dressing's ability to monitor pH fluctuations in a simulated wound environment. In another study, Pooria Mostafalu et al. reported a smart wound dressing that can monitor and transmit wound oxygen content in real time (2015). They used polyparaxylene as the soft

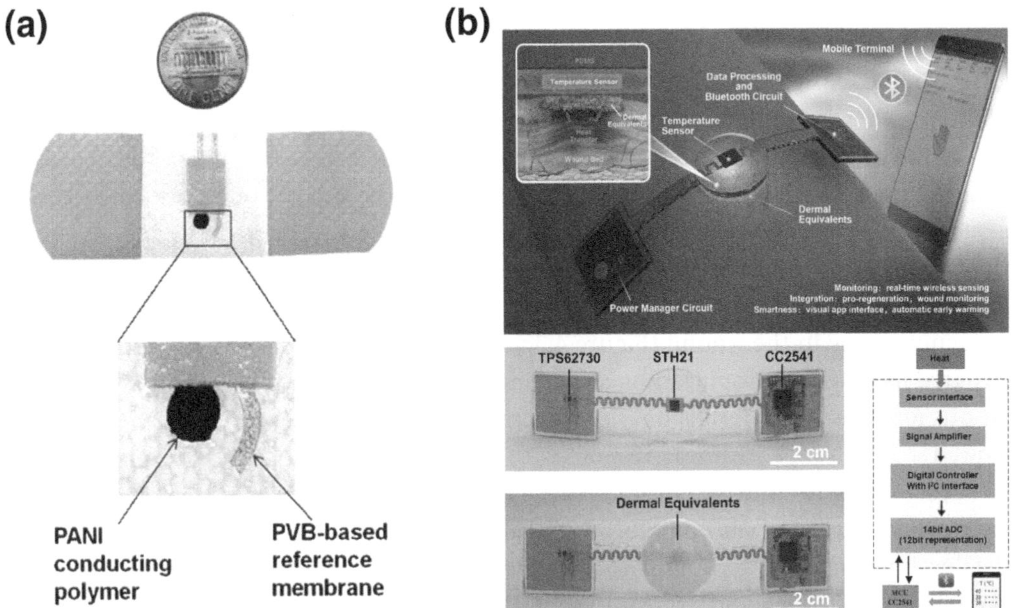

FIGURE 4.2 Wound dressing with physiological indicator monitoring function. (a) Optical image of an adhesive bandage with an embedded pH sensor. (b) Schematic diagram of the working scene of temperature monitoring dressing (top) and its optical pictures and system block diagram (bottom). ([a] Copyright 2014, Wiley-VCH. Adapted with permission (Guinovart et al., 2014); [b] Adapted with permission (Lou et al., 2020). Copyright 2020, Elsevier.)

substrate, silver and zinc as the cathode and anode, potassium hydroxide gel as the electrolyte, and PDMS film as the oxygen-selective membrane to prepare a soft galvanic oxygen sensor. They then connected the sensor to an integrated circuit system and built it into a bandage printed with an elastic material. Finally, they also verified the oxygen-sensing capabilities of the wound dressing in a simulated wound environment. Smart wound dressings for wound temperature sensing have also received widespread attention. For example, Lou et al. reported a smart wound dressing that can achieve wound temperature monitoring and infection early warning (2020). They used a snake-shaped structure to fabricate commercially available micro temperature sensors, power management circuits, and data processing circuits into a PDMS substrate and built a dermal equivalent of collagen-chitosan on the bottom so that the device could be directly attached to the wound. Through a dedicated application installed on a smartphone, they can accurately understand the temperature information of the wound (deviation < 0.1°C) (Figure 4.2b). In the treatment of a porcine full-thickness wound infection model using this smart wound dressing, they found that when the wound temperature fluctuated between 39°C and 39.5°C, the wound was in an infected state. It can be seen that smart wound dressings with temperature-sensing capabilities can provide early warning of infection and excessive inflammation during treatment.

In addition, there are many studies that have achieved monitoring of multiple parameters in wounds. For example, Pal's group reported a disposable smart wound dressing that can simultaneously monitor the pH and UA values of the wound (2018). They printed flexible electrodes on fully hydrophobic paper and fabricated polyaniline and uricase onto the surface of the sensing electrode for sensing pH and UA, respectively (Figure 4.3a). It is then connected to a wearable potentiostat, allowing the pH and uric acid levels of the wound can be quantitatively monitored simultaneously. The data can be sent wirelessly to medical staff (Figure 4.3b). In the study, they successfully used the smart wound dressing to assess tissue damage in closed chronic wounds (pressure ulcers). Recently, Liu and colleagues reported a smart wound dressing with powerful sensing capabilities that integrates a multiple sensor array to enable real-time monitoring of sodium, potassium, calcium, pH, UA, and temperature in the wound (Figure 4.3c) (2021). The electrodes of the sensor array are prepared by magnetron sputtering, and then electrochemical methods are used to deposit various ion-sensing materials onto the electrode surface. The sensor array they prepared showed a wide range of linear responses to the above physiological indicators and had excellent selectivity and stability. Further, in vivo experiments also demonstrated that smart wound dressing can monitor wound status in real time and predict early infection. The development of these wound dressings with sensing capabilities provides quantitative tools for the complex and diverse wound healing process, which is of great significance for guiding wound treatment.

However, ideal wound dressings are integrated and multifunctional, have both diagnostic and therapeutic capabilities, and work in a Closed-loop (Wang et al., 2022a; Zhu et al., 2023). An ideal smart wound dressing should be able to simultaneously monitor multiple biochemical parameters of the wound, quantify wound information, communicate with smart terminals in real time, and actively treat the wound on demand. With these advantages, they can provide patients with accurate and personalized diagnosis and treatment services, accelerate wound healing, reduce pain during treatment, and avoid problems such as antibiotic abuse (Ge et al., 2023; Jiang et al., 2023b; Xu et al., 2021). Therefore, in recent years, the research on multifunctional closed-loop wound dressings has attracted widespread attention from scientific research and medical circles. For example, Xu et al. developed a fully integrated smart wound dressing for closed-loop wound management (2021). They fabricated a battery-free, wireless, and flexible circuit platform and then integrated multiple wound monitoring modules and electronically controlled drug release modules onto the platform (Figure 4.4a). Among them, the multiple wound monitoring module includes temperature, pH, and UA value sensing. They used a commercial sensor chip (LMT70) directly in the circuit as a temperature sensor. The pH and UA sensors are fabricated using electrochemical methods. First, the electrode array was constructed on a PDMS substrate through screen printing. Then, the rGO/AuNP composite and PANI were deposited on the surfaces of the two working electrodes, respectively, through electrochemical modification methods for UA and pH sensing. Similarly, using electrochemical modification methods, polypyrrole and the anti-infective drug ceftezole were constructed onto drug-controlled release electrodes. During the treatment process, the controlled release of the antibacterial drug cefazolin can be achieved by simply changing the voltage on the drug electrode through the drug delivery module. Both in vitro experiments and original animal experiments have shown

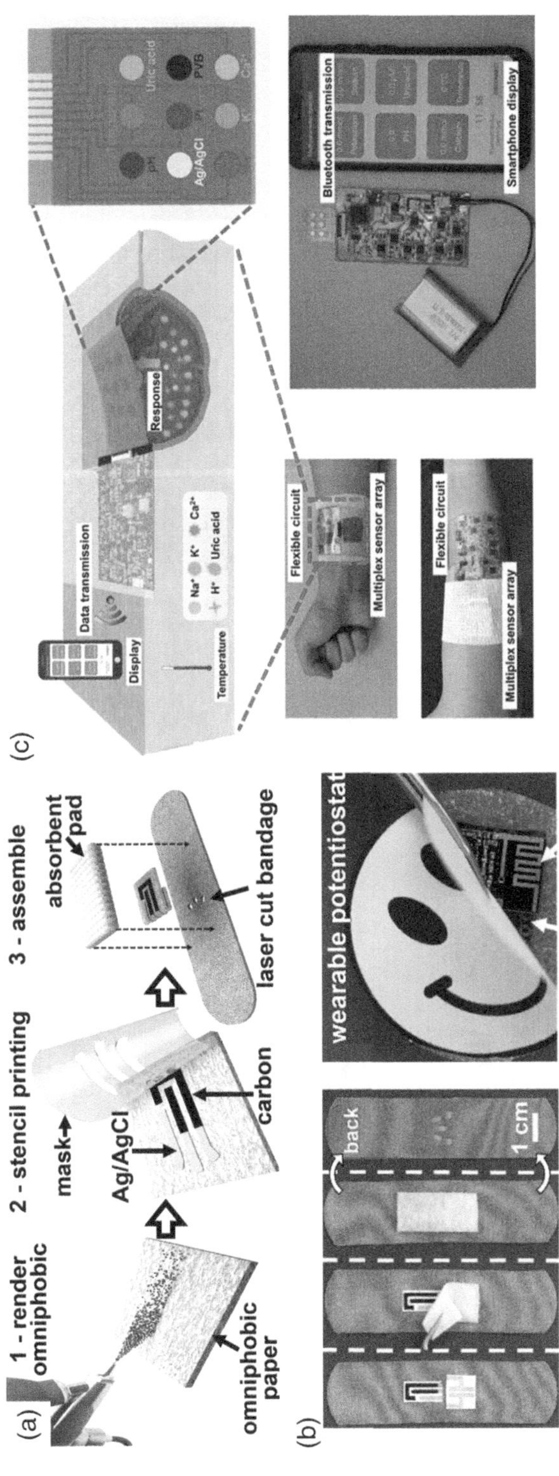

FIGURE 4.3 Smart dressing with integrated multiple sensors (a, b) Schematic diagram (a) of paper-based wound dressing preparation for pH and uric acid monitoring and its optical images (b). (c) Diagram of the working principle of a wound dressing with multiple sensing capabilities (top), and an optical image of its components (bottom). ([a, b] Adapted with permission (Pal et al., 2018). Copyright 2020, Elsevier; [c] Adapted with permission (Liu et al., 2021). Copyright 2021, American Chemical Society.)

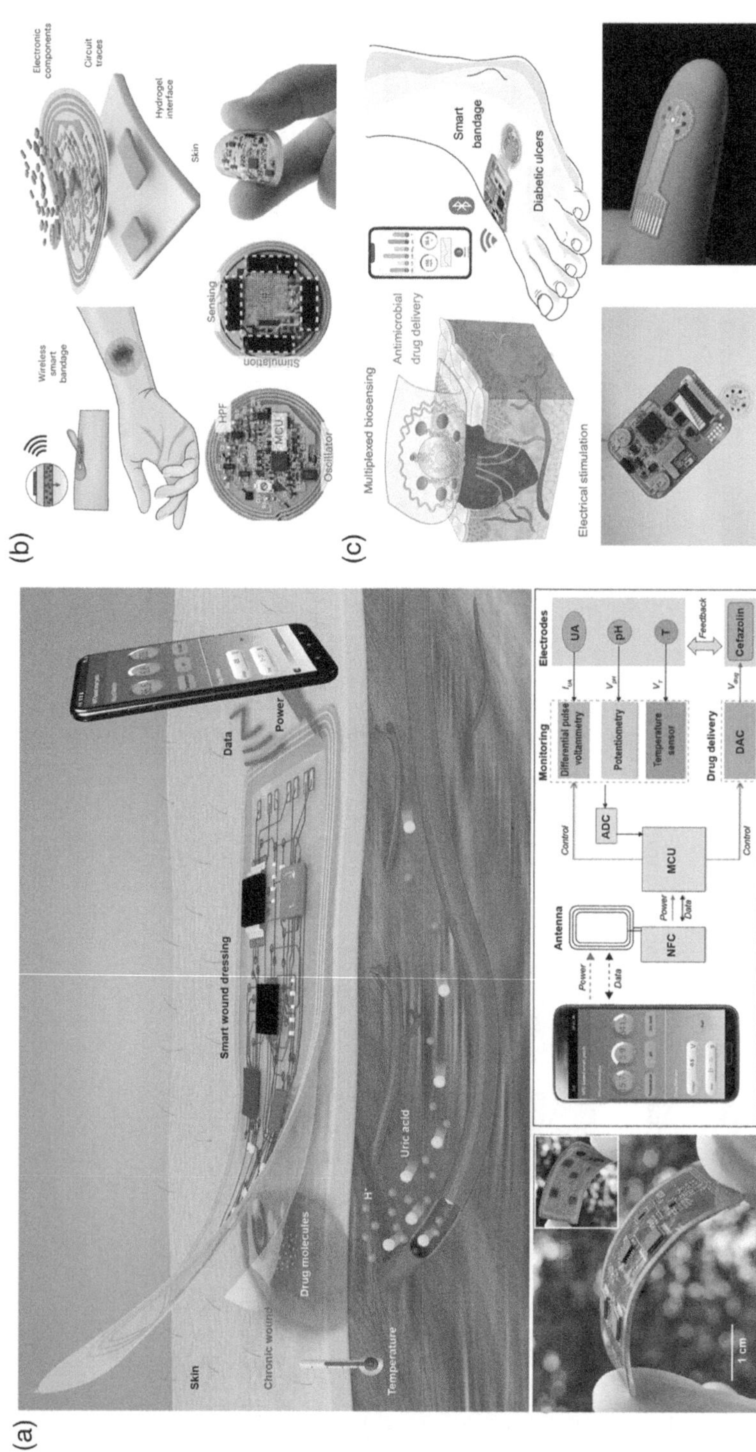

FIGURE 4.4 Smart wound dressing for closed-loop diagnosis and treatment. (a) Schematic diagram of smart wound dressing for wound sensing and electronically controlled on-demand drug delivery (top) and its optical picture and system block diagram (bottom). (b) Schematic and exploded view of a wireless smart bandage containing a flexible printed circuit board and adhesive conductive hydrogel (top) and its optical image (bottom). (c) Schematic diagram of using smart wound dressings with multiple sensing and combined treatment functions to treat diabetic foot (top), and optical pictures of smart wound dressings (bottom). ([a] Adapted with permission (Xu et al., 2021). Copyright 2021, Wiley-VCH; [b] Adapted with permission (Y. W. Jiang et al., 2023b). Copyright 2023, Springer Nature; [c] Adapted with permission (Sani et al., 2023). Copyright 2019, AAAS.)

that this multifunctional intelligent wound dressing can accurately monitor the wound status, provide effective antibacterial treatment, and significantly accelerate wound healing. In addition to the therapeutic strategy of controlled drug release, many researchers are also trying to achieve chronic treatment of wounds through electrical stimulation. For example, Jiang et al. developed a wireless intelligent wound dressing that integrates sensors and electrical stimulators (2023b). First, they designed a miniaturized flexible printed circuit system containing an energy-harvesting antenna, a microcontroller, an oscillator, and a filter, through which wound impedance and temperature can be continuously monitored. On the other hand, they designed a low-resistance adhesive hydrogel electrode based on poly (3,4-ethylenedioxythiophene): polystyrenesulfonate (PEDOT: PSS). One side of the hydrogel electrode is connected to the electrical stimulation circuit in the flexible printed circuit board and the other side of the hydrogel electrode fits tightly into the wound (Figure 4.4b). In animal experiments, they successfully achieved continuous monitoring of physiological signals at burn wounds in mice. It also expedited wound closure by employing targeted electrical signal stimulation, fostering increased cardiovascular formation, and enhancing dermal recovery. In another study, Sani et al. proposed a wound dressing with more comprehensive functions (2023). They designed a fully integrated wireless wearable bioelectronic system that can continuously monitor and analyze multiple biomarkers at the wound site to determine the condition of the wound and make appropriate diagnostic and therapeutic responses based on the wound condition (Figure 4.4c). Through customized electrochemical biosensor arrays, wound temperature, pH, ammonia, glucose, lactate, and UA can be selectively and accurately monitored in real time. In addition, the smart dressing has multiple treatment modes. It can jointly treat wounds through electrically modulated antibiotic release and electrical stimulation. This treatment mode can not only inhibit wound infection but also promote tissue regeneration at the wound site. Multi-modal bio-chemical information monitoring and treatment systems can provide more comprehensive and personalized diagnostic and treatment services for patients with chronic wounds. In vivo experiments showed that the integrated smart wound dressing successfully accelerated wound healing in diabetic rats.

The development of intelligent wound dressings based on soft bioelectronics has brought revolutionary progress to wound treatment, especially the management of chronic wounds. This is a development field full of prospects and opportunities. However, it is undeniable that there are still many challenges that need to be solved. For example, changes in early biomarkers of wound infection are very subtle, so the sensitivity and accuracy of sensors in wound dressings need to be further improved. In particular, for the treatment of chronic wounds, the durability and comfort of smart wound dressings and the minimization of damage during dressing replacement are all difficult problems that need to be solved. In addition, large-scale and low-cost manufacturing of intelligent wound dressings is also one of the main problems currently. Overall, smart wound dressings based on flexible electronics have shown great application potential in wound management, especially comprehensive, scientific, and personalized closed-loop diagnosis and treatment capabilities. We believe that with the deepening and progress of research, future intelligent wound dressings based on soft electronic devices will provide advanced and reliable solutions for the diagnosis and treatment of wounds, especially chronic wounds.

4.3 BIOELECTRONIC PATCH FOR TRANSDERMAL AND EPIDERMAL TREATMENTS

Skin is the largest organ of the human body and an important barrier that isolates the inside of the human body from the outside world. This barrier can not only protect the organs and tissues in the body from external physical, chemical, and pathogenic microorganisms but also prevent the loss of water, electrolytes, and nutrients in the body (Venus et al., 2010). However, skin is much more than a barrier. The physiological structure of the skin also contains complex appendages such as hair follicles and sweat glands. The dermis layer of the skin contains a significant network of blood vessels, lymphatic vessels, and nerves that connect to various distant organs within the body (Figure 4.5). Therefore, the skin is regarded as an ideal therapeutic surface (Liu et al., 2017). The skin provides a noninvasive means to extract a wealth of valuable medical information from the body. The skin can also be used to deliver drugs and physical stimulation to all parts of the body to treat diseases (Someya & Amagai, 2019).

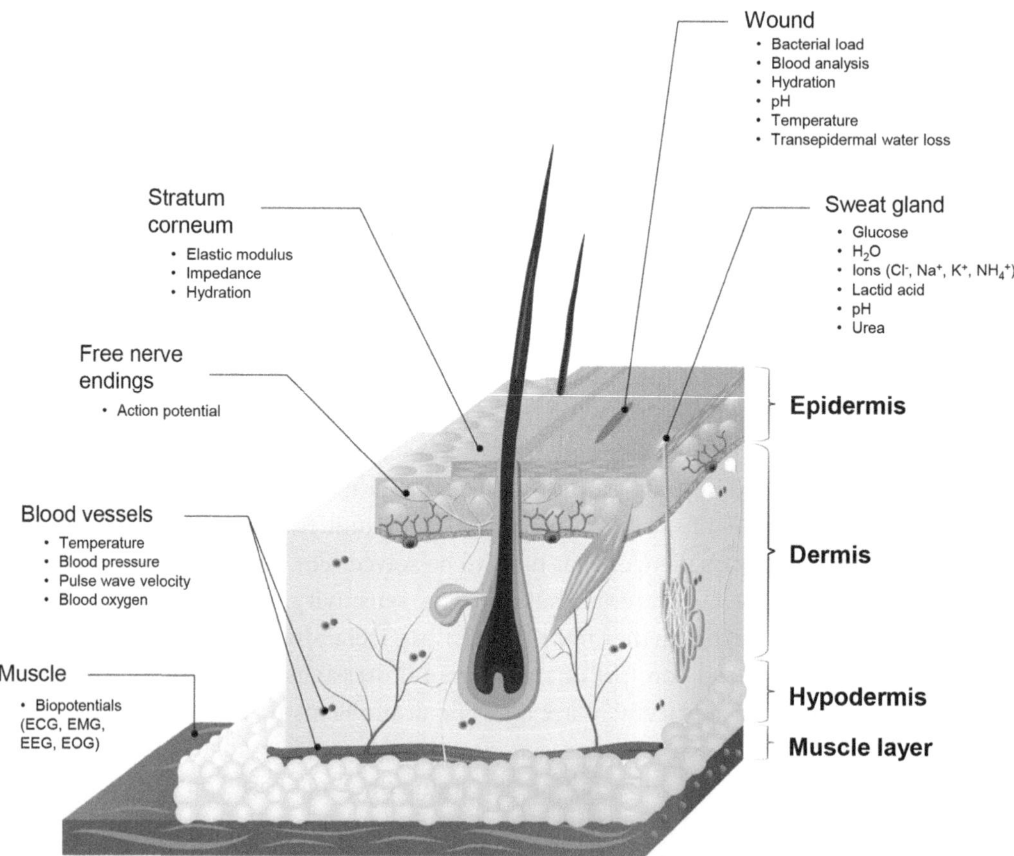

FIGURE 4.5 Schematic diagram of the structure of the skin and the physiological information it carries. (Adapted with permission (Liu et al., 2017). Copyright 2017, American Chemical Society.)

In fact, the use of skin to treat physical ailments has a long history, dating back to the oldest surviving medical records (Pastore et al., 2015). For example, in China, over 2000 BC, plasters containing a variety of herbal ingredients were dispersed in a sticky gum base and applied to a fabric backing, the precursor to today's transdermal patches (Chien, 1987). Today, medical skin patches have become one of the most basic and versatile tools in disease treatment. They are widely used in medical work such as drug delivery, wound dressings, stoma stents, medical equipment fixation, and adhesion monitoring devices (Hwang et al., 2018). Although medical skin patches have been hugely successful in the past, research into their development has never stopped. Since the beginning of the 21st century, the development of information technology, nanotechnology, and flexible electronic technology has been driving traditional medical patches to become intelligent (Someya & Amagai, 2019). A new generation of soft electronic medical patches has attracted widespread attention. Compared with traditional medical patches, bioelectronic patches have successfully integrated complex diagnosis and treatment systems and functions into a thin and soft integrated patch, giving them convenient, intelligent, and personalized treatment advantages in medical applications (Hwang et al., 2018). In this section, we summarize recent efforts in bioelectronic devices for transdermal and epidermal therapies and look ahead to the future development of bioelectronic medical patches.

Transdermal drug delivery is one of the most widespread applications of skin patches and a classic transdermal treatment strategy. Transdermal drug delivery patches adhere to the surface of the skin and deliver the loaded drug through the skin into the body's circulation to treat systemic diseases (Bird & Ravindra, 2020). Transdermal drug delivery has many advantages over oral or subcutaneous injection of drugs. For example, it requires a lower dose than oral drugs and can avoid first-pass metabolism and adverse reactions when the drug passes through the gastrointestinal tract and liver. Compared with injections, it is convenient and non-invasive, improving patients' medication compliance (Lee et al., 2018; Prausnitz & Langer, 2008). However, transdermal drug delivery is not a perfect drug delivery technology. The stratum corneum in the skin, while acting as a protective barrier, also hinders drug transport, making it difficult to achieve transdermal delivery of most therapeutic-level compounds (Brown et al., 2006). Therefore, in the past few decades, researchers have developed various physical and chemical auxiliary means to improve the efficiency of transdermal drug delivery and expand the types of drugs that can be delivered. These adjuncts include ultrasound, microneedling, electroporation, iontophoresis, and chemical enhancers. However, the external stimulation used in these technical solutions still requires additional instruments and circuits, thus reducing the convenience and compliance of transdermal drug delivery to a certain extent (Ogawa et al., 2015; Sun et al., 2023). Fortunately, the development of soft electronics technology quickly brought solutions to these problems. By integrating advanced soft electronic systems with transdermal drug delivery patches into one platform, a multifunctional, diagnostic, and therapeutic bioelectronic drug delivery patch has been developed. These bioelectronic patches can be conveniently and comfortably worn on the surface of human skin. The small and precise circuit system can assist transdermal drug delivery, realize intelligent management of drug delivery, and improve the controllability, efficiency, convenience, and patient compliance of drug delivery (Zhang et al., 2023a).

The soft electronic transdermal drug delivery patch based on iontophoresis technology is a typical representative. Iontophoresis is a technology based on the delivery of therapeutic agents deep into the skin through the stratum corneum via electrophoretic and electro-osmotic flow methods based on mild electrical current (Dhote et al., 2012). Since its working mechanism involves applying an external electric field to the skin surface to change the local potential, it is more suitable for combination with soft electronic devices than other auxiliary technologies (Sun et al., 2023). Iontophoretic drug delivery technology based on soft electronic patches has been extensively studied in the past period. For example, Yang et al. developed an iontophoretic microneedle array patch (Yang et al., 2020a). They integrated solid microneedles with iontophoresis therapy into a transdermal patch that can be controlled by a smartphone, successfully achieving one-step insulin delivery of "penetration, diffusion and iontophoresis" (Figure 4.6a). The patch is composed of medical tape (containing electrodes and anti-leakage pads), the microneedle array, and a medical sponge stacked together. The iontophoresis drive circuit is powered through the charging port of the smartphone. Using this soft electronic patch, they successfully regulated blood sugar in type I diabetic rats, effectively avoiding the side effects of hypoglycemia. In the experiment, the normal blood sugar state of rats was successfully maintained for up to 6.8 hours, which was 3.1 times that of the injection group. In another research work, Li et al. proposed a closed-loop iontophoretic microneedle patch with both sensing and therapeutic functions (2021b). In this study, they designed two-module microneedle modules to achieve sensing and drug delivery functions, respectively. They are mesoporous microneedle reverse iontophoresis glucose-sensing components and microneedle iontophoresis insulin-delivery components. The two microneedle modules are connected to the flexible printed circuit system in the middle, which realizes electrical modulation and delivery control (Figure 4.6b). This bioelectronic patch can accurately track blood sugar fluctuations and release insulin responsively to achieve closed-loop regulation of blood sugar. In experimental animal studies, this treatment strategy successfully regulated blood sugar in a diabetic rat model. For example, Lim et al. developed a functionalized hydrogel bioelectronic patch for transdermal treatment (2021). This is a conductive polymer-functionalized hydrogel film based on polyacrylamide that has the advantages of high-quality permeability and low impedance (Figure 4.6c). Using this hydrogel patch, they successfully implemented medical diagnosis and treatment research on transcutaneous oxygen pressure sensing, impedance sensing, iontophoretic drug delivery, and transcutaneous electrical nerve stimulation.

In addition to patches for iontophoresis, there are also various other stimulation types for transdermal delivery of electronic patches. For example, Lee et al. developed a patch for sweat glucose monitoring and heat-responsive transdermal drug delivery (Figure 4.7a) (2016a). The patch provides highly sensitive monitoring of pH and glucose levels in sweat, calibrating glucose concentration by temperature and pH. Hyperglycemia triggers thermal activation of bioabsorbable microneedles, inducing thermal dissolution of the phase change material and release of metformin (Figure 4.7b). At the same time, sensors in the thermal stimulation device will also monitor skin temperature in real time to prevent drug overdose and low-temperature burns. In animal trials, the patch demonstrated its ability to

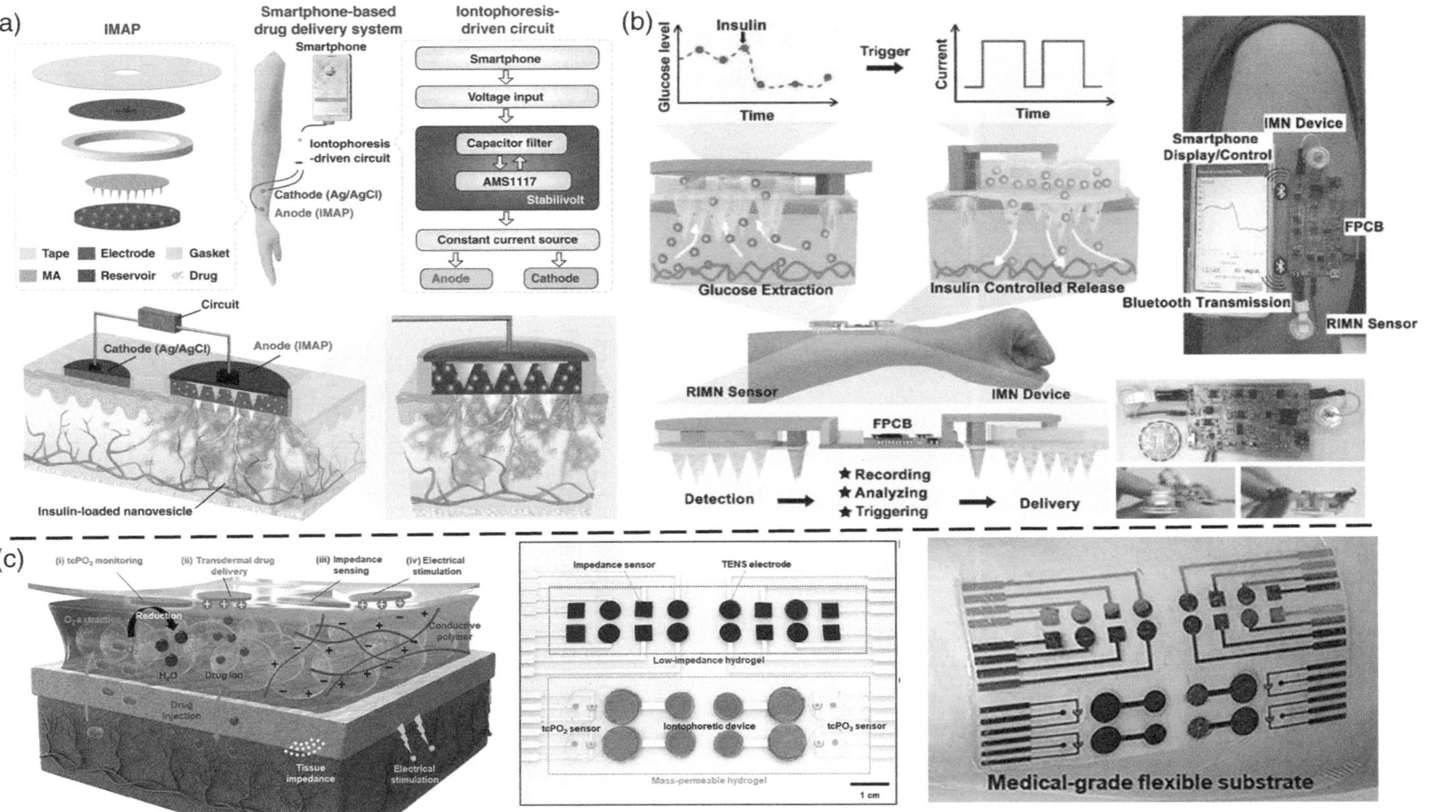

FIGURE 4.6   Bioelectronic patches for iontophoretic drug delivery. (a) Schematic diagram of a smartphone-driven transdermal drug delivery patch (top) and an explanation diagram of its drug delivery mechanism (bottom). (b) A schematic diagram of an intelligent closed-loop transdermal drug delivery patch based on a microneedle platform for real-time diabetes monitoring and treatment (left) and an optical picture of its system (right). (c) Illustration of the multifunctional hydrogel interface and optical images of the bioelectronic patch with integrated hydrogel electrodes. ([a] Adapted with permission (J. B. Yang et al., 2020a). Copyright 2020, Springer Nature, [b] Adapted with permission (X. L. Li et al., 2021b). Copyright 2021, Wiley-VCH, [c] Adapted with permission (Lim et al., 2021). Copyright 2021, AAAS.)

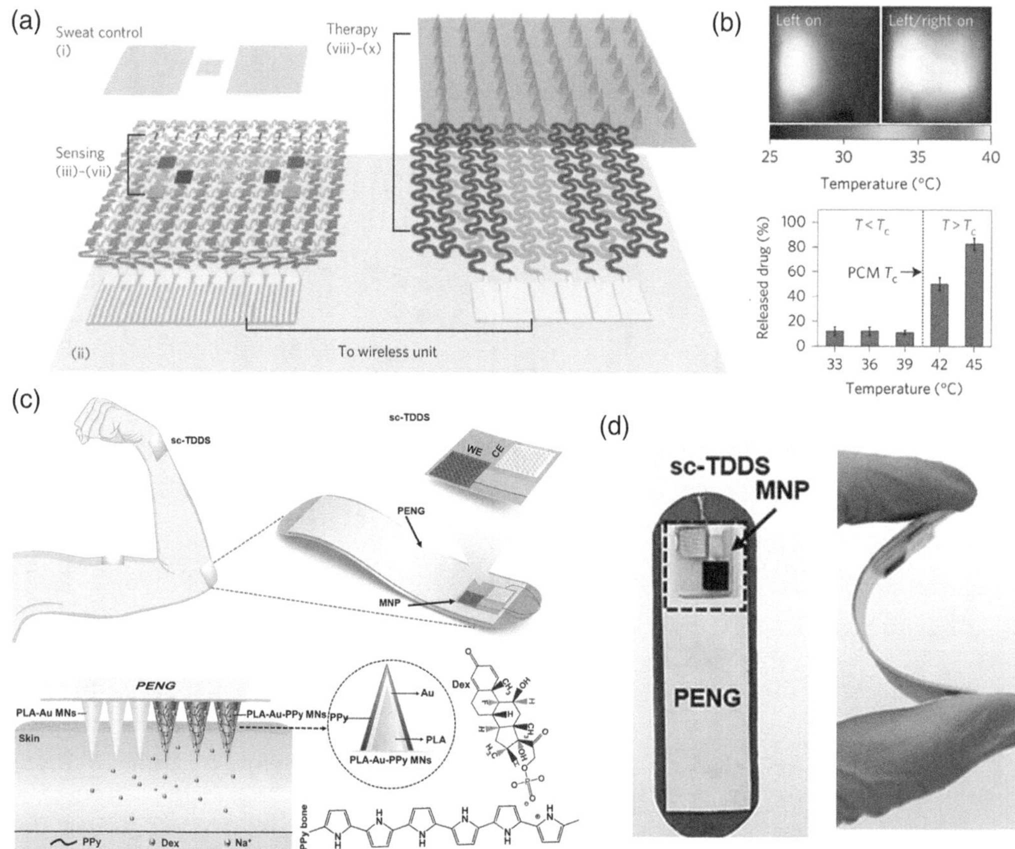

FIGURE 4.7   Bioelectronic patches for thermal and electrical stimulation transdermal drug delivery. (a) Schematic diagram of a diabetes treatment patch integrating electrochemical sensing and thermally responsive drug delivery functions. (b) Infrared images during patch heating and the results of temperature-promoted drug release. (c, d) Schematic diagram of the working principle of the self-powered controllable transdermal drug delivery patch (c) and its optical image (d). ([a, b] (Adapted with permission (H. Lee et al., 2016a). Copyright 2016, Springer Nature.); [b, c] Adapted with permission (Yang et al., 2021). Copyright 2021, Wiley-VCH.)

deliver metformin via heat actuation and reduce blood sugar levels in diabetic mice. Yuan and colleagues proposed a self-powered drug-controlled release patch (Figure 4.7c) (Yang et al., 2021). In this study, they used polypyrrole as a carrier for controlled drug release. As a smart electrically responsive material, polypyrrole can load and release drug molecules through conversion between oxidation and reduction states. Drug-loaded microneedle patches and piezoelectric nanogenerators were integrated to form a self-powered drug delivery platform (Figure 4.7d). In in-vivo experiments, they successfully used this light-weight, battery-free patch to achieve on-demand transdermal drug delivery treatment for psoriasis in mice.

On the other hand, soft bioelectronic patches are also widely used in epidermal treatments. These treatments are mainly based on physical stimulation outside the body. They are mainly used to treat injuries or lesions of the skin, muscles, and nervous system

(Ma et al., 2020; Wu et al., 2017). For example, for the treatment of muscle fatigue, Song et al. developed a breathable and sweat-resistant MXene epidermal patch, which can reliably collect electrophysiological signals and perform low-voltage hyperthermia through Joule heating (2022). Researchers use the signals collected by the patch to analyze and infer muscle fatigue and then use electrical stimulation and electric heating to relieve muscle fatigue (Figure 4.8a). This integrated muscle therapy diagnostic patch has a guiding value for both muscle health care and rehabilitation training. In addition, electronic patches with electric heating functions are also useful in the treatment of joint diseases. Choi et al. used silver

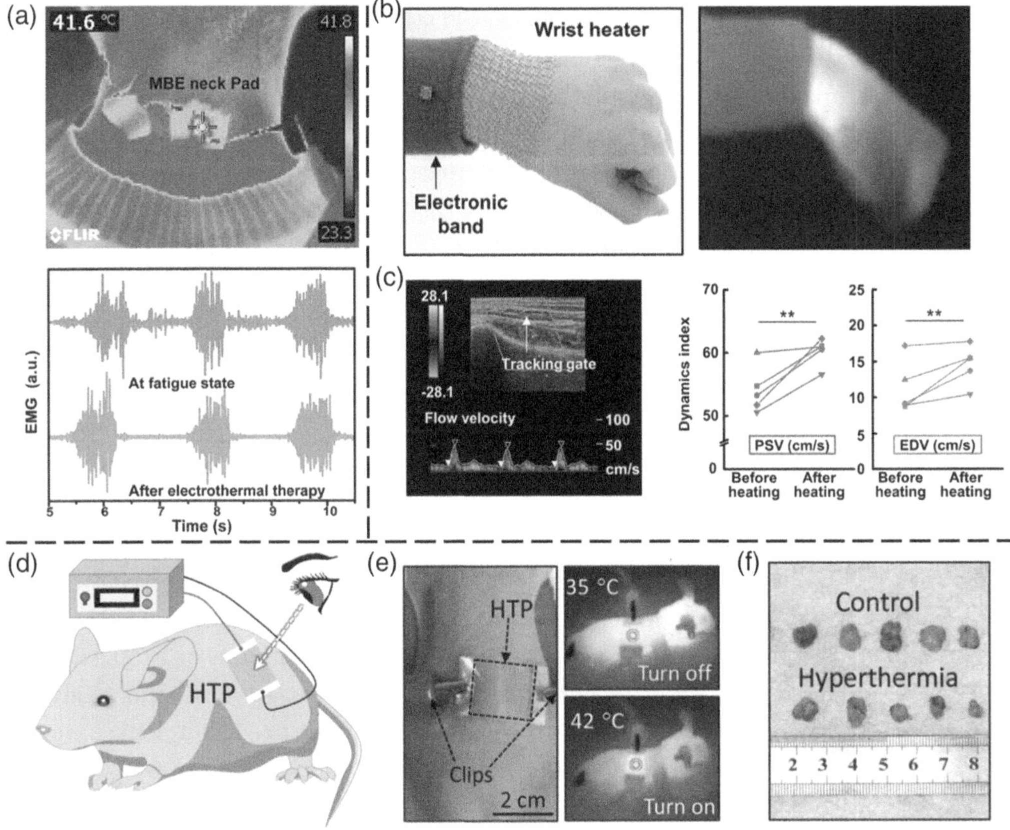

FIGURE 4.8 Bioelectronic patch for epidermal thermal therapy. (a) Infrared images of thermal stimulation and electrical stimulation patches used to treat muscle fatigue when heated (top) and comparison of electromyographic signals of fatigued muscles before and after thermal treatment (bottom). (b) Optical images (left) and infrared images (right) of the patch used for arthritis hyperthermia treatment. (c) B-mode ultrasound color Doppler imaging (left) and flow velocity statistics (right) of the blood flow in the radial artery of the forearm during the experiment. (d–f) Schematic diagram (d), optical picture (e), and tumor inhibition results (f) in animal experiments when the transparent thermotherapy electronic patch is used for subcutaneous tumor treatment. ([a] Adapted with permission (Song et al., 2022). Copyright 2022, American Chemical Society; [b, c] Adapted with permission (Choi et al., 2015). Copyright 2015, American Chemical Society; [d–f] Adapted with permission (Q. Wang et al., 2022b). Copyright 2022, Wiley-VCH.)

nanowires and SBS thermoplastic elastomer to develop a soft heating patch that can be used for arthritis treatment (Figure 4.8b) (2015). The high electrical conductivity of the AgNW/SBS nanocomposite allows the patch to operate at low voltages powered by a small battery. They tested the patch's therapeutic effects on five volunteers. As the patch worked, Doppler color imaging showed an increase in pulsatile blood flow in the volunteers' radial arteries, which may lead to less arthritis pain and muscle relaxation (Figure 4.8c). An appropriate and controllable temperature range can not only be used to treat conventional diseases but it can also be used to kill tumor cells. Therefore, bioelectronic patches for hyperthermia also have application potential in the treatment of superficial tumors. For example, Wang et al. developed a transparent electronic patch that can inhibit the growth of subcutaneous tumors (2022b). The patch uses PDMS as the packaging material, and the middle layer of the patch is a directional silver nanofiber network. The arranged silver nanofiber network not only ensures the optical transparency of the patch but also exerts an excellent Joule heating effect. The transparent thermal therapy patch allows medical staff to treat subcutaneous tumors under a clear viewing angle, improving treatment efficiency while ensuring the safety of other normal tissues (Figure 4.8d). The heat therapy ability of the patch has been verified in animal experiments (Figure 4.8e). Only gentle (42 °C) heating at ultra-low voltage (0.7 V) can significantly inhibit tumor growth (Figure 4.8f). This Joule heat-based mild hyperthermia bioelectronic patch is expected to provide a new strategy for the treatment of superficial tumors.

In addition to electrical and thermal stimulation, ultrasound therapeutic patches have also been studied. For example, Zhou et al. studied an ultrasound patch for the treatment of neurological diseases, which consists of multiple ultrasound transducers stimulated by low-frequency, low-intensity pulsed ultrasound (Zhou et al., 2019). They wore it on the heads of mice suffering from acute Parkinson's disease to stimulate the motor cortex of the mice. The experimental results showed that the treatment successfully improved the mice's Parkinson's motor defects. The therapeutic properties of bioelectronic patches have been widely studied and proven, but most of these patches require batteries or external power sources, which are not friendly to chronic diseases that require long-term treatment. Therefore, bioelectronic patches based on wearable self-powering technology have also received attention and research. For example, Yao et al. developed a self-powered omnidirectional activated electrical stimulation patch based on TENG to treat hair loss (2019). The patch consists of an omnidirectional triboelectric generator (OTG) that acts as an electrical pulse generator and a pair of interdigitated dressing electrodes (Figure 4.9a). When worn on a rat, the electrical pulses generated by the rat's movement can promote the proliferation of its hair follicles and the secretion of vascular endothelial growth factor and keratinocyte growth factor, thereby alleviating hereditary keratin disorders in hair and ultimately promoting hair regeneration (Figure 4.9b).

Over the past period of time, the progress made by bioelectronic devices in transdermal and epidermal treatments is obvious to all. With many advantages such as softness, conformal contact, and stretchability, bioelectronic patches are likely to become a key tool in personalized and intelligent healthcare in the future. However, there are still many difficult challenges that need to be overcome before bioelectronic patches can be truly used in

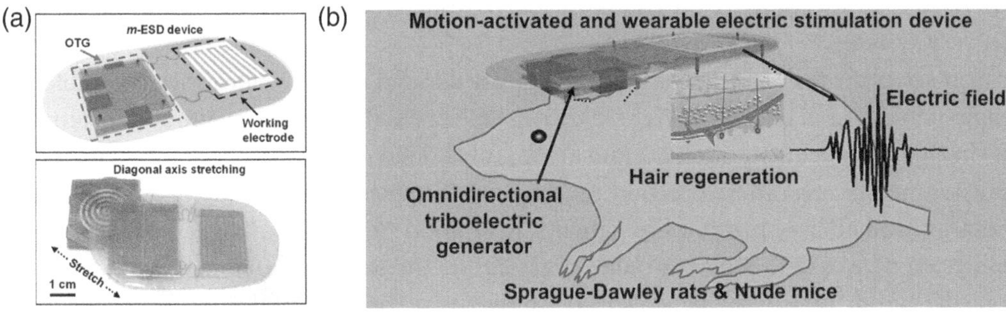

FIGURE 4.9 Bioelectronic patches with ultrasound or electrical stimulation therapy functions. (a) Optical image of an electrical stimulation hair loss treatment patch based on an omnidirectional triboelectric generator. (b) Schematic of using self-activating electrical stimulation patches to promote hair regeneration in mice. ([a, b] Adapted with permission (Yao et al., 2019). Copyright 2019, American Chemical Society.)

clinical treatments. For example, most of the currently proven therapeutic systems are based on small animal studies, but before being translated into clinical practice, they must be validated in large animal and human experiments and the treatment procedures must comply with relevant medical standards. Moreover, the long-term biocompatibility and reliability of these bioelectronic patches must also be thoroughly reviewed and tested before they can be approved by government agencies such as the Food and Drug Administration. In addition, further integration of therapeutic systems and economical large-scale manufacturing capabilities remains one of the issues that must be considered. Of course, with the advancement of materials chemistry, medicine, information science, and in-depth research on the application of bioelectronic patches, we believe that these challenges will be overcome one by one. Soft bioelectronic patches will surely become an important component in transdermal and epidermal therapeutic technologies.

4.4 SOFT ACTUATORS FOR DRUG DELIVERY

Drugs are the most critical tools in medicine, which relies on them to control and treat disease. The effectiveness of a drug is directly related to its administration and delivery method. Drug delivery affects a drug's pharmacokinetics, absorption, distribution, metabolism, duration of efficacy, and toxicity (Tibbitt et al., 2016). Various strategies have been developed to improve drug delivery systems, such as stimulus response, co-delivery, biomimetic delivery, and targeted delivery (Li et al., 2019). There are still many challenges and room for improvement in drug delivery, such as rapid response release, precise and controllable delivery, long-term continuous administration, improved patient compliance, and compliance with chronobiological laws (Smolensky & Peppas, 2007; Tibbitt et al., 2016). Ideal drug delivery systems should be intelligent and controllable, and they can accurately deliver drugs to therapeutic targets at precise times (Jain, 2020). Many emerging strategies are being developed to achieve this goal, and soft electronic systems are one of the promising solutions (Tan et al., 2022). In the previous chapters, we have introduced the intelligent cases of soft electronic devices in assisting wound treatment and transdermal drug delivery. In this section, we present more recent research efforts on soft electronics in drug delivery systems.

Soft actuators for drug delivery can be mainly divided into two categories: wearable and implantable (Kar et al., 2022). Wearable drug delivery soft actuators play an important role in chronic therapeutic treatments and are mainly adhered to the surface of human skin or mucous membranes. Therefore, they must be comfortable to wear for a long time, not cause irritation and allergic reactions to patients, have good sustained or triggered release capabilities, and be easy to replace (Yadav et al., 2019). The smart wound dressings and smart transdermal drug delivery patches in the previous section both fall into this category. In addition to wearable soft actuators for drug delivery on the skin, soft actuators for drug delivery in the eye and oral cavity have been studied. Keum and colleagues have developed a smart contact lens that can be used for diabetes diagnosis and treatment (Figure 4.10a) (Keum et al., 2020). The smart contact lens contains five parts: a chemical sensor for monitoring glucose concentration, an on-demand drug delivery system, a wireless energy transmission system, a microcontroller with a power management unit, and a long-range radio frequency communication system. Therapeutic drugs are stored in drug reservoirs that can be selectively released via voltage control. In animal experiments, the team constructed a diabetic rabbit model and used the smart contact lens to measure glucose levels in tears, verified it with traditional blood glucose testing technology (Figure 4.10b), and then released drugs on demand to treat retinopathy in diabetic rabbits (Figure 4.10c). In another recent study, Shi et al. reported a wireless, battery-free dental patch for intraoral sensing and drug delivery (Figure 4.10d) (2022). The patch consists of a control circuit and an array of electrodes. The electrochemical potential sensor on the patch can monitor local acidic environment fluctuations caused by microbial metabolism on the tooth surface, thereby issuing an early warning of potential dental caries lesions. In this study, polypyrrole was modified on the electrode and used as a carrier for electroresponsive drugs and the fluoride therapeutic agent loaded on it could achieve local delivery by applying a negative potential on the electrode (Figure 4.10e). This integrated treatment strategy combines *in situ* diagnosis and drug delivery, offering potential avenues for the future development of wearable personalized diagnosis and treatment systems within the oral cavity.

Implantable drug delivery soft actuators are mainly placed under body tissues through surgery, which can bring non-negligible improvements to treatment effects.[15] Because the implantable drug soft actuator can be conformably attached to the surface of the organ, the drug it carries does not need to penetrate the organ and cell barriers and can directly act on the target. Coupled with the advantage of controllable drug release, it can maximize the treatment rate, improve treatment effects, and reduce drug side effects (Jiang et al., 2023a). Therefore, research on implantable soft actuators for drug delivery has also attracted widespread interest. For example, implantable drug delivery soft actuators could play an important role in the on-site treatment of epilepsy. Joo et al. developed a life-threatening epilepsy treatment device that combines a wearable wireless module with a soft implantable drug delivery actuator (2021). In their design, a soft implantable drug delivery actuator is implanted into the subcutaneous area near the wrist, with a corresponding wearable power transmitter on the outside and a wearable electrophysiological sensor mounted on the

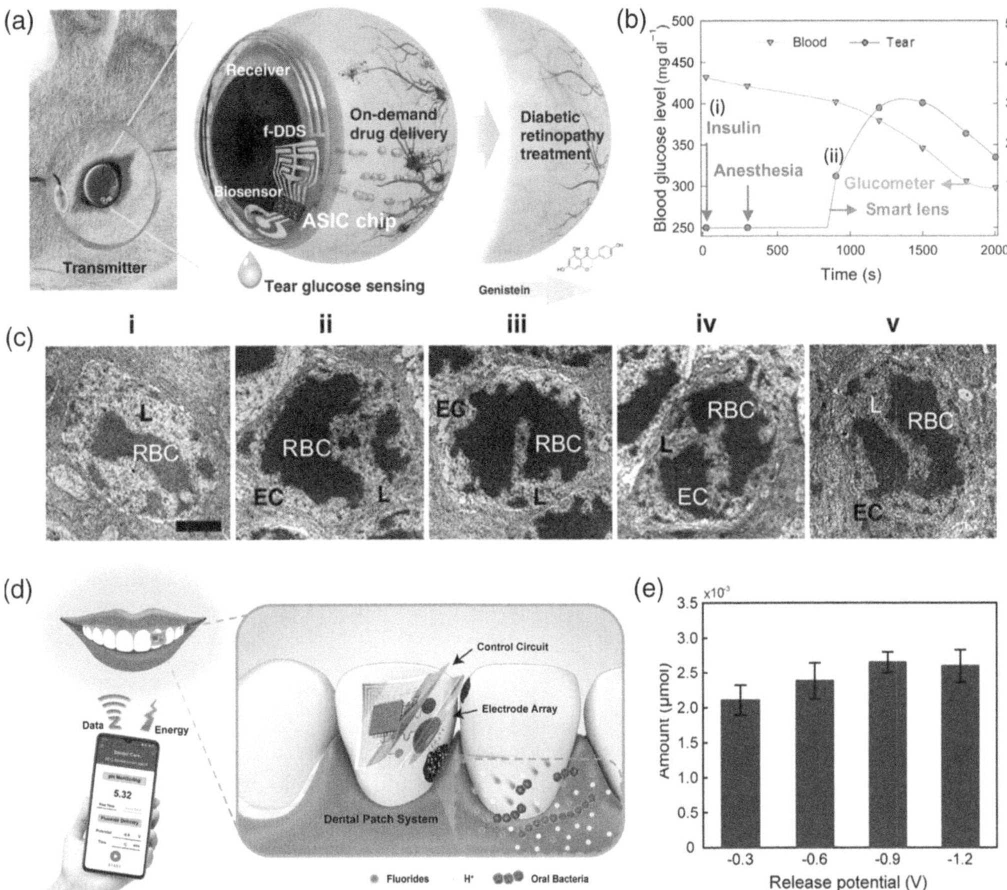

FIGURE 4.10 Contact lenses and oral patches for drug delivery. (a) Schematic diagram of smart contact lenses used in diabetes diagnosis and treatment. (b) Comparison of tear blood glucose monitoring results using wireless smart glasses and conventional methods. (c) Transmission electron microscopy image of retinal blood vessels illustrating the therapeutic effect of genistein released from smart contact lenses on retinopathy: (i) an eye drop of PBS (control), (ii) an eye drop of genistein, (iii) intravitreal injection of genistein, (iv) intravitreal injection of Avastin, and (v) genistein released from the smart contact lens. L, lumen of vessel; EC, endothelial cell; RBC, red blood cell. (d) Schematic of a dental patch for intraoral diagnosis and treatment. (e) Effect of different potentials on drug release from smart oral patches. ([a–c] Adapted with permission (Keum et al., 2020). Copyright 2020, AAAS; [d, e] Adapted with permission (Shi et al., 2022). Copyright 2022, Springer Nature.)

patient's head to monitor brain electrical signals (Figure 4.11a). Animal experiments with the device demonstrated that prompt treatment of fatal epilepsy can reduce brain damage and improve survival rates (Figure 4.11b). Sung et al. also proposed a drug delivery soft actuator that can be used for epilepsy treatment (Figure 4.11c) (2018). The soft actuator is implanted directly into the cerebral cortex and delivers drugs precisely through a micro-storage layer mechanism and electrochemical dissolution of the gold seal (Figure 4.11d). The team has successfully used the soft actuator to deliver two neural tracers to the brain and use anti-epileptic drugs to prevent epileptic seizures.

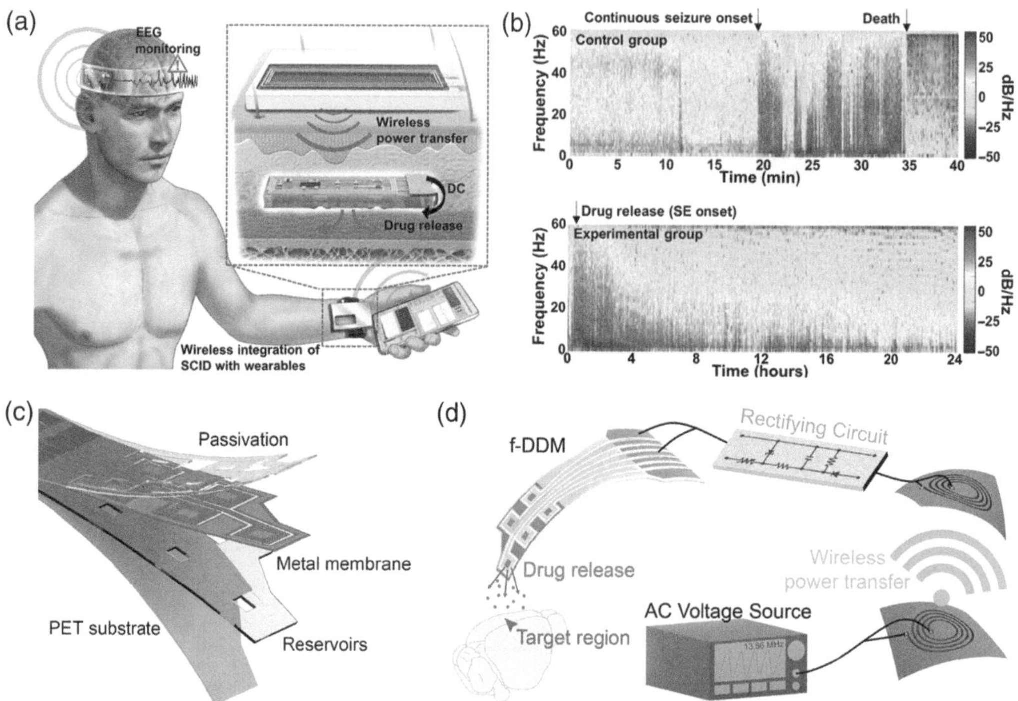

FIGURE 4.11 Implantable soft drug actuator for treating epileptic seizures. (a) Schematic diagram of wireless integration of implantable drug soft actuators and wearable devices for epilepsy treatment. (b) EEG signal spectrograms of the control group (top) and the treatment group (bottom) during epileptic seizures in mice. (c, d) Structural diagram (c) and working schematic diagram (d) of an implantable cerebral cortex drug delivery soft actuator to prevent epileptic seizures through wireless electrical controlled drug delivery. ([a, b] Adapted with permission (Joo et al., 2021). Copyright 2021, AAAS; [c, d] Adapted with permission (Sung et al., 2018). Copyright 2018, Elsevier.)

In situ drug delivery is extremely attractive in the treatment of neoplastic diseases. Li et al. designed a biodegradable soft actuator for controlled drug release for cancer treatment (2021a). The soft actuator is powered by an external alternating magnetic field and triggers the internal heating coil to generate heat to control the *in situ* heat release of the anti-cancer drug paclitaxel (Figure 4.12a). Its good biodegradability can avoid secondary surgery for patients. Cell experiments verified its highly controllable drug release and inhibitory effect on cancer cells (Figure 4.12b). Lee and colleagues proposed a flexible, adhesive, and biodegradable soft actuator for brain tumor drug delivery (2019). The soft actuator can conformally adhere to the curved brain surface, achieve drug release during gentle thermal actuation, minimize unnecessary drug leakage, and extend the time of drug delivery (Figure 4.12c). Using this system, they controllably delivered anti-tumor drugs to deep brain tumors and verified the inhibition of tumor growth and improvement of survival rate in animal experiments (Figure 4.12d). The designed intracranial biocompatible absorbable soft actuator reduces potential side effects. The materials and technologies proposed by this research will play a positive role in the development of intracranial treatment of brain tumors.

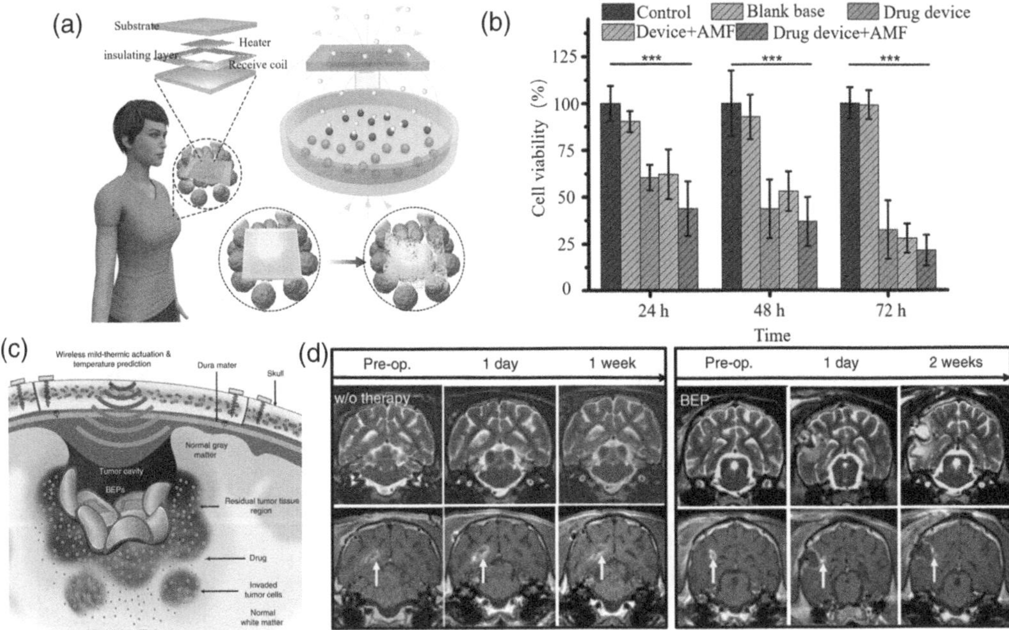

FIGURE 4.12 Implantable soft actuators for drug delivery treatment of oncological diseases. (a) Schematic diagram of a degradable drug controlled-release soft actuator for breast cancer treatment. (b) Live and dead cell staining results from in vitro experiments demonstrate the inhibitory effect of this strategy on breast cancer cells. (c) Schematic of drug delivery into deep glioblastoma tissue via a wireless, gentle, thermally driven drug delivery soft actuator. (d) Magnetic resonance images demonstrating significant suppression of canine brain tumors compared with controls growth. ([a, b] Adapted with permission (Li et al., 2021a). Copyright 2021, American Chemical Society; [c, d] Adapted with permission (Lee et al., 2019). Copyright 2019, Springer Nature.)

For abdominal hernias, Kaveti et al. proposed a soft, long-lasting, bioabsorbable electronic surgical mesh with wireless pressure monitoring and on-demand drug delivery capabilities (Figure 4.13a) (Kaveti et al., 2023). A poly(L-lactide-co-ε-caprolactone)-based mesh can provide mechanical strength over time and potentially prevent hernia recurrence, and a resistive microheater integrated with an induction coil provides a thermoresponsive drug delivery system for antibacterial agents (Figure 4.13b). In the study, they used an abdominal defect model to evaluate the effectiveness of the electronic surgical mesh in hernia repair. The experimental results confirmed the reliability of the system, which enhanced the healing process and reduced side effects such as tissue adhesion and postoperative complications. Huang et al. reported a bioabsorbable implantable microneedle device integrating wireless electrical stimulation and drug delivery (Figure 4.13c) (2022). The device combines a radio frequency wireless power transmission system and drug-loaded microneedles to achieve a combined treatment of electrical stimulation and drugs (Figure 4.13d). As a verification, they used the device to treat skeletal muscle injury in rats. Through periodic electrical stimulation, they modulated cell behavior and tissue regeneration. The release of anti-inflammatory drugs prevented inflammation and ultimately enhanced skeletal muscle regeneration (Figure 4.13e).

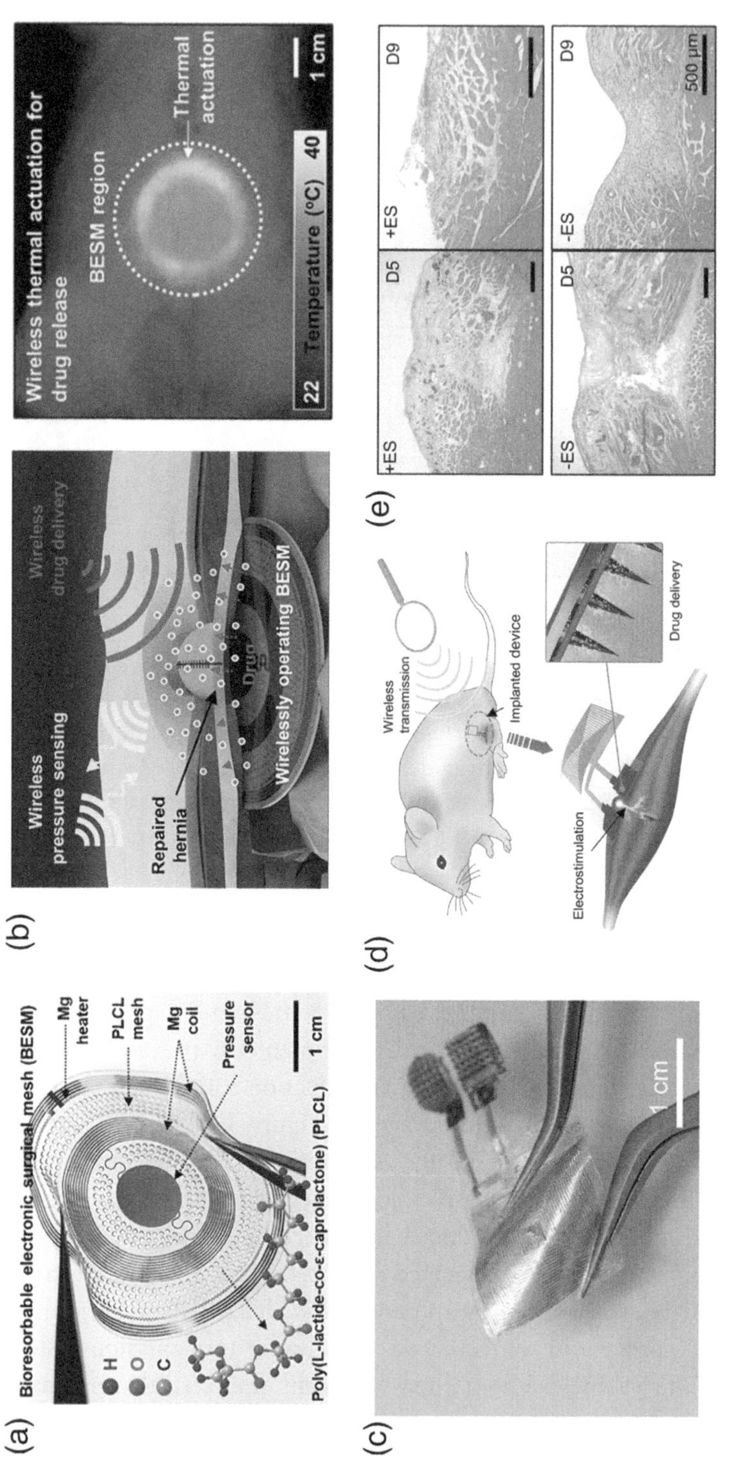

FIGURE 4.13 Implantable soft actuators for drug delivery treatment of oncological diseases. (a) Optical pictures of degradable electronic surgical mesh. (b) Schematic diagram of surgical implantation of degradable electronic surgical mesh to heal weak areas of the abdominal wall (left) and its infrared imaging when heated to release drugs (right). (c) Optical image of the implantable drug delivery microneedle device. (d) Schematic illustration of wireless electrical stimulation and drug delivery using implantable microneedles in rats. (e) Tissue staining experiments confirmed that the therapeutic device can promote muscle fiber regeneration and suppress inflammation. ([a, b] Adapted with permission (Kaveti et al., 2023). Copyright 2022, American Chemical Society; [c–e] Adapted with permission (Huang et al., 2022). Copyright 2023, Wiley-VCH.)

The integration of bioelectronics and drug delivery technology opens up new avenues for drug delivery and provides a high degree of operability for the directed and controlled release of drugs. However, the research on soft actuators for drug delivery is not extensive and in-depth enough, especially for implantable drug delivery systems. Related reports have just appeared in the past few years. Therefore, there are still many problems that need to be solved. For example, soft actuators usually have a limited amount of drug loading, and drug refilling is a problem that needs to be solved, especially for implantable devices. A safe and stable energy supply is an important guarantee for the long-term continuous operation of soft actuators. Existing solutions are mostly based on wireless power supply strategies, which still need to be improved. Secondly, the long-term stability and reliability of drug delivery systems still need to be fully experimentally verified in large animals and humans before they can be recognized. For degradable implantable soft actuators, they have to face the complex internal environment of the human body, which means that they must prevent unnecessary leakage of drugs while degrading. In addition, during the operation of implantable soft actuators, it is also necessary to study how to minimize the trauma caused during the implantation process. At the same time, after the implant is removed, the biological activity of the site must also be paid attention to. In short, the future progress of soft actuators for drug delivery can be achieved through improvements in drug storage, energy supply, equipment reliability verification, and non-destructive treatment.

4.5 OTHER SOFT ELECTRONICS FOR MEDICAL TREATMENT

Soft electronic devices have been widely explored for medical applications. In addition to the above-mentioned treatment methods and applications, soft electronic devices have shown extraordinary potential in the fields of heart disease, neurological disease, obesity, bladder regulation, bone and joint treatment and other fields (Koo et al., 2018; Mickle et al., 2019; Ouyang et al., 2019; Xu et al., 2015; Yamagishi et al., 2019; Yao et al., 2021, 2018). Different from the cases in the previous chapters, these treatment methods are mainly based on implantable non-drug stimulation methods.

In recent years, many soft implantable electronic devices have been developed for the diagnosis and treatment of heart diseases, especially arrhythmias. Li et al. designed a 3D multifunctional outer envelope with cardiac electrotherapy function (Xu et al., 2015). The core component of the membrane is an eight-electrode array that is conformally distributed on the heart surface through a fractal structure design. These electrodes provide spatially and temporally programmed electrical stimulation on the epicardium, and they are connected to external electrical devices via flexible cables. They demonstrated the device's ability to diagnose and treat cardiac arrhythmias through animal experiments on Langendorff-perfused rabbit hearts (Figure 4.14a). Power supply is crucial for implantable pacemakers, and traditional battery-powered models face limitations due to their battery life. Therefore, combining self-power technology or wireless power technology with soft implantable pacemakers is very promising (Sheng et al., 2021). To this end, Ouyang et al. proposed a symbiotic pacemaker based on an implantable triboelectric nanogenerator (Ouyang et al., 2019). The symbiotic pacemaker consists of three parts: an energy collection unit, a power management unit, and a pacemaker unit. This symbiotic system uses triboelectric nanogenerators to collect energy from the beating heart and then uses a pacemaker to generate pacing electrical pulses to control the rate of heart contraction (Figure 4.14b). To achieve treatment of cardiac arrhythmias in a large animal model, they applied the symbiotic pacemaker system to adult Yorkshire pigs. In the experiment, they used ice cubes to cause sinoatrial node hypothermia, and after observing typical arrhythmias on the electrocardiogram, treatment was initiated immediately. When the symbiotic pacemaker was turned on, sinus arrhythmia was converted to a paced rhythm and blood pressure began to return to its previous level. After about 1 minute, the power supply voltage dropped, the symbiotic pacemaker stopped working, and the pacing rhythm returned to a normal heart rhythm. Their study demonstrates the potential of symbiotic pacing systems for the correction of sinus arrhythmias. In another study, Choi et al. developed a soft, biodegradable, and closed-loop wireless MEMS system for heart rate monitoring and control (Figure 4.14c) (2022). The system has a set of soft skin sensor interfaces for capturing physiological information such as electrocardiogram, heart rate, and respiration. Utilizing a handheld device with a software application allows real-time visualization of heart rate information and functionality of an implanted degradable stretchable epicardial pacemaker via a wireless module. Demonstrated in rat, canine, and human heart studies, this transient closed-loop system can provide a range of autonomous, rate-adaptive cardiac pacing capabilities.

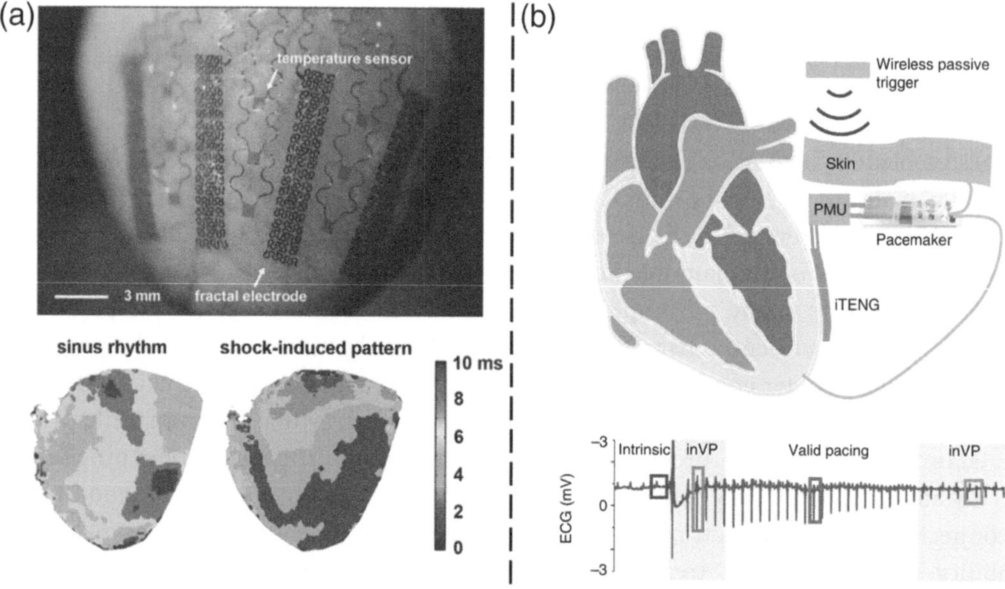

FIGURE 4.14 Implantable soft pacemaker. (a) Image of the epicardial membrane integrated with 3D multifunctional electrotherapy on a Langendorff-perfused rabbit heart (Top) and its activation map created by light signals on the epicardial side during sinus beat and when subjected to 50 V shock (bottom). (b) Schematic diagram of turning on the symbiotic pacemaker system via a wireless passive trigger (Top) and electrocardiogram of a pig heart during its activation (bottom). ([a] Adapted with permission (Xu et al., 2015). Copyright 2015, Wiley-VCH; [b] Adapted with permission (Ouyang et al., 2019). Copyright 2019, Springer Nature.)

Neurological disorders can affect the brain, spinal cord, and peripheral nerve function. Electrical stimulation has been shown to play a key role in the treatment of a variety of neurological diseases (Nag & Thakor, 2016). Compared with traditional rigid nerve treatment electrodes, soft implantable electrodes have more treatment advantages, such as being ultra-thin, soft, and conformable, which can improve treatment effects while minimizing side effects (Lee et al., 2016b). Therefore, soft implantable bioelectronic devices have broad prospects in the treatment of neurological diseases. Koo et al. reported a wireless bioabsorbable electronic system for sustained non-drug neuroregeneration therapy (2018). The system uses a bioabsorbable wireless electrical stimulator as an implantable device to promote nerve regeneration and wirelessly powers the stimulator through a coil (Figure 4.15a). They verified the therapeutic effect of this system on rat sciatic nerve crush injury and transection injury models. The results showed that the regeneration and functional recovery of injured nerves are enhanced through therapeutic electrical stimulation provided by this system (Figure 4.15b). Ejneby et al. developed an implantable organic photocapacitance converter that can use deep infrared light to perform chronic electrical stimulation of peripheral nerves (2022). Their wireless neurostimulation solution uses thin films of organic molecules to effectively convert light pulses into electrolytic currents, thereby modulating the activity of excitable cells (Figure 4.15c). Compared with traditional stimulation methods, photocapacitor stimulation equipment does not require additional power sources or coils, which can reduce the occurrence of complications and facilitate long-term safe stimulation. Moreover, both the timing and amplitude of stimulation can be flexibly adjusted through the intensity and timing of light pulses. In animal experiments, the stimulator was fixed around the sciatic nerve of rats and successfully achieved electrical stimulation for more than 100 days (Figure 4.15d). In addition, Jiang and Burton also proposed different construction plans for implantable neural electrical stimulation soft electronic systems and conducted detailed in vitro and in vivo experimental verifications (Burton et al., 2021; Jiang et al., 2022). Their research demonstrates the great potential of soft electronic devices for long-term neurostimulation to treat diseases and assist in motor rehabilitation.

There is also some interesting research into diseases that use implantable electrical nerve stimulation to modulate other body functions. For example, Yao et al. designed an implantable self-powered vagus nerve stimulation device to treat obesity (2018). Food intake affects gastric motility, and they respond to gastric peristalsis via a flexible friction nanogenerator attached to the stomach surface. Biphasic electrical pulse signals generated by frictional nanogenerators are used to stimulate the vagus nerve, thereby reducing food intake and ultimately achieving weight control (Figure 4.16a). They successfully tested this strategy in rats, which lost 38% of their body weight without regaining weight within 15 days of implanting the device (Figure 4.16b). This case demonstrates that some diseases can be effectively treated through self-response and real-time peripheral nerve modulation. In another study, Mickle et al. developed an implantable wireless neuromodulation system for monitoring and regulating bladder function (Figure 4.16c) (2019). They used low-modulus strain sensors to monitor bladder filling or voiding and then combined them with tiny inorganic light-emitting diodes to activate an optical stimulation interface of opsins to

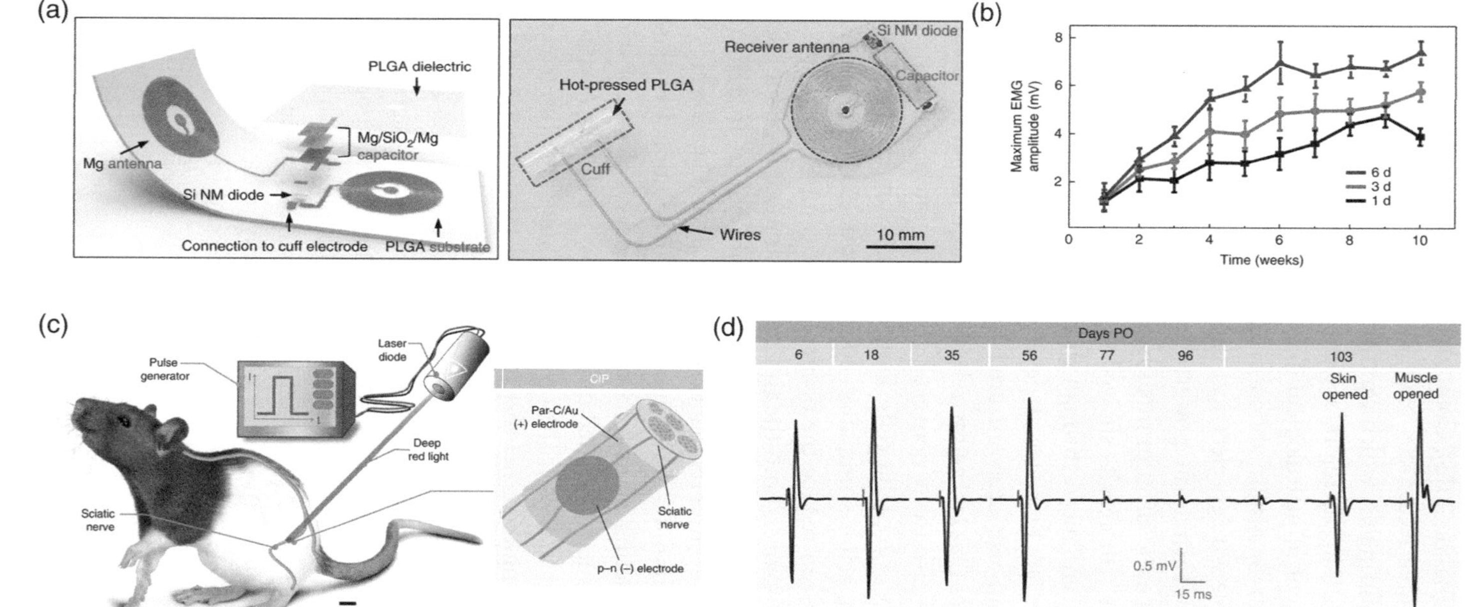

FIGURE 4.15   Electrical stimulation implantable soft electronics for neurotherapy. (a) Structural diagram (left) and optical picture (right) of a wireless implantable device for electrical stimulation of nerve regeneration. (b) Maximum amplitude recording of myoelectric signals during electrical stimulation treatment of sciatic nerve injury in mice. (c) Schematic illustration of photoelectric signal conversion of deep infrared light through implanted organic photocapacitors to stimulate the sciatic nerve of rats. (d) Implanted organic photocapacitors enable electrical stimulation to induce compound muscle action potentials in a rat for up to 103 days. ([a, b] Adapted with permission (Koo et al., 2018). Copyright 2018, Springer Nature; [c, d] Adapted with permission (Ejneby et al., 2022). Copyright 2022, Springer Nature.)

modulate bladder function. Further, by using data analysis algorithms to identify patho-
logical behaviors, this implantable optogenetic neuromodulation successfully normalized
bladder function in the setting of acute cystitis (Figure 4.16d).

In addition to the above-mentioned diseases, more diseases are being tried to be treated
using soft electronic devices. Yao et al. developed a self-powered, bioabsorbable implantable electrical stimulation device to promote rapid fracture healing (2021). The soft electronic device mainly consists of a triboelectric nanogenerator that generates electrical
pulses and a pair of interdigitated dressing electrodes that provide a spatially distributed
electric field. The island bridge and serpentine connection forms improve the structural
solidity, reduce the overall modulus, and maximize the flexibility of the equipment. They
demonstrated the device's therapeutic ability in fracture healing in rats. The experimental
results showed that the optimized electric field can activate relevant growth factors, regulate the bone microenvironment, and promote bone formation and bone remodeling
(Figure 4.17). Yamagishi et al. constructed a tissue-adhesive wireless optoelectronic device
for local anti-tumor therapy (2019). The device can be fixed to the surface of internal tissue
without suturing, and through the wireless power supply, it can achieve on–off control of
the implanted optoelectronic devices externally. In animal tests, the device was implanted
under the skin of mice with subcutaneously transplanted tumors and irradiated for 10 days

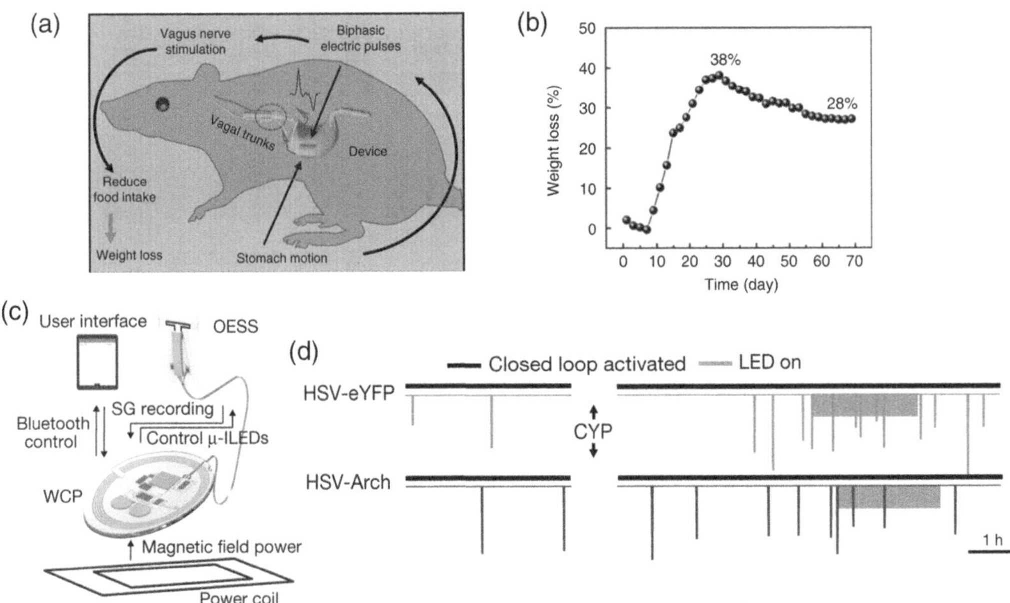

FIGURE 4.16 Soft electronic device to treat obesity and bladder disease through electrical neurostimulation. (a) Schematic diagram of implanting a self-powered vagus nerve stimulation device
to treat obesity. (b) Recording of weight loss rate in rats after implantation of a self-powered vagus
nerve stimulation device. (c) Schematic diagram of the automated closed-loop optogenetic neuromodulation device. (d) Recording of modulated urinary behavior in rats using an optogenetic
neurostimulation device. ([a, b] Adapted with permission (Yao et al., 2018). Copyright 2018, Springer
Nature; [c, d] Adapted with permission (Mickle et al., 2019). Copyright 2019, Springer Nature.)

at an intensity about 1,000 times lower than traditional photodynamic therapy, which produced a good anti-tumor effect.

It is obvious that soft electronic devices have shown application potential in the treatment of various diseases, especially in the treatment of long-term, chronic, and complex diseases, which have unique advantages. But there are still many unanswered questions such as safety, comfort, long-term reliability, and commercialization. Most biocompatibility and implantation experiments are based on small animal models, which still have a long way to go before they can be truly used in clinical applications. Undoubtedly, research in this field is in its nascent stage, brimming with vitality. We have reason to believe that in the future, the breadth and depth of soft electronic devices in medical treatment will continue to increase, becoming a powerful tool in the treatment of human diseases.

4.6 CONCLUSION AND OUTLOOK

In this chapter, we introduce recent advances in soft electronic devices for medical treatments. In past research, soft electronic devices have led to exciting advances in medical treatments. From wearable therapies to implanted therapies, from drug delivery to physical stimulation, various types of treatment cases demonstrate the extraordinary potential

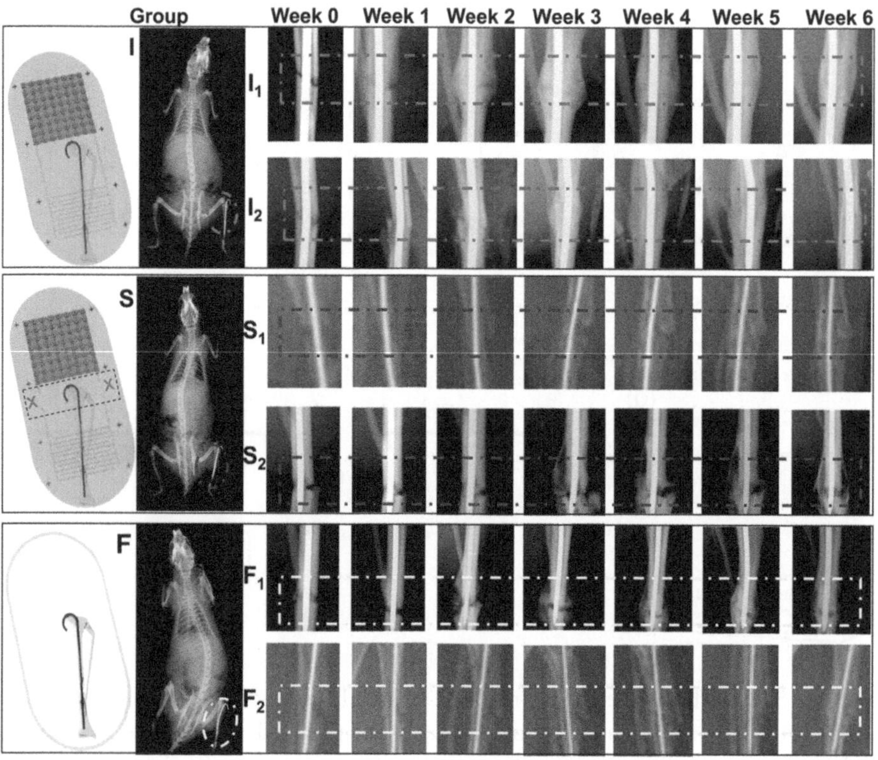

FIGURE 4.17 X-ray images of the recovery process of right tibia fracture in rats under different experimental groups: implantable self-powered electrical stimulation device (I), sham operation group (S), and sham implant group (F). (Adapted with permission (Yao et al., 2021). Copyright 2021, National Academy of Sciences.)

of soft electronics. Compared with traditional rigid therapeutic devices, soft electronic devices have many advantages, such as being lightweight, soft, compliant, biocompatible, and patient compliant. However, as an emerging field, its research has not yet been in-depth, and actual clinical trials have not yet been widely carried out. It still faces many common challenges that require breakthroughs in the future. Here we outline these challenges and propose possible solutions.

For the construction of intelligent and accurate closed-loop treatment systems, it is necessary to improve the accuracy and long-term stability of sensors and actuators, especially to accurately distinguish target physiological signals from background noise. This places higher requirements on equipment design, manufacturing, and signal processing. The triggering of treatment mechanisms cannot rely solely on self-response or human judgment, because the mechanisms and influencing factors of many diseases are complex. In the future, artificial intelligence technology can be combined to assist signal processing and provide diagnostic suggestions to improve the efficiency and accuracy of diagnosis and treatment.

In addition, the comfort and biocompatibility of soft electronic therapeutic devices should be fully verified. Especially for implantable soft electronic devices, the trauma caused during the implantation process and its long-term impact on the bioactivity of the implanted site must be closely followed and studied. In the research of degradable implantable soft electronic devices, we also need to balance the relationship between degradation time and effective working time, which involves systematic research on biology and materials science.

Undoubtedly, addressing energy-related challenges remains an inevitable aspect of this endeavor. Soft electronic devices used for treatment must build an efficient and precise energy supply management system to meet long-term and stable work requirements. Recently, the development of self-powered technology and wireless energy supply technology is expected to provide solutions for this.

Finally, before moving toward commercialization and clinical application, cost-effective materials and technological pathways must be developed to lay the foundation for large-scale production. Furthermore, these devices must undergo comprehensive and systematic evaluation testing on large animals and humans, and treatment procedures must follow relevant medical protocols and obtain approval from relevant regulatory authorities.

In summary, soft electronic devices, as an emerging multidisciplinary electronic technology, have demonstrated great potential and advantages in medical treatment, and many recent studies have also made encouraging progress. However, there are still many challenges to be overcome on the way to clinical application. Nonetheless, as technology advances, researchers in various fields work together. The prospect of soft electronics in the field of medical diagnosis and treatment is certain and full of hope. It will bring revolutionary development to traditional medicine and become a core tool in future medical diagnosis and treatment.

REFERENCES

Bird, D., & Ravindra, N. M. (2020). Transdermal drug delivery and patches—An overview. *Medical Devices & Sensors, 3*(6), e10069.

Brett, D. W. (2006). A review of moisture-control dressings in wound care. *Journal of Wound Ostomy & Continence Nursing, 33*, 3–8.

Brown, M. B., Martin, G. P., Jones, S. A., & Akomeah, F. K. (2006). Dermal and transdermal drug delivery systems: Current and future prospects. *Drug Delivery, 13*(3), 175–187.

Brumberg, V., Astrelina, T., Malivanova, T., & Samoilov, A. (2021). Modern wound dressings: Hydrogel dressings. *Biomedicines, 9*(9), 1235.

Burton, A., Won, S. M., Sohrabi, A. K., Stuart, T., Amirhossein, A., Kim, J. U., Park, Y., Gabros, A., Rogers, J. A., Vitale, F., Richardson, A. G., & Gutruf, P. (2021). Wireless, battery-free, and fully implantable electrical neurostimulation in freely moving rodents. *Microsystems & Nanoengineering, 7*(1), 62.

Castaño, O., Pérez-Amodio, S., Navarro-Requena, C., Mateos-Timoneda, M. A., & Engel, E. (2018). Instructive microenvironments in skin wound healing: Biomaterials as signal releasing platforms. *Advanced Drug Delivery Reviews, 129*, 95–117.

Castilla, D. M., & Velazquez, O. C. (2012). Oxygen: Implications for wound healing. *Advances in Wound Care, 1*(6), 225–230.

Chanmugam, A., Langemo, D., Thomason, K., Haan, J., Altenburger, E. A., Tippett, A., Henderson, L., & Zortman, T. A. (2017). Relative temperature maximum in wound infection and inflammation as compared with a control subject using long-wave infrared thermography. *Advances in Skin & Wound Care, 30*(9), 406–414.

Cheng, Y. F., Ma, Y. A., Li, L. Y., Zhu, M., Yue, Y., Liu, W. J., Wang, L. F., Jia, S. F., Li, C., Qi, T. Y., Wang, J. B., & Gao, Y. H. (2020). Bioinspired microspines for a high-performance spray TiC_2T_x MXene-based piezoresistive sensor. *Acs Nano, 14*(2), 2145–2155.

Chien, Y. W. (1987). Development of transdermal drug delivery systems. *Drug Development and Industrial Pharmacy, 13*(4–5), 589–651.

Choi, S., Park, J., Hyun, W., Kim, J., Kim, J., Lee, Y. B., Song, C., Hwang, H. J., Kim, J. H., Hyeon, T., & Kim, D. H. (2015). Stretchable heater using ligand-exchanged silver nanowire nanocomposite for wearable articular thermotherapy. *Acs Nano, 9*(6), 6626–6633.

Choi, Y. S., Jeong, H., Yin, R. T., Avila, R., Pfenniger, A., Yoo, J., Lee, J. Y., Tzavelis, A., Lee, Y. J., Chen, S. W., Knight, H. S., Kim, S., Ahn, H. Y., Wickerson, G., Vázquez-Guardado, A., Higbee-Dempsey, E., Russo, B. A., Napolitano, M. A., Holleran, T. J., Razzak, L. A., Miniovich, A. N., Lee, G., Geist, B., Kim, B., Han, S. L., Brennan, J. A., Aras, K., Kwak, S. S., Kim, J., Waters, E. A., Yang, X. X., Burrell, A., Chun, K. S., Liu, C., Wu, C. S., Rwei, A. Y., Spann, A. N., Banks, A., Johnson, D., Zhang, Z. J., Haney, C. R., Jin, S. H., Sahakian, A. V., Huang, Y. G., Trachiotis, G. D., Knight, B. P., Arora, R. K., Efimov, I. R., & Rogers, J. A. (2022). A transient, closed-loop network of wireless, body-integrated devices for autonomous electrotherapy. *Science, 376*(6596), 1006–1012.

Derakhshandeh, H., Kashaf, S. S., Aghabaglou, F., Ghanavati, I. O., & Tamayol, A. (2018). Smart bandages: The future of wound care. *Trends in Biotechnology, 36*(12), 1259–1274.

Derwin, R., Patton, D., Strapp, H., & Moore, Z. (2023). The effect of inflammation management on pH, temperature, and bacterial burden. *International Wound Journal, 20*(4), 1118–1129.

Dhote, V., Bhatnagar, P., Mishra, P. K., Mahajan, S. C., & Mishra, D. K. (2012). Iontophoresis: A potential emergence of a transdermal drug delivery system. *Scientia Pharmaceutica, 80*(1), 1–28.

Dong, R. N., & Guo, B. L. (2021). Smart wound dressings for wound healing. *Nano Today, 41*, 101290.

Ejneby, M. S., Jakesová, M., Ferrero, J. J., Migliaccio, L., Sahalianov, I., Zhao, Z. F., Berggren, M., Khodagholy, D., Derek, V., Gelinas, J. N., & Glowacki, E. D. (2022). Chronic electrical stimulation of peripheral nerves via deep-red light transduced by an implanted organic photocapacitor. *Nature Biomedical Engineering, 6*(6), 741–753.

Emaminejad, S., Gao, W., Wu, E., Davies, Z. A., Nyein, H. Y. Y., Challa, S., Ryan, S. P., Fahad, H. M., Chen, K., Shahpar, Z., Talebi, S., Milla, C., Javey, A., & Davis, R. W. (2017). Autonomous sweat extraction and analysis applied to cystic fibrosis and glucose monitoring using a fully integrated wearable platform. *Proceedings of the National Academy of Sciences of the United States of America, 114*(18), 4625–4630.

Falanga, V., Isseroff, R. R., Soulika, A. M., Romanelli, M., Margolis, D., Kapp, S., Granick, M., & Harding, K. (2022). Chronic wounds. *Nature Reviews Disease Primers, 8*(1), 50.

Farahani, M., & Shafiee, A. (2021). Wound healing: From passive to smart dressings. *Advanced Healthcare Materials, 10*(16), 2100477.

Fernandez, M. L., Upton, Z., Edwards, H., Finlayson, K., & Shooter, G. K. (2012). Elevated uric acid correlates with wound severity. *International Wound Journal, 9*(2), 139–149.

Gao, W., Emaminejad, S., Nyein, H. Y. Y., Challa, S., Chen, K. V., Peck, A., Fahad, H. M., Ota, H., Shiraki, H., Kiriya, D., Lien, D. H., Brooks, G. A., Davis, R. W., & Javey, A. (2016). Fully integrated wearable sensor arrays for multiplexed perspiration analysis. *Nature, 529*(7587), 509–514.

Ge, Z. Y., Guo, W. S., Tao, Y., Sun, H. X., Meng, X. Y., Cao, L. Y., Zhang, S. G., Liu, W. Y., Akhtar, M. L., Li, Y., & Ren, Y. K. (2023). Wireless and closed-loop smart dressing for exudate management and on-demand treatment of chronic wounds. *Advanced Materials, 35*(47), 2304005.

Ghomi, E. R., Khalili, S., Khorasani, S. N., Neisiany, R. E., & Ramakrishna, S. (2019). Wound dressings: Current advances and future directions. *Journal of Applied Polymer Science, 136*(27), 47738.

Guinovart, T., Valdés-Ramírez, G., Windmiller, J. R., Andrade, F. J., & Wang, J. (2014). Bandage-based wearable potentiometric sensor for monitoring wound pH. *Electroanalysis, 26*(6), 1345–1353.

Guo, X., Avila, R., Huang, Y., & Xie, Z. (2021). Flexible electronics with dynamic interfaces for biomedical monitoring, stimulation, and characterization. *International Journal of Mechanical System Dynamics, 1*(1), 52–70.

Haller, H. L., Sander, F., Popp, D., Rapp, M., Hartmann, B., Demircan, M., Nischwitz, S. P., & Kamolz, L. P. (2021). Oxygen, pH, lactate, and metabolism-how old knowledge and new insights might be combined for new wound treatment. *Medicina-Lithuania, 57*(11), 1190.

Huang, Y., Li, H., Hu, T. L., Li, J., Yiu, C. K., Zhou, J. K., Li, J. Y., Huang, X. C., Yao, K. M., Qiu, X., Zhou, Y., Li, D. F., Zhang, B. B., Shi, R., Liu, Y. M., Wong, T. H., Wu, M. G., Jia, H. L., Gao, Z., Zhang, Z. B., He, J. H., Zheng, M. J., Song, E. M., Wang, L. D., Xu, C. J., & Yu, X. E. (2022). Implantable electronic medicine enabled by bioresorbable microneedles for wireless electrotherapy and drug delivery. *Nano Letters, 22*(14), 5944–5953.

Hwang, I., Kim, H. N., Seong, M., Lee, S. H., Kang, M., Yi, H., Bae, W. G., Kwak, M. K., & Jeong, H. E. (2018). Multifunctional smart skin adhesive patches for advanced health care. *Advanced Healthcare Materials, 7*(15), 1800275.

Jain, K. K. (2020). An overview of drug delivery systems. *Drug Delivery Systems,* 1–54. https://doi.org/10.1007/978-1-4939-9798-5_1

Jiang, X. R., Wu, H., Xiao, A., Huang, Y., Yu, X. G., & Chang, L. Q. (2023a). Recent advances in bioelectronics for localized drug delivery. *Small Methods, 8,* 202301068.

Jiang, Y. W., Trotsyuk, A. A., Niu, S. M., Henn, D., Chen, K., Shih, C. C., Larson, M. R., Mermin-Bunnell, A. M., Mittal, S., Lai, J. C., Saberi, A., Beard, E., Jing, S., Zhong, D. L., Steele, S. R., Sun, K. F., Jain, T., Zhao, E., Neimeth, C. R., Viana, W. G., Tang, J., Sivaraj, D., Padmanabhan, J., Rodrigues, M., Perrault, D. P., Chattopadhyay, A., Maan, Z. N., Leeolou, M. C., Bonham, C. A., Kwon, S. H., Kussie, H. C., Fischer, K. S., Gurusankar, G., Liang, K., Zhang, K. L., Nag, R., Snyder, M. P., Januszyk, M., Gurtner, G. C., & Bao, Z. N. (2023b). Wireless, closed-loop, smart bandage with integrated sensors and stimulators for advanced wound care and accelerated healing. *Nature Biotechnology, 41*(5), 652–662.

Jiang, Y. W., Zhang, Z. T., Wang, Y. X., Li, D. L., Coen, C. T., Hwaun, E., Chen, G., Wu, H. C., Zhong, D. L., Niu, S. M., Wang, W. C., Saberi, A., Lai, J. C., Wu, Y. L., Wang, Y., Trotsyuk, A. A., Loh, K. Y., Shih, C. C., Xu, W. H., Liang, K., Zhang, K. L., Bai, Y. H., Gurusankar, G., Hu, W. P., Jia, W., Cheng, Z., Dauskardt, R. H., Gurtner, G. C., Tok, J. B. H., Deisseroth, K., Soltesz, I., & Bao, Z. N. (2022). Topological supramolecular network enabled high-conductivity, stretchable organic bioelectronics. *Science, 375*(6587), 1411–1417.

Joo, H., Lee, Y., Kim, J., Yoo, J. S., Yoo, S., Kim, S., Arya, A. K., Kim, S., Choi, S. H., Lu, N., Lee, H. S., Kim, S., Lee, S. T., & Kim, D. H. (2021). Soft implantable drug delivery device integrated wirelessly with wearable devices to treat fatal seizures. *Science Advances, 7*(1), eabd4639.

Kang, M., Jeong, H., Park, S. W., Hong, J., Lee, H., Chae, Y., Yang, S., & Ahn, J. H. (2022). Wireless graphene-based thermal patch for obtaining temperature distribution and performing thermography. *Science Advances, 8*(15), eabm6693.

Kar, A., Ahamad, N., Dewani, M., Awasthi, L., Patil, R., & Banerjee, R. (2022). Wearable and implantable devices for drug delivery: Applications and challenges. *Biomaterials, 283*, 121435.

Kaveti, R., Lee, J. H., Youn, J. K., Jang, T.-M., Han, W. B., Yang, S. M., Shin, J.-W., Ko, G.-J., Kim, D.-J., Han, S., Kang, H., Bandodkar, A. J., Kim, H.-Y., & Hwang, S.-W. (2023). Soft, long-lived, bioresorbable electronic surgical mesh with wireless pressure monitor and on-demand drug delivery. *Advanced Materials, 36*, 2307391.

Keum, D., Kim, S. K., Koo, J., Lee, G. H., Jeon, C., Mok, J. W., Mun, B. H., Lee, K. J., Kamrani, E., Joo, C. K., Shin, S., Sim, J. Y., Myung, D., Yun, S. H., Bao, Z. N., & Hahn, S. K. (2020). Wireless smart contact lens for diabetic diagnosis and therapy. *Science Advances, 6*(17), eaba3252.

Kim, J., Ghaffari, R., & Kim, D. H. (2017). The quest for miniaturized soft bioelectronic devices. *Nature Biomedical Engineering, 1*(3), 0049.

Koo, J., MacEwan, M. R., Kang, S. K., Won, S. M., Stephen, M., Gamble, P., Xie, Z. Q., Yan, Y., Chen, Y. Y., Shin, J., Birenbaum, N., Chung, S. J., Kim, S. B., Khalifeh, J., Harburg, D. V., Bean, K., Paskett, M., Kim, J., Zohny, Z. S., Lee, S. M., Zhang, R. Y., Luo, K. J., Ji, B. W., Banks, A., Lee, H. M., Huang, Y. G., Ray, W. Z., & Rogers, J. A. (2018). Wireless bioresorbable electronic system enables sustained nonpharmacological neuroregenerative therapy. *Nature Medicine, 24*(12), 1830–1836.

Koo, J. H., Song, J. K., Kim, D. H., & Son, D. (2021). Soft implantable bioelectronics. *ACS Materials Letters, 3*(11), 1528–1540.

Kruse, C. R., Nuutila, K., Lee, C. C. Y., Kiwanuka, E., Singh, M., Caterson, E. J., Eriksson, E., & Sorensen, J. A. (2015). The external microenvironment of healing skin wounds. *Wound Repair and Regeneration, 23*(4), 456–464.

Kus, K. J. B., & Ruiz, E. S. (2020). Wound dressings – A practical review. *Current Dermatology Reports, 9*(4), 298–308.

Lee, H., Choi, T. K., Lee, Y. B., Cho, H. R., Ghaffari, R., Wang, L., Choi, H. J., Chung, T. D., Lu, N. S., Hyeon, T., Choi, S. H., & Kim, D. H. (2016a). A graphene-based electrochemical device with thermoresponsive microneedles for diabetes monitoring and therapy. *Nature Nanotechnology, 11*(6), 566–572.

Lee, H., Song, C., Baik, S., Kim, D., Hyeon, T., & Kim, D. H. (2018). Device-assisted transdermal drug delivery. *Advanced Drug Delivery Reviews, 127*, 35–45.

Lee, J., Cho, H. R., Cha, G. D., Seo, H., Lee, S., Park, C. K., Kim, J. W., Qiao, S. T., Wang, L., Kang, D., Kang, T., Ichikawa, T., Kim, J., Lee, H., Lee, W., Kim, S., Lee, S. T., Lu, N. S., Hyeon, T., Choi, S. H., & Kim, D. H. (2019). Flexible, sticky, and biodegradable wireless device for drug delivery to brain tumors. *Nature Communications, 10*, 5205.

Lee, J. H., Kim, H., Kim, J. H., & Lee, S. H. (2016b). Soft implantable microelectrodes for future medicine: Prosthetics, neural signal recording and neuromodulation. *Lab on a Chip, 16*(6), 959–976.

Li, C., Wang, J. C., Wang, Y. G., Gao, H. L., Wei, G., Huang, Y. Z., Yu, H. J., Gan, Y., Wang, Y. J., Mei, L., Chen, H. B., Hu, H. Y., Zhang, Z. P., & Jin, Y. G. (2019). Recent progress in drug delivery. *Acta Pharmaceutica Sinica B, 9*(6), 1145–1162.

Li, H. F., Gao, F., Wang, P., Yin, L., Ji, N., Zhang, L. W., Zhao, L. Y., Hou, G. H., Lu, B. W., Chen, Y., Ma, Y. J., & Feng, X. (2021a). Biodegradable flexible electronic device with controlled drug release for cancer treatment. *Acs Applied Materials & Interfaces, 13*(18), 21067–21075.

Li, M. X., Xia, W. Z., Khoong, Y. M., Huang, L. J., Huang, X., Liang, H., Zhao, Y., Mao, J. Y., Yu, H. J., & Zan, T. (2023). Smart and versatile biomaterials for cutaneous wound healing. *Biomaterials Research, 27*(1), 87.

Li, X. L., Huang, X. S., Mo, J. S., Wang, H., Huang, Q. Q., Yang, C., Zhang, T., Chen, H. J., Hang, T., Liu, F. M., Jiang, L. L., Wu, Q. N., Li, H. B., Hu, N., & Xie, X. (2021b). A fully integrated closed-loop system based on mesoporous microneedles-iontophoresis for diabetes treatment. *Advanced Science, 8*(16), 2100827.

Lim, C., Hong, Y. J., Jung, J., Shin, Y., Sunwoo, S. H., Baik, S., Park, O. K., Choi, S. H., Hyeon, T., Kim, J. H., Lee, S., & Kim, D. H. (2021). Tissue-like skin-device interface for wearable bioelectronics by using ultrasoft, mass-permeable, and low-impedance hydrogels. *Science Advances*, *7*(19), eabd3716.

Liu, Y., Pharr, M., & Salvatore, G. A. (2017). Lab-on-skin: A review of flexible and stretchable electronics for wearable health monitoring. *Acs Nano*, *11*(10), 9614–9635.

Liu, Z. Q., Liu, J. Q., Sun, T. C., Zeng, D. K., Yang, C. D., Wang, H., Yang, C., Guo, J., Wu, Q. N., Chen, H. J., & Xie, X. (2021). Integrated multiplex sensing bandage for in situ monitoring of early infected wounds. *Acs Sensors*, *6*(8), 3112–3124.

Lou, D., Pang, Q., Pei, X. C., Dong, S. R., Li, S. J., Tan, W. Q., & Ma, L. (2020). Flexible wound healing system for pro-regeneration, temperature monitoring and infection early warning. *Biosensors & Bioelectronics*, *162*, 112275.

Luo, Y. F., Wang, M., Wan, C. J., Cai, P. Q., Loh, X. J., & Chen, X. D. (2020). Devising materials manufacturing toward lab-to-fab translation of flexible electronics. *Advanced Materials*, *32*(37), 2001903.

Ma, Y. J., Zhang, Y. C., Cai, S. S., Han, Z. Y., Liu, X., Wang, F. L., Cao, Y., Wang, Z. H., Li, H. F., Chen, Y. H., & Feng, X. (2020). Flexible hybrid electronics for digital healthcare. *Advanced Materials*, *32*(15), 1902062.

Maliyar, K., Persaud-Jaimangal, R., & Sibbald, R. G. (2020). Associations among skin surface pH, temperature, and bacterial burden in wounds. *Advances in Skin & Wound Care*, *33*(4), 180–185.

McLister, A., McHugh, J., Cundell, J., & Davis, J. (2016). New developments in smart bandage technologies for wound diagnostics. *Advanced Materials*, *28*(27), 5732–5737.

Meng, K. Y., Chen, J., Li, X. S., Wu, Y. F., Fan, W. J., Zhou, Z. H., He, Q., Wang, X., Fan, X., Zhang, Y. X., Yang, J., & Wang, Z. L. (2019). Flexible weaving constructed self-powered pressure sensor enabling continuous diagnosis of cardiovascular disease and measurement of cuffless blood pressure. *Advanced Functional Materials*, *29*(5), 1806388

Metcalf, D. G., Haalboom, M., Bowler, P. G., Gamerith, C., Sigl, E., Heinzle, A., & Burnet, M. W. M. (2019). Elevated wound fluid pH correlates with increased risk of wound infection. *Wound Medicine*, *26*(1), 100166.

Mickle, A. D., Won, S. M., Noh, K. N., Yoon, J., Meacham, K. W., Xue, Y. G., McIlvried, L. A., Copits, B. A., Samineni, V. K., Crawford, K. E., Kim, D. H., Srivastava, P., Kim, B. H., Min, S., Shiuan, Y., Yun, Y., Payne, M. A., Zhang, J. P., Jang, H., Li, Y. H., Lai, H. H., Huang, Y. G., Park, S. I., Gereau, R. W., & Rogers, J. A. (2019). A wireless closed-loop system for optogenetic peripheral neuromodulation. *Nature*, *565*(7739), 361–365.

Mostafalu, P., Lenk, W., Dokmeci, M. R., Ziaie, B., Khademhosseini, A., & Sonkusale, S. R. (2015). Wireless flexible smart bandage for continuous monitoring of wound oxygenation. *Ieee Transactions on Biomedical Circuits and Systems*, *9*(5), 670–677.

Nag, S., & Thakor, N. V. (2016). Implantable neurotechnologies: Electrical stimulation and applications. *Medical & Biological Engineering & Computing*, *54*(1), 63–76.

Ogawa, Y., Kato, K., Miyake, T., Nagamine, K., Ofuji, T., Yoshino, S., & Nishizawa, M. (2015). Organic transdermal iontophoresis patch with built-in biofuel cell. *Advanced Healthcare Materials*, *4*(4), 506–510.

Ouyang, H., Liu, Z., Li, N., Shi, B. J., Zou, Y., Xie, F., Ma, Y., Li, Z., Li, H., Zheng, Q., Qu, X. C., Fan, Y. B., Wang, Z. L., Zhang, H., & Li, Z. (2019). Symbiotic cardiac pacemaker. *Nature Communications*, *10*, 1821.

Pal, A., Goswami, D., Cuellar, H. E., Castro, B., Kuang, S. H., & Martinez, R. V. (2018). Early detection and monitoring of chronic wounds using low-cost, omniphobic paper-based smart bandages. *Biosensors & Bioelectronics*, *117*, 696–705.

Pastore, M. N., Kalia, Y. N., Horstmann, M., & Roberts, M. S. (2015). Transdermal patches: History, development and pharmacology. *British Journal of Pharmacology*, *172*(9), 2179–2209.

Prausnitz, M. R., & Langer, R. (2008). Transdermal drug delivery. *Nature Biotechnology*, *26*(11), 1261–1268.

Qiao, Z., Chen, S., Fan, S., Xiong, Z., & Lim, C. T. (2023). Epidermal bioelectronics for management of chronic diseases: Materials, devices and systems. *Advanced Sensor Research, 2*(8), 2200068.

Sani, E. S., Xu, C. H., Wang, C. R., Song, Y., Min, J. H., Tu, J. B., Solomon, S. A., Li, J. H., Banks, J. L., Armstrong, D. G., & Gao, W. (2023). A stretchable wireless wearable bioelectronic system for multiplexed monitoring and combination treatment of infected chronic wounds. *Science Advances, 9*(12), eadf7388.

Sen, C. K. (2021). Human wound and its burden: Updated 2020 compendium of estimates. *Advances in Wound Care, 10*(5), 281–292.

Sheng, H. W., Zhang, X. T., Liang, J., Shao, M. J., Xie, E. Q., Yu, C. J., & Lan, W. (2021). Recent advances of energy solutions for implantable bioelectronics. *Advanced Healthcare Materials, 10*(17), 2100199.

Shi, Z. H., Lu, Y. L., Shen, S. Y., Xu, Y., Shu, C., Wu, Y., Lv, J. J., Li, X., Yan, Z. P., An, Z. J., Dai, C. B., Su, L. K., Zhang, F. N., & Liu, Q. J. (2022). Wearable battery-free theranostic dental patch for wireless intraoral sensing and drug delivery. *Npj Flexible Electronics, 6*(1), 49.

Singer, A. J., & Clark, R. A. (1999). Cutaneous wound healing. *New England journal of medicine, 341*(10), 738–746.

Smolensky, M. H., & Peppas, N. A. (2007). Chronobiology, drug delivery, and chronotherapeutics. *Advanced Drug Delivery Reviews, 59*(9), 828–851.

Someya, T., & Amagai, M. (2019). Toward a new generation of smart skins. *Nature Biotechnology, 37*(4), 382–388.

Song, D. K., Ye, G., Zhao, Y., Zhang, Y., Hou, X. C., & Liu, N. (2022). An all-in-one, bioderived, air-permeable, and sweat-stable MXene epidermal electrode for muscle theranostics. *Acs Nano, 16*(10), 17168–17178.

Sun, C., Bu, N., & Hu, X. (2023). Recent trends in electronic skin for transdermal drug delivery. *Intelligent Pharmacy, 1*(4), 183–191.

Sun, H., Saeedi, P., Karuranga, S., Pinkepank, M., Ogurtsova, K., Duncan, B. B., Stein, C., Basit, A., Chan, J. C., & Mbanya, J. C. (2022). IDF diabetes atlas: Global, regional and country-level diabetes prevalence estimates for 2021 and projections for 2045. *Diabetes Research and Clinical Practice, 183*, 109119.

Sung, S. H., Kim, Y. S., Joe, D. J., Mun, B. H., You, B. K., Keum, D. H., Hahn, S. K., Berggren, M., Kim, D., & Lee, K. J. (2018). Flexible wireless powered drug delivery system for targeted administration on cerebral cortex. *Nano Energy, 51*, 102–112.

Tan, M. H., Xu, Y., Gao, Z. Q., Yuan, T. J., Liu, Q. J., Yang, R. S., Zhang, B., & Peng, L. H. (2022). Recent advances in intelligent wearable medical devices integrating biosensing and drug delivery. *Advanced Materials, 34*(27), 2108491.

Tibbitt, M. W., Dahlman, J. E., & Langer, R. (2016). Emerging frontiers in drug delivery. *Journal of the American Chemical Society, 138*(3), 704–717.

Trinh, X. T., Long, N. V., Anh, L. T. V., Nga, P. T., Giang, N. N., Chien, P. N., Nam, S. Y., & Heo, C. Y. (2022). A comprehensive review of natural compounds for wound healing: Targeting bioactivity perspective. *International Journal of Molecular Sciences, 23*(17), 9573.

Vaghasiya, J. V., Mayorga-Martinez, C. C., & Pumera, M. (2023). Wearable sensors for telehealth based on emerging materials and nanoarchitectonics. *Npj Flexible Electronics, 7*(1), 26.

Venus, M., Waterman, J., & McNab, I. (2010). Basic physiology of the skin. *Surgery (Oxford), 28*(10), 469–472.

Wang, C. R., Sani, E. S., & Gao, W. (2022a). Wearable bioelectronics for chronic wound management. *Advanced Functional Materials, 32*(17), 2111022.

Wang, Q., Sheng, H., Lv, Y., Liang, J., Liu, Y., Li, N., Xie, E., Su, Q., Ershad, F., Lan, W., Wang, J., & Yu, C. (2022b). A skin-mountable hyperthermia patch based on metal nanofiber network with high transparency and low resistivity toward subcutaneous tumor treatment. *Advanced Functional Materials, 32*(21), 2111228.

Wu, H., Gao, W., & Yin, Z. P. (2017). Materials, devices and systems of soft boelectronics for precision therapy. *Advanced Healthcare Materials, 6*(10), 1700017.

Xu, G., Lu, Y. L., Cheng, C., Li, X., Xu, J., Liu, Z. Y., Liu, J. L., Liu, G., Shi, Z. H., Chen, Z. T., Zhang, F. N., Jia, Y. X., Xu, D. F., Yuan, W., Cui, Z., Low, S. S., & Liu, Q. J. (2021). Battery-free and wireless smart wound dressing for wound infection monitoring and electrically controlled on-demand drug delivery. *Advanced Functional Materials, 31*(26), 2100852.

Xu, L. Z., Gutbrod, S. R., Ma, Y. J., Petrossians, A., Liu, Y. H., Webb, R. C., Fan, J. A., Yang, Z. J., Xu, R. X., Whalen, J. J., Weiland, J. D., Huang, Y. G., Efimov, I. R., & Rogers, J. A. (2015). Materials and fractal designs for 3D multifunctional integumentary membranes with capabilities in cardiac electrotherapy. *Advanced Materials, 27*(10), 1731–1737.

Yadav, K. S., Kapse-Mistry, S., Peters, G. J., & Mayur, Y. C. (2019). E-drug delivery: A futuristic approach. *Drug Discovery Today, 24*(4), 1023–1030.

Yamagishi, K., Kirino, I., Takahashi, I., Amano, H., Takeoka, S., Morimoto, Y., & Fujie, T. (2019). Tissue-adhesive wirelessly powered optoelectronic device for metronomic photodynamic cancer therapy. *Nature Biomedical Engineering, 3*(1), 27–36.

Yamamoto, Y., Yamamoto, D., Takada, M., Naito, H., Arie, T., Akita, S., & Takei, K. (2017). Efficient skin temperature sensor and stable gel-less sticky ECG sensor for a wearable flexible healthcare patch. *Advanced Healthcare Materials, 6*(17), 1700495.

Yang, J. B., Li, Y. J., Ye, R., Zheng, Y., Li, X. L., Chen, Y. Z., Xie, X., & Jiang, L. L. (2020a). Smartphone-powered iontophoresis-microneedle array patch for controlled transdermal delivery. *Microsystems & Nanoengineering, 6*(1), 112.

Yang, Y., Xu, L. L., Jiang, D. J., Chen, B. Z., Luo, R. Z., Liu, Z., Qu, X. C., Wang, C., Shan, Y. Z., Cui, Y., Zheng, H., Wang, Z. W., Wang, Z. L., Guo, X. D., & Li, Z. (2021). Self-powered controllable transdermal drug delivery system. *Advanced Functional Materials, 31*(36), 2104092.

Yang, Y. R., Song, Y., Bo, X. J., Min, J. H., Pak, O. S., Zhu, L. L., Wang, M. Q., Tu, J. B., Kogan, A., Zhang, H. X., Hsiai, T. K., Li, Z. P., & Gao, W. (2020b). A laser-engraved wearable sensor for sensitive detection of uric acid and tyrosine in sweat. *Nature Biotechnology, 38*(2), 217–224.

Yao, G., Jiang, D., Li, J., Kang, L., Chen, S., Long, Y., Wang, Y., Huang, P., Lin, Y., Cai, W., & Wang, X. (2019). Self-activated electrical stimulation for effective hair regeneration via a wearable omnidirectional pulse generator. *Acs Nano, 13*(11), 12345–12356.

Yao, G., Kang, L., Li, C. C., Chen, S. H., Wang, Q., Yang, J. Z., Long, Y., Li, J., Zhao, K. N., Xu, W. N., Cai, W. B., Lin, Y., & Wang, X. D. (2021). A self-powered implantable and bioresorbable electrostimulation device for biofeedback bone fracture healing. *Proceedings of the National Academy of Sciences of the United States of America, 118*(28), e2100772118.

Yao, G., Kang, L., Li, J., Long, Y., Wei, H., Ferreira, C. A., Jeffery, J. J., Lin, Y., Cai, W. B., & Wang, X. D. (2018). Effective weight control via an implanted self-powered vagus nerve stimulation device. *Nature Communications, 9*, 5349.

Zhang, H. J., Pan, Y. P., Hou, Y., Li, M. H., Deng, J., Wang, B. C., & Hao, S. L. (2023a). Smart physical-based transdermal drug delivery system: Towards intelligence and controlled release. *Small, 2023*, 2306944.

Zhang, T., Liu, N., Xu, J., Liu, Z., Zhou, Y., Yang, Y., Li, S., Huang, Y., & Jiang, S. (2023b). Flexible electronics for cardiovascular healthcare monitoring. *Innovation (Camb), 4*(5), 100485.

Zhang, Z. M., Zhu, Z. T., Zhou, P. C., Zou, Y. F., Yang, J. W., Haick, H., & Wang, Y. (2023c). Soft bioelectronics for therapeutics. *Acs Nano, 17*(18), 17634–17667.

Zheng, H., Pu, Z. H., Wu, H., Li, C. C., Zhang, X. G., & Li, D. C. (2023). Reverse iontophoresis with the development of flexible electronics: A review. *Biosensors & Bioelectronics, 223*, 115036.

Zhou, H., Niu, L., Xia, X., Lin, Z., Liu, X., Su, M., Guo, R., Meng, L., & Zheng, H. (2019). Wearable ultrasound improves motor function in an MPTP mouse model of parkinson's disease. *IEEE Transactions on Biomedical Engineering, 66*(11), 3006–3013.

Zhu, J., Zhou, H. L., Gerhard, E. M., Zhang, S. H., Rodríguez, F. I. P., Pan, T. S., Yang, H. B., Lin, Y., Yang, J., & Cheng, H. Y. (2023). Smart bioadhesives for wound healing and closure. *Bioactive Materials, 19*, 360–375.

CHAPTER 5

Soft Electronics for Neural Engineering

Fan Zhang, Shurong Dong, and Shaomin Zhang

5.1 INTRODUCTION

The brain comprises an extensive network of synapses and 100 billion interconnected neurons that form the basis of its communication mechanism, facilitating the transmission of chemical and electrical signals (Herculano-Houzel, 2009, 2012). Brain–computer interfaces (BCIs) enable direct communication between external devices, usually computers, and the complex brain network, with bidirectional signaling (Fouad et al., 2015; Hughes et al., 2020). BCIs have revolutionized nervous system disease diagnosis, cognitive enhancement, medical rehabilitation, and neuroprosthetics (Abdulkader et al., 2015; López-Larraz et al., 2018). Advanced BCI applications such as communication aids (Widge et al., 2018), motor control (Birbaumer, 2006), and neuromodulation strategies like deep brain stimulation (Widge et al., 2018) depend on continuous brain monitoring and neural modulation. Implanted neural interfaces serve as the primary means to continuously measure tiny neural signals or stimulate the central nervous system with high accuracy. However, traditional implanted neural interfaces face limitations such as tissue damage, inflammation, and limited lifetime that impede long-term neural stimulation and recording (Jeong et al., 2015; Woeppel et al., 2017).

Soft electronics represent a transformative development in BCI, revolutionizing the approach to interfacing with the intricate circuitry of the brain (Tang et al., 2023). This budding field merges electronics, neuroscience, and materials science to produce flexible, biocompatible devices that blend in with neural tissues. This chapter explores both the breakthroughs and limitations in soft neural electronics, focusing specifically on their applications in multimodal interfaces, neural recording, and electrical neuromodulation. The chapter delves into recent advancements, materials, and applications, outlining the potential transformative power of soft neural electronics in BCI.

DOI: 10.1201/9781003493631-5

5.2 SOFT NEURAL ELECTRONICS FOR NEURAL RECORDING

5.2.1 Neural Signals and Interfaces

Neural signals can be classified into different types based on the electrode placement locations, including electroencephalogram (EEG), electrocorticogram (ECoG), local field potential (LFP), and single-neuron cellular signals. Although these signals all originate from neuronal activity within the same brain, their recording methods result in significant differences between their frequency and amplitude (Im & Seo, 2016), as shown in Table 5.1. The amplitude of neural signals is inversely proportional to the square of the distance between the neuron and the recording site (Buzsáki et al., 2012). Thus, implanted neural interfaces provide more precise representations of neuronal activity than EEG since these interfaces bypass the attenuation caused by long-distance neural signal transmission and signal propagation through the skull. However, implanted neural probes have problems such as insufficient spatial resolution, tissue damage, limited recording region and neuron count, restricted effective operation life, and so on. The advancements in soft electronics provide a promising solution for optimizing the implanted neural interfaces for BCI applications.

A simplified equivalent circuit from Rivnay et al. has been utilized to elucidate the electrode–tissue interface concerning the recording of neural probes, as exemplified in Figure 5.1 (2017). Here, the signal of the neuron is abstracted as a low-impedance voltage source V_e. R_{spread}, also known as R_{media}, represents the resistance of signal transmission in the electrolyte solution outside the neurons and its magnitude depends on the geometry of the recording site. Within this simplified model, R_e is employed to designate the leakage resistance encountered at the electrode–tissue interface, while C_e embodies the Helmholtz or double-layer capacitance positioned at the same interface. Concurrently, R_s signifies the resistance inherent in the interconnection pathway leading to an amplifier, typically identified as the headstage within the neural signal recording system. Remarkably, in scenarios involving metal wire interconnections, R_s is customarily disregarded.

5.2.2 Conductive Material in Soft Neural Electronics for Neural Recording

Various conductive materials have been employed in neural recording electrodes, characterized by different charge transfer mechanisms and electrode/tissue interface properties.

TABLE 5.1 Types and Characteristics of Neural Signals

Type of Neural Signals	Position of Electrodes	Amplitude	Frequency Band
EEG	Scalp	5–300 μV	<100 Hz
ECoG	Dura or sub-dura	0.01–5 mV	<200 Hz
LFP	Intracortical microelectrodes	<1 mV	<250 Hz
Action potentials	Intracortical microelectrodes	≈500 μV	>250 Hz

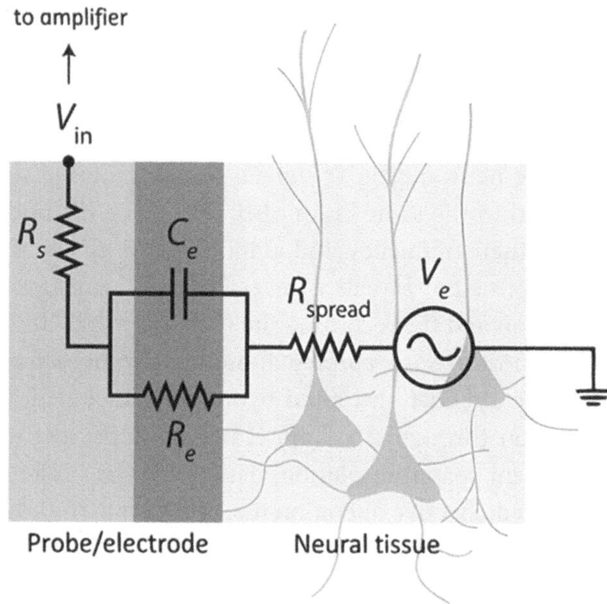

FIGURE 5.1 The equivalent circuit of neural electrode–tissue interface. (Adapted with permission. (Rivnay et al., 2017) Copyright 2017, AAAS.)

5.2.3 Metals

To date, the prevailing choice of conductive materials for neural probes predominantly encompasses metals and metal composites, notably including platinum, iridium, gold, silver, tungsten, stainless steel, and platinum–iridium alloys (Campbell et al., 1991; Cogan et al., 2004; Dalrymple et al., 2020; Dong et al., 2017; McClain et al., 2011), among others. For instance, the Utah array, which stands as both the most extensively employed and the sole FDA-approved neural electrode designed for human implantation, incorporates platinum and sputtered iridium oxide as conductive materials (Leber et al., 2019; Maynard et al., 1997; Nordhausen et al., 1994; Rousche & Normann, 1998). As shown in Figure 5.2, microwire electrodes, utilizing insulated metal wires, and flexible electrode arrays formed through metal deposition on flexible substrates, are also widely employed for recording neuroelectrophysiological activity from the cortex or within its various layers.

Metals have excellent electrical conductivity; however, their interface impedance with brain tissue is hindered by their low electrochemical active area (Boehler et al., 2020). To overcome this challenge, researchers have employed the use of electrode coating layers to increase the surface area between metal electrodes and brain tissue. This approach aims to improve the acquisition of high-quality neural signals. Various coating materials have been suggested, including metal and alloy nano-coatings, carbon nanotubes, graphene, conductive polymers, and others (Aqrawe et al., 2019; Baranauskas et al., 2011; Bourrier et al., 2019; Zhao et al., 2016). For instance, the PEDOT: PSS-coated gold microelectrode displayed in Figure 5.3, has proven to be effective in enhancing the surface area of neural electrodes (Pranti et al., 2017).

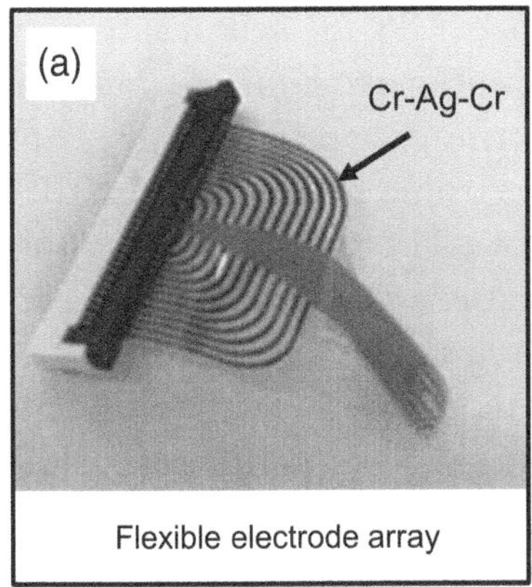
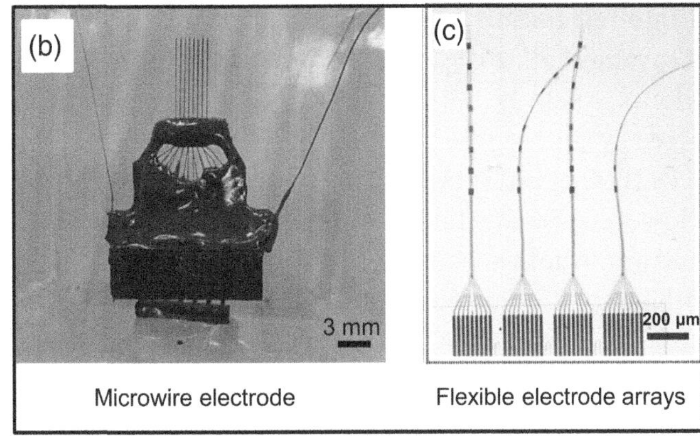

FIGURE 5.2 Several types of metal-based electrodes for neuroelectrophysiology. (a) ECoG electrode array. (b) Microwire electrode array and (c) Flexible electrode arrays for recording intracortical neural signals. ([a] Adapted with permission. (Xie et al., 2017) Copyright 2017, Springer Nature; [b, c] Adapted with permission. (Wei et al., 2018) Copyright 2018, Wiley-VCH.)

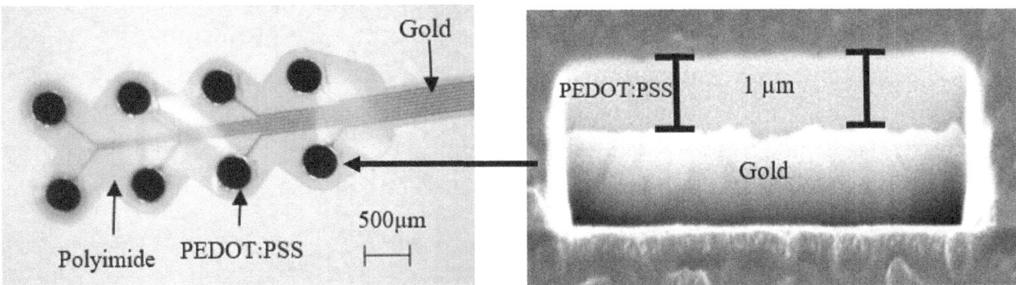

FIGURE 5.3 Gold microelectrodes coated with PEDOT: PSS for electrochemical high surface area. (Adapted with permission. (Pranti et al., 2017) Copyright 2017, MDPI.)

5.2.4 Conductive Polymers

Conductive polymers (CPs) function differently from metals in terms of their conductive mechanism. They possess a unique structure with a conjugated backbone and are electroactive organic polymers that enable charge carriers to move within them after they are doped (Deslouis et al., 1996; Heeger, 2001). Among CPs, poly (3, 4-ethylene dioxythiophene) (PEDOT) and polypyrrole (PPy) are commonly used for neural interfaces (Green et al., 2008). Due to their biocompatibility, they can make direct contact with tissues (Guo & Ma, 2018). Moreover, their special structure makes them bulk conductive, thereby increasing the electrochemical surface area of the electrode. As a result, they minimize the impedance of the electrode–tissue interface and provide high signal-to-noise ratio (SNR) electrophysiological signals (Liang et al., 2021). PEDOT-doped polymers, such as PEDOT-doped with poly (sodium 4-styrene sulfonate) (PEDOT: PSS), are widely used as conductive materials for electrodes or biocompatible coatings due to their high electronic and ionic conductivities and mechanical flexibility (Aqrawe et al., 2018; Green et al., 2008).

Various fabrication methods have been developed by researchers to address the substrate integration and high-resolution patterning issues of CPs for neural interfaces (Ouyang et al., 2015; Zhang & Travas-Sejdic, 2021). Conventional manufacturing techniques, such as inkjet printing, electrochemical patterning, aerosol printing, and screen printing, are commonly used for fabricating electronic devices based on the CPs (Feig et al., 2019; Garma et al., 2019; Sinha et al., 2017; Thompson & Yoon, 2013). However, these techniques are limited by their low resolution, which typically exceeds 100 μm. Another popular method for fabricating CP-based neural interfaces is photolithography (Ouyang et al., 2015). Unfortunately, this technique is often costly and complex to carry out. An alternative to these methods is additive manufacturing, which provides a highly cost-effective solution for producing high-resolution neural probes based on CPs. This approach enables the production of multiple probes in high volume while maintaining the necessary resolution for effective neural interface applications. In 2020, Zhao et al. developed a 3D printable CP ink capable of high resolution (over 30 microns), high aspect ratio (over 20 layers), and high conductivity (over 155 S cm^{-1} after dry annealing, up to 28 S cm^{-1} for hydrogel). The resulting printable ink displayed high repeatability and was easily integrated into other 3D printing materials. As illustrated in Figure 5.4, they utilized this method to print a flexible electrode array capable of single-unit recording in vivo (Yuk et al., 2020). In 2022, Zheng et al. proposed a new PEDOT:PSS 3D printing method based on room-temperature coagulation bath direct ink writing technology. This approach produced a component with high resolution ($\approx$20 μm) and high conductivity ($\approx$35 S cm^{-1}) while maintaining stable electrochemical properties. They used this approach to prepare flexible electrode arrays and conduct electrical cortical stimulation in mice (Zheng et al., 2022).

5.2.5 Carbon-Based Materials

Carbon-based materials, such as graphene and carbon nanotubes, have been widely used in the development of flexible, high-resolution neural electrodes (Devi et al., 2021). This is primarily attributed to their remarkable electrical, mechanical, and stable electrochemical properties, and high biocompatibility (Kim et al., 2018).

5.2.6 Graphene

Graphene is a two-dimensional carbon-based material with superior mechanical and chemical stability due to its strong sp2 bonds (Soldano et al., 2010). It also boasts excellent physical properties, featuring a fracture strength of 42 N m^{-1} and Young's modulus of 1 Tpa (Lee et al., 2008). Additionally, graphene has exceptional electrical conductivity, with a high mobility of up to 1×10^5 cm^2/Vs, surpassing both metals and semiconductors in electron transport rate (Hwang & Sarma, 2008). Its significant specific surface area enhances charge transfer and neuron attachment, elevating the recording and stimulation capabilities of neural electrodes (Kostarelos et al., 2017). Graphene fibers and planar-grown graphene are employed to fabricate neural electrodes. Researchers have used thin platinum-coated graphene fibers to construct flexible and free-standing microelectrode arrays that capture single neuronal signals in the rat cerebral cortex, achieving a high

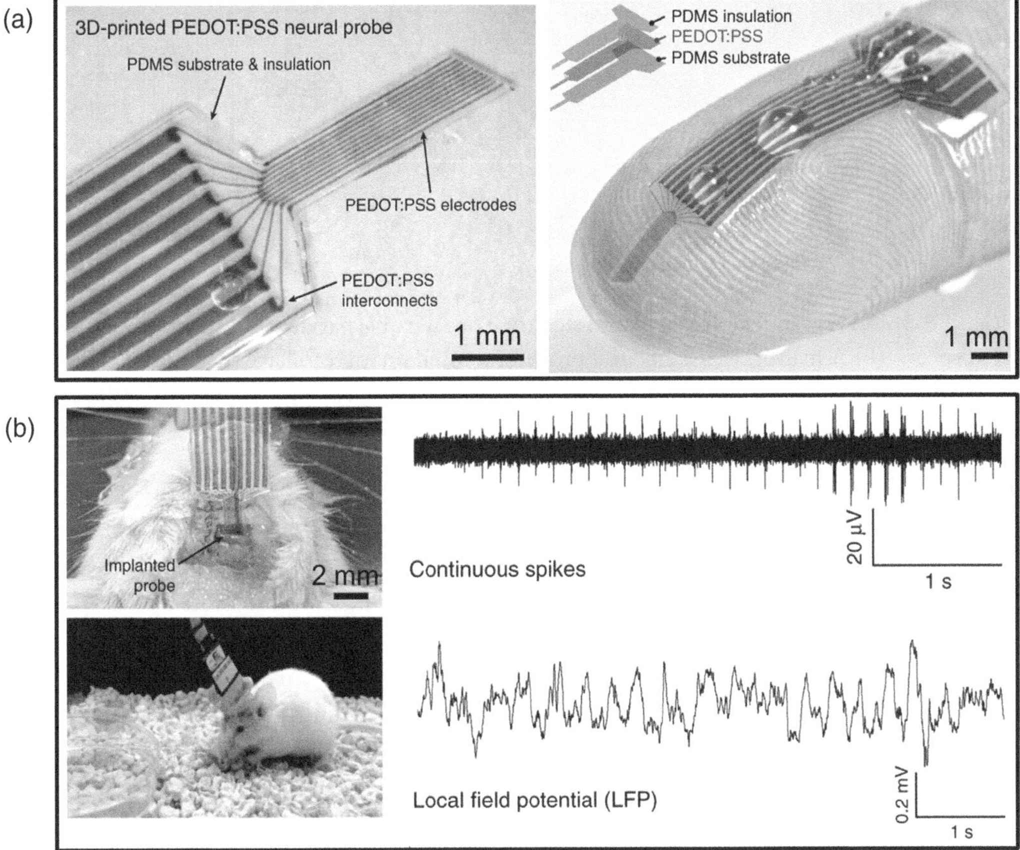

FIGURE 5.4 Conductive polymer-based neural electrodes. (a) 3D-printed PEDOT:PSS neural electrodes. (b) The implanted 3D-printed soft neural probe recorded LFP and continuous spikes from a freely moving rat. ([a, b] Adapted with permission. (Yuk et al., 2020) Copyright 2023, Springer Nature.)

SNR of 9.2 dB. The porous structure of the graphene fibers improves electrode surface area and charge transform capacity, and platinum coating modification transmits the collected signal effectively (Wang et al., 2019). This combination results in electrodes that have low impedance, a generous surface area, and outstanding electrochemical performance. Lasers have been used to produce graphene directly on flexible substrates, such as the direct creation of porous graphene electrode arrays by laser pyrolysis on polyimide (PI) substrates (Lu et al., 2016), or the formation of graphite-carbon coatings on metal electrodes by laser carbonization of parylene-C (Vomero et al., 2018). Nevertheless, limited by the resolution of the laser, the graphene traces tend to have larger widths, resulting in relatively large electrode sizes (ranging from 200 to 700 µm) (Xin Sally Zheng et al., 2021a). This does not align with the ongoing trend toward miniaturization and high-density neural electrodes. Presently, chemical vapor deposition (CVD) represents the most effective approach for developing graphene-based neural electrodes (Kumar et al., 2021; Lu et al., 2018). Due to the high growth temperature

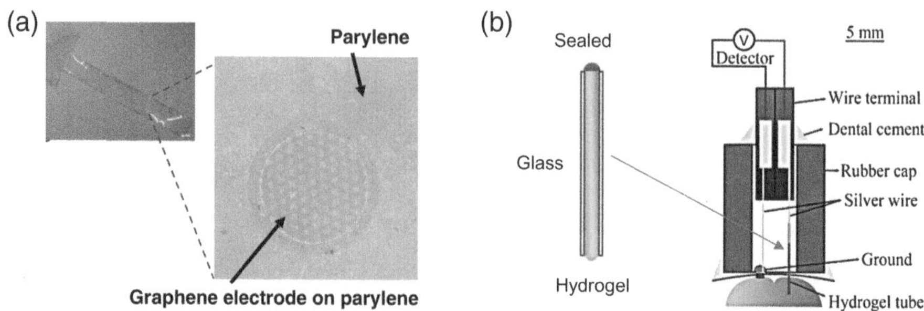

FIGURE 5.5　(a) A graphene-based neural electrode on a flexible parylene substrate using a transfer-free process. (b) A hydrogel-based neural probe in a fused quartz capillary tube. ([a] Adapted with permission. (Bakhshaee Babaroud et al., 2022) Copyright 2023, Springer Nature; [b] Adapted with permission. (Liang et al., 2022) Copyright 2022, Wiley-VCH.)

($\geq$900°C) required for CVD graphene (Weatherup et al., 2012) and the low melting point of the polymer, the planar graphene electrode array is typically pre-prepared by CVD on a substrate and subsequently transferred to the desired flexible substrate before patterning. In this manner, graphene can function as a conductive layer or as a modification for flexible neural electrodes (Bakhshaee Babaroud et al., 2022; Chen et al., 2013; Kuzum et al., 2014). This method enables the fabrication of single or multilayer graphene electrodes with excellent light transmittance (Nair et al., 2008; Thunemann et al., 2018). As shown in Figure 5.5a, Giagka et al. developed a CVD multilayer graphene-based electrode using a process that bypasses the need for transfer, thereby rendering it more compatible with conventional wafer-scale fabrication and subsequent post-processing technologies (Bakhshaee Babaroud et al., 2022).

5.2.7 Carbon Nanotubes

Carbon nanotubes (CNTs), which consist of rolled-up graphene sheets into tubular structures, are classified as one-dimensional nanomaterials (Iijima, 1991). CNTs exhibit several key attributes, including a high surface area-to-volume ratio, exceptional electrical conductivity, remarkable biocompatibility, flexibility, high mechanical strength, and outstanding affinity for neuron adhesion (Chen et al., 2013; Iijima et al., 1996; Peigney et al., 2001; Salvetat et al., 1999; Smart et al., 2006). Similar to graphene, carbon nanotubes can serve in the construction of both fibrous neural probes and planar electrodes (Alvarez et al., 2020; Lin et al., 2009). The substantial surface area of carbon nanotubes significantly reduces tissue contact impedance in CNT fiber electrodes compared to metal wire electrodes of equivalent dimensions. This feature makes CNT fiber electrodes particularly well-suited for recording the activity of single neurons without requiring additional surface treatments (Vitale et al., 2015). Additionally, CNT electrodes elicit a milder inflammatory response compared to their metal counterparts and can sustain neural activity recording for several weeks (Hejazi et al., 2021). In a study by Duan et al., soft neural electrodes employing CNT fibers precisely targeted specific brain regions and facilitated the tracking of individual neuron units in the rat brain for extended periods, up to 4–5 months

(Lu et al., 2019). This approach resulted in a notable reduction in brain inflammation when contrasted with conventional metal electrodes. In addition, CNTs can serve as an electrode coating layer and act as conductive layers for planar, transparent neural electrodes (Zhang et al., 2018).

5.2.8 Hydrogels

Hydrogels can absorb ions dissolved in electrolyte solutions, generating ionic currents (Yang & Suo, 2018). Their porous structure allows the incorporation of various conductive materials like metal nanomaterials, CNTs, graphene, and CPs (Peng et al., 2020). This combination enables the hydrogels to facilitate collaborative charge transport mechanisms involving both electrons and ions. This unique property renders hydrogels highly suitable for electrode–tissue interfaces, serving as coatings for neural electrodes to enhance interface impedance and as conductive materials for electrodes (Dong-Hwan Kim et al., 2010b; Liang et al., 2023). However, using hydrogels as conductive layers for electrodes raises the challenge of patterning or encapsulating them effectively. Techniques such as 3D printing and photolithography are employed to achieve precise patterning of hydrogel neural electrodes (Yang et al., 2023; Yuk et al., 2020). For encapsulation, Liang et al. utilized free radical polymerization to create a pure ionic conducting hydrogel. As depicted in Figure 5.5b, they encapsulated this hydrogel within a flexible PI-coated fused quartz capillary tube with an inner diameter of 320 μm. This method ensured that the hydrogel electrode could acquire nerve signals effectively from its tip. Consequently, the electrode successfully recorded LFP and neuronal spikes, demonstrating its functionality in neural signal detection (Liang et al., 2022).

5.3 SOFT NEURAL ELECTRONICS FOR ELECTRICAL NEUROMODULATION

The objective of neural electrical stimulation (NES) is to alter the depolarization threshold of neurons, consequently influencing their activity (Brocker & Grill, 2013). NES of the brain can be categorized into different types based on the location of the stimulation electrodes: transcranial electrical stimulation, cortical electrical stimulation, and deep brain stimulation (DBS) (Fertonani & Miniussi, 2017; Gordon et al., 1990). Among them, DBS electrodes have been used to treat various movement disorders, including Parkinson's disease and essential tremors (Sironi, 2011).

5.3.1 Evaluation of NES Electrodes Performance

Compared to neural recording electrodes, stimulating electrodes encounter more rigorous constraints. On one hand, under the Shannon criterion (Shannon, 1992), the charge density and charge per phase must be strictly limited to prevent tissue damage resulting from electrical stimulation. On the other hand, an excess of charge density can lead to the degradation of the electrode (Sandeep Negi et al., 2010b). Therefore, assessing the electrical stimulation capability of the electrode material becomes imperative to determine the electrode size and establish the parameters of electrical stimulation within the confines of safety.

The charge injection in NES typically takes the form of a biphasic charge-balanced signal. During this process, solid-state electron carriers on the electrode surface exchange charge with the ions present in the electrolyte solution within the tissue. This exchange can be entirely reversible, as seen in capacitive charging/discharging on the electric double layer and reversible faradaic reactions, such as REDOX reactions at Pt electrodes (Cogan, 2008). On the other hand, irreversible reactions often stem from changes in the concentration of reactants, such as volatile substances, at the surface during faraday reactions, leading to a disruption in the reaction's equilibrium in the forward and reverse directions (Boehler et al., 2020). NES electrodes typically involve a combination of capacitive sensing and faraday reactions.

Ideally, electrodes should be capable of indefinitely exchanging charge with the tissue's electrolyte during NES. Nevertheless, irreversible reactions can lead to changes in the electrode's chemical composition or the surrounding environment, potentially causing gradual corrosion or degradation of the electrode interface (Robblee et al., 1983; Shepherd et al., 2021). Given that all NES electrodes experience the same irreversible faraday reaction, namely the electrolysis of water, the voltage of hydrolysis is considered a voltage threshold (Brummer & Turner, 1975). The maximum amount of charge that can be injected before the anode or cathode phase triggers hydrolysis is defined as the charge injection capacity (CIC) of electrodes (Cogan et al., 2006). During NES, it is crucial to ensure that the charge delivered during a single-phase stimulation does not exceed the CIC of the electrode.

5.3.2 The CIC of Various Materials

Titanium nitride (TiN) electrodes are capable of undergoing charging only through the electric double layer between the electrode and electrolyte (Janders et al., 1996; Weiland et al., 2002). Roughening the surface of TiN can augment the surface area, consequently enhancing the capacitance of the electrode (Guyton & Terry Hambrecht, 1974; Rose et al., 1985). Although the capacitances of Pt and PtIr electrodes are typically considered to range between 0.3 and 0.35 mC cm^{-2} for low current intensities and extended pulse durations (<0.45 A cm^{-2}, >0.6 ms) (Brummer & Turner, 1977a; Brummer & Turner, 1977b), certain studies have proposed that in NES, the CIC should be reconsidered for high current density and brief pulse durations (0.2 ms), ranging in a span of 50–150 µC cm^{-2} (Rose & Robblee, 1990). Additionally, it has been observed that platinum dissolves under low-intensity stimulation (20–50 µC cm^{-2}) (Robblee et al., 1983), limiting its utilization in NES, especially for small electrode areas.

Compared to Pt, iridium oxide (IrOx) demonstrated superior corrosion resistance and CIC (Cogan et al., 2004; S Negi et al., 2010a). Anodic iridium oxide films (AIROFs) exhibit the ability to facilitate ion absorption or release in the electrolyte through a series of reversible redox reactions involving the transformation of multiple valence oxides (Mozota & Conway, 1983). AIROFs, comprising polymer-insulated iridium wires, have been applied in intracortical or spinal cord stimulation (Grill et al., 1999; McCreery et al., 1986; McCreery et al., 2002). Likewise, sputtered iridium oxide films (SIROFs) generated through the sputtering of metallic iridium have similar capacitance to that of

TABLE 5.2   The CIC Values of Various Conductive Materials for NES

Conductive Materials	CIC (mc cm^{-2})	Ref.
TiN	0.87	(Weiland et al., 2002)
Pt/PtIr	0.3–0.35	(Brummer & Turner, 1977b)
SIROF/AIROF	1.7–5.1	(Cogan et al., 2009)
PEDOT:PSS	6.3	(Zheng et al., 2022)
PEDOT:PSS/Au	2.71	(Ganji et al., 2017)
PEDOT:PSS/Pt	1.9	(Ganji et al., 2017)
CNTs	1–1.6	(Wang et al., 2006)

AIROF, with approximately 5 mC cm^{-2} registered during pulses of 0.4 ms for electrodes that measured 2000 µm^2 (Cogan, 2008; Slavcheva et al., 2004).

The conductive conjugated main chains within CPs can absorb ions within the material and establish electrostatic interactions with them, creating a pseudo-capacitor within the CPs capable of transferring charges (Bobacka et al., 2000). Especially, PEDOT:PSS exhibits larger CIC compared to Pt and Au; for instance, photolithographically patterned PEDOT:PSS electrodes with a diameter of 200 µm demonstrated a threefold increase in CIC compared to an Au electrode with the same size (Cui et al., 2021). Furthermore, the CIC of the 3D-printed PEDOT:PSS electrode, as reported by Zheng et al. is 6.366 mC cm^{-2} (2022).

The geometry and area of the electrode, along with the thickness of the conductive layer also play a crucial role in influencing the CIC of the NES electrode (Brocker & Grill, 2013; Chakraborty et al., 2022; Ganji et al., 2017). Smaller electrodes exhibit higher CIC values during transient voltage. For instance, considering SIROF with a consistent thickness, the CIC measures 5.1 mC cm^{-2} for an electrode size of 1960 µm^2, whereas it diminishes to 1.7 mC cm^{-2} as the electrode area extends up to 125,600 µm^2 (Cogan et al., 2009).

Adding coating layers to NES electrodes improves their stimulation capability. For instance, spin-coating PEDOT:PSS onto Au and Pt electrodes increased their CIC values by 9.5 and 3.2 times, respectively (Ganji et al., 2017). Microelectrodes composed of PtIr or Au and modified with PEDOT:PSS showed a CIC of 15 mC cm^{-2}, about three times greater than similar AIROF or SIROF electrodes (Cogan et al., 2007). Other materials, including Pt-black and CNTs, are also used to augment CIC (Arcot Desai et al., 2010; Zhou et al., 2013). Figure 5.6 shows microelectrodes modified with composite materials, incorporating PEDOT/CNTs-coated surface. The modified electrodes display a CIC of 5.68 mc cm^{-2}, exceeding that of the IrOx electrode (1 mc cm^{-2}) (Zheng et al., 2021b). This substantial difference notably enhances the energy efficiency for applications involving electrical stimulation.

5.4 MECHANICAL PROPERTIES FOR SOFT NEURAL INTERFACES

Rigid neural probes, such as silicon-based ones, are known to inflict damage on brain tissue and elicit chronic biological responses during long-term implantation. As depicted in Figure 5.7a, the initial phase involves the implantation of the probe into the brain, which triggers acute injury, activating microglia and astrocytes and resulting in tissue edema (Marin & Fernández, 2010). This acute response is characterized by a swift increase in

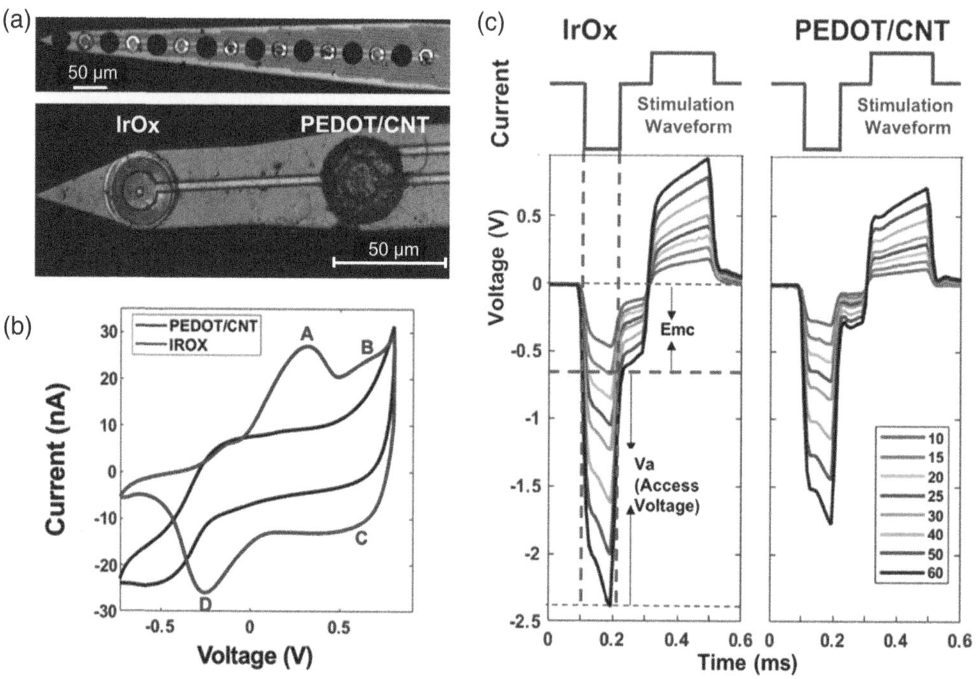

FIGURE 5.6   (a) IrOx-coated electrodes and PEDOT/CNT-coated electrodes for neural stimulation. CV curves (b) and CIC measurements (c) for both types of electrodes. Va represents access voltage and Emc indicates the electrode polarization voltage for calculating the CIC. (Adapted with permission. (Zheng et al., 2021b) Copyright 2021, Wiley-VCH.)

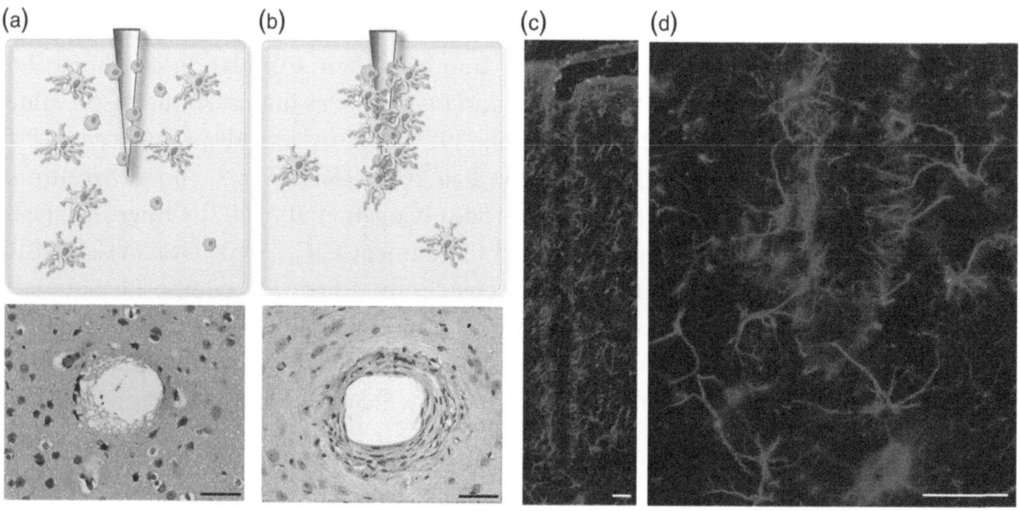

FIGURE 5.7   Inflammatory response of intracortical microelectrode. (a) Acute neural injury. Activated astrocytes and microglial cells migrate to the injury site. (b) Chronic response leads to the formation of a dense sheath around implanted probes, comprising fibroblasts, macrophages, and astrocytes. (c, d) The immunohistochemically labeled reactive astrocytes, identified by GFAP labeling, encapsulate the neural probes, forming a tightly packed cellular sheath. Scale bar: 50 μm. (Adapted with permission. (Marin & Fernández, 2010) Copyright 2010, Frontiers.)

electrode impedance within 1–3 weeks post-implantation (Polikov et al., 2005). During long-term implantation periods, micro-movements ensue between the probe and brain tissue due to mechanical property mismatches, transforming the inflammatory response into a persistent chronic phase (Nguyen et al., 2014), as shown in Figure 5.7b. This prolonged inflammation can lead to the formation of a glial scar around the electrode, insulating it (McConnell et al., 2009), as illustrated in Figure 5.7c and d. Additionally, it may cause neuronal death and migration around the electrode, increasing the distance between the electrode and neurons, and ultimately deteriorating neural signal quality (Campbell & Wu, 2018; Kozai et al., 2015).

Young's modulus is an intrinsic mechanical property of the material while bending stiffness dictates the mechanical interactions between the electrode and brain tissue during prolonged implantation (Renz et al., 2018). Bending stiffness is contingent on Young's modulus of the material and the material's shape, with thickness serving as the primary determinant (He et al., 2020). The bending stiffness is primarily determined by the substrate and encapsulation layers of neural electrodes, as the thickness of the conductive layer is considerably smaller. Reduced bending stiffness in ECoG electrode arrays implies a more conformal contact with the uneven brain surface (Alahi et al., 2021; Lacour et al., 2010), while for intracortical electrodes, it signifies diminished micromotion between the electrode and tissue, resulting in reduced chronic inflammation and glial scarring (Stiller et al., 2018).

5.4.1 Soft Substrate Materials

Flexible substrate materials, such as polydimethylsiloxane (PDMS), PI, parylene-C, SU-8, polyethylene terephthalate (PET), and hydrogels, exhibit Young's modulus that is more closely aligned with that of brain tissue (0.1–16 kPa) compared to rigid materials like silicon or metals (Alahi et al., 2021; Fekete & Pongrácz, 2017; Hong et al., 2018). These flexible substrates are used as thin-film substrate layers for neural electrodes. Table 5.3 summarizes the mechanical properties of these flexible materials employed in neural electrode substrates.

PI is a flexible polymer known for its high-temperature resistance and insulation properties (Liu et al., 2022). While the thickness of PI can be precisely controlled through spincoating, its tensile properties are less robust. Nevertheless, PI is a preferred soft substrate for neural electrodes due to its commendable chemical stability and biocompatibility (Constantin et al., 2019; Degenhart et al., 2016). Neuralink utilize ultrathin PI as the substrate for their flexible neural threads, with the total thickness ranging from 4–6 μm and width spanning 5 to 50 μm, enabling efficient implantation into the brain with robotic assistance (Musk & Neuralink, 2019).

PDMS, an elastomer material, is biocompatible, highly air permeable, and possesses an exceptionally low Young's modulus compared to PI, parylene-C, or SU-8 (Ariati et al., 2021; Wolf et al., 2018). While PDMS offers advantageous mechanical properties, it may deform when heated and is relatively incompatible with silicon-based micromachining processes. Additionally, its volume expansion post-implantation, due to increased temperature, can cause the metal layer to peel off from the substrate (Lacour et al., 2003). To address these challenges, a PDMS-based electrode array with an additional parylene-C layer between the

TABLE 5.3　Mechanical Properties of Substrate Materials

Materials	Young's Modulus (MPa)	Tensile Strength (MPa)	Elongation (%)	Ref.
Silicon	1.9×10^5	165	—	(Petersen, 1982)
PI[a]	8540	350	25	(Stieglitz et al., 2000)
PDMS[b]	1.32–2.97	3.51–7.65	140	(Johnston et al., 2014)
Parylene-C	2900	77	24.7	(Von Metzen & Stieglitz, 2013)
SU-8[c]	2000	60	6.5	(Abgrall et al., 2007)
PET	2000–2700	50	90–120	(Gupta et al., 2009; Kunugi et al., 1986)
SBS	45	1.4	18.2	(Imai et al., 2023)
Silk hydrogel	1.2–10.7	4.4	350	(Cui et al., 2021)

[a]　PI (PYRALIN 2611)

[b]　PDMS (SYLGARD 184)

[c]　SU-8 (Microchem 2000 Series)

PDMS and the metal layer was developed, enhancing mechanical and thermal strength while maintaining the inherent flexibility and consistency of PDMS. This approximately 80-μm thick electrode array is robust enough to be self-supporting and remains flexible, ensuring conformal contact with the brain (Lee et al., 2020).

Parylene-C, an FDA-approved polymer known for its high biocompatibility, is widely used as a coating for various biological applications (Hassler et al., 2010; Von Metzen & Stieglitz, 2013). However, its low tensile strength and susceptibility to layering compared to other materials limit its long-term in vivo use. Researchers employed pinhole-free 2-μm thick parylene-C as a substrate and encapsulation to create an ultra-thin (4-μm thickness) NeuroGrid, which successfully recorded the LFP and action potentials of cortical neurons on the cerebral cortex (Khodagholy et al., 2015).

SU-8, a negative photoresist with a high aspect ratio, meets biocompatibility standards (ISO 10993) and boasts high chemical and mechanical stability, light transmittance (>400 nm), and ease of fabrication (Altuna et al., 2013; Nemani et al., 2013; Nordström et al., 2008). Xie et al. utilized SU-8 to construct insulation and encapsulation layers, creating ultra-thin (a few microns thick, minimum 1-μm thick) film neural electrode interfaces. The subcellular size and ultra-flexibility result in reliable, glial scarring-free neural integration (Luan et al., 2017; Wei et al., 2018; Zhao et al., 2023).

Additionally, PET, polystyrene-*block*-polybutadiene-*block*-polystyrene (SBS), and hydrogels find application as substrate materials for neural electrodes (Imai et al., 2023; Kunori & Takashima, 2015; Oribe et al., 2019). PET film, recognized for its stable thermal and chemical properties, biocompatibility, high light transmittance, and compatibility with micro-processing technology, is frequently chosen as the substrate material for neural electrodes, particularly transparent neural electrodes (Kumar et al., 2019; Seo et al., 2020; Sin & Tueen, 2022). SBS, a thermoplastic elastomer boasting a lower Young's modulus compared to PI, parylene-C, or SU-8, has been effectively utilized to prepare a flexible electrode array, approximately 8-μm thick (Imai et al., 2023). This array was successfully implanted on the cortical surface of rats for in vivo ECoG recording and electrical stimulation, with no severe inflammatory reactions observed even after six weeks of implantation. Young's modulus of hydrogels is considerably lower than that of other flexible materials, approaching the elasticity of brain tissue (Huang et al., 2018). The mechanical strength of silk hydrogels was enhanced through the incorporation of PEGylated silk protein with poly(ethylene glycol) diglycidyl ether, resulting in the fabrication of silk hydrogel-based transparent PEDOT:PSS neural electrodes (Cui et al., 2021).

5.4.2 Implantation Strategies

The inherent flexibility of intracortical probes poses challenges in direct insertion into the cortex without bending (Apollo et al., 2020; Sharafkhani et al., 2022). Various strategies contribute to facilitating the implantation of flexible probes, with two primary approaches commonly used (Patel et al., 2015). One method involves using a rigid guide shuttle (Guo et al., 2022; Musk & Neuralink, 2019; Zhao et al., 2019), as shown in Figure 5.8a and b, which enables the precise positioning of a flexible probe. Another approach focuses on dynamically altering the hardness of the electrode itself. For example, electrodes can be enveloped with biodegradable or soluble materials, such as PEG, silk, carboxymethylcellulose, and maltose, before implantation (Kozai et al., 2014; Lecomte et al., 2015; Tien et al., 2013; Xiang et al., 2014). These coatings undergo degradation or dissolution within the tissue after implantation. Alternatively, as illustrated in Figure 5.8c, hydrogel-coated electrodes can undergo a temporary hardening process by dehydration prior to implantation and subsequently absorb water from the surrounding tissue and revert to a softened state after implantation (Park et al., 2021). This dual-state characteristic aids in the ease of insertion while maintaining the required flexibility for optimal performance after implantation. Moreover, freezing can also impart adaptive bending stiffness to some neural probes (Xie et al., 2015).

5.4.3 Structure Design

In addition to thin-film electrode arrays and micro-wires, mesh electronics have gained widespread use for achieving enhanced conformability within the cerebral cortex and deep brain regions. Hole mesh and finger mesh configurations (Kaiju et al., 2017; Dae-Hyeong Kim et al., 2010a) are employed to intricately cover complex brain surfaces, while 3D mesh structures are utilized for recording activities within the deep brain (Liu et al., 2015; Xie et al., 2015). Sub-micrometer-thick, centimeter-scale macroporous mesh electronics were introduced into the brains of mice using a needle with a diameter as small as 100 μm. These mesh electronic devices, once injected into the brains of mice, seamlessly integrate with the neural tissue, exhibiting low chronic immune reactivity, and reliably monitor brain activity (Liu et al., 2015). Moreover, certain design strategies, such as incorporating papercut structures and serpentine wiring, not only maintain the intrinsic flexibility of the array but also introduce additional stretchability to accommodate deformations caused by the pulsation of the brain (Ji et al., 2020; Morikawa et al., 2018).

5.5 SOFT ELECTRONICS FOR MULTIMODAL NEURAL INTERFACES

The artifacts stemming from NES pose significant challenges when attempting simultaneous NES and electrophysiological recording (Gnadt et al., 2003). The advancement and

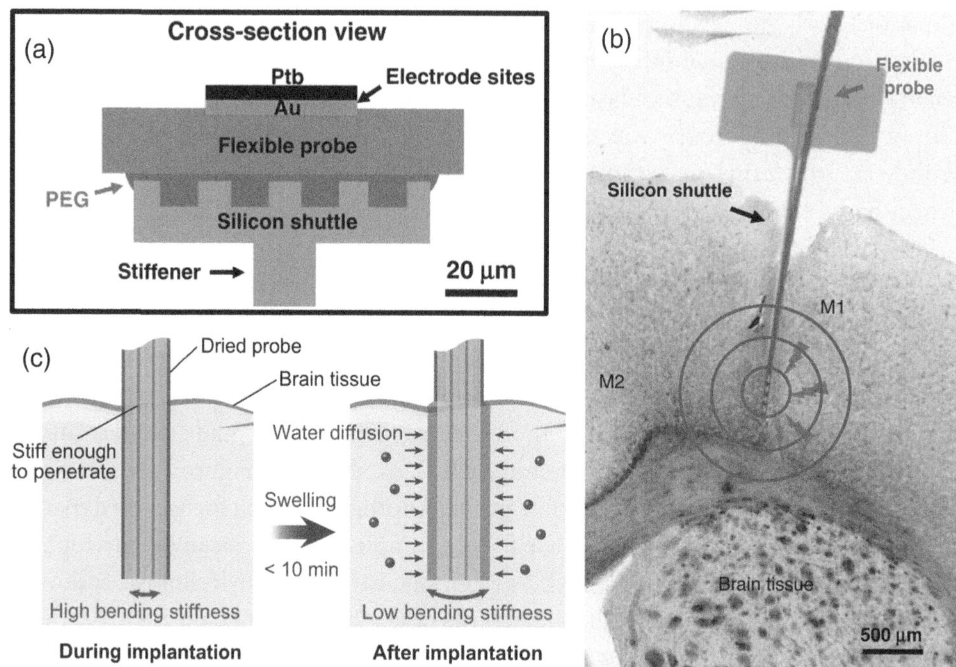

FIGURE 5.8   Implantation strategies. (a) A flexible probe connected to a silicon-based shuttle integrated with PEG to augment bending stiffness. (b) Implantation of the probe in (a) into the targeted brain region facilitated by the shuttle. (c) The adaptation of hydrogel-wrapped electrodes to bending stiffness through water absorption post-implantation. ([a] Adapted with permission. (Guo et al., 2022) Copyright 2023, Springer Nature; [b, c] Adapted with permission. (Park et al., 2021) Copyright 2023, Springer Nature.)

refinement of optical brain imaging and optogenetics provide an alternative path for brain observation and modulation (Hong & Lieber, 2019). Optical imaging of the brain compensates for the spatial resolution limitations inherent in electrophysiological recording, and when combined with electrophysiological recordings, it yields more comprehensive information for brain observation. Combining optical recording with NES effectively avoids the artifacts associated with the latter. Furthermore, unlike spatially dispersed NES, light stimulation is both localized and cell-specific. Its integration with electrophysiological recordings becomes a valuable tool for studying neural circuits (Chen et al., 2017). Integrating electrophysiology with magnetic resonance imaging (MRI) addresses the constraint of localized electrophysiological recording, enabling observation across various brain regions (Pan et al., 2023). This section further explores the soft electronic devices for multimodal neural interfaces, ensuring compatibility with electrical, optical, or magnetic modalities.

5.5.1 Flexible Transparent Electrodes

Transparent neural electrodes enable simultaneous light modulation (optogenetics) and electrophysiology or simultaneous electrical stimulation and optical imaging of the brain (Cho, Lim, et al., 2022b; Park et al., 2016). High transmittance of neural electrodes is crucial for light penetration, stimulating, or imaging neurons or blood vessels beneath the electrode. Various transparent conductive materials have been utilized to concurrently observe and modulate the brain by integrating optical and electrical approaches.

As a carbon-based material, graphene boasts over 97% visible light transmittance and high transmittance (90%) in the UV and IR bands (Nair et al., 2008). Transparent neural electrodes were fabricated using CVD graphene transferred onto parylene-C, achieving transmittance exceeding 90% at 470 nm and 570 nm. These electrodes have been effectively utilized in applications such as fluorescence imaging, OCT imaging, and optogenetics (Park et al., 2018; Park et al., 2014). Several studies have successfully demonstrated the effectiveness of utilizing graphene neural electrodes on PET films to produce an optoelectronic artifact-free signal by using complex transfer techniques to create the electrodes (Thunemann et al., 2018). Ultimately, these electrodes have been applied for deep 2P calcium imaging, angiography, and optogenetics (Figure 5.9). CNTs also demonstrated superior light transmittance. Duan et al. produced a stretchable transparent electrode array of CNT mesh films on PDMS with 70–90% light transmittance (at 550 nm), demonstrating photoelectric artifact-free properties and usage in optogenetic and 2P calcium imaging (Zhang et al., 2018).

The conductive polymer PEDOT:PSS is widely used for transparent neural interfaces. Integrating PEDOT:PSS with silk hydrogels produces a transparent neural electrode characterized by exceptional stretchability and electrical properties (>85% transparency from visible to near-infrared) (Cui et al., 2021). This electrode facilitates electrophysiological tracking concurrently with light stimulation of blood vessels. Moreover, it enables electrical stimulation in conjunction with simultaneous OISI and OCT imaging. Another study patterned PEDOT:PSS-based electrodes on a PET substrate, achieving 85% transmittance in the visible light range, utilized for optogenetics (Cho, Lee, et al., 2022a).

Additionally, metal oxides like ITO have been used but are limited by brittleness (Kunori & Takashima, 2015; Ledochowitsch et al., 2015). Strategies, including adding metal interconnects or metal conductive layers (ultra-thin metal layer, metal grid), are adopted to prevent ITO fragmentation on flexible substrates (Chen et al., 2020; Jimbo et al., 2017). In a study, fully transparent microelectrode arrays of hybrid PEDOT: PSS-ITO-Ag-ITO

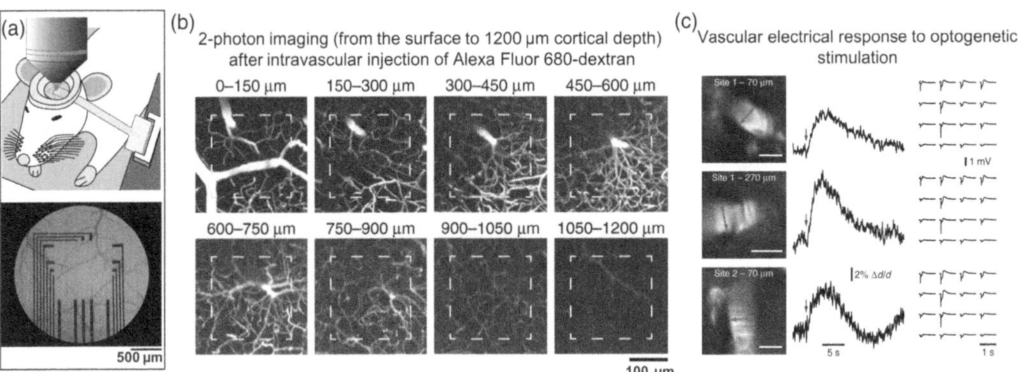

FIGURE 5.9 Artifact-free transparent graphene microelectrode arrays (a) for deep brain (at a depth of 1,200 μm) two-photon imaging (b), optogenetics, and electrophysiological recording (c). (Adapted with permission. (Thunemann et al., 2018) Copyright 2023, Springer Nature.)

assemblies on thin parylene-C films achieved a maximum light transmittance of 91%, used for recording light-evoked ECoG oscillations from a rat cortex (Yang et al., 2021). Indium zinc oxide (IZO) and AgNWs were also used for neural interfaces, yielding 74% light transmittance (at 550 nm) (Neto et al., 2021).

Metals can improve their transparency beyond their inherent limitations on light transmittance through nanometer-thick films, grids, and nanowires (Tian et al., 2021). The duty cycle of the gold metal grid was optimized, resulting in the attainment of the highest light transmittance, approximately 69% (Lee et al., 2017). The Au/PEDOT:PSS nanomesh microelectrode array on flexible parylene-C achieved a maximum light transmittance of 70%, utilized for simultaneous two-photon Ca^{2+} imaging and electrophysiological recording of an awake mouse (Qiang et al., 2017).

5.5.2 Soft Electronics for Optogenetics

Flexible neural electrode arrays, integrating microscale inorganic light-emitting diodes (μ-ILEDs) or optical fiber through soft electronic technology, can be utilized for synchronous light stimulation and neural electrophysiological recording (Scharf et al., 2016; Tian et al., 2022). In a groundbreaking approach, Rogers et al. integrated several independently addressable μ-ILEDs with microelectrodes, photodetectors, and thermometer sensors in a multilayer configuration, forming a multifunctional optoelectronic system with a total thickness of approximately 20 μm (Kim et al., 2013). The slim and flexible design of the device mitigates neuronal loss, glioma formation, and immune reactivity. Following injection into the mice brain via a microneedle, the probe with integrated μ-ILEDs maintained functional integrity in freely moving animals for several months. Anikeeva and Zhao et al. incorporated a microscale optical fiber, a microelectrode array with seven insulated tin microwires, and polyethyleneimine tubes for microfluidic channels into a soft hydrogel matrix. The hydration-dependent flexural stiffness of the hydrogel matrix facilitates easy implantation, reduces stress on surrounding brain tissues, and enhances overall biocompatibility (Park et al., 2021). Leveraging elastomeric stamp transfer printing technology, Huang et al. transferred a flexible microelectrode array with PI as the substrate to the optical fiber. Featuring a total of four optical fibers, each microelectrode array on the fiber has eight channels, providing four selectable wavelengths and distributed high-throughput electrophysiological sensing (Yu et al., 2021). The neural probe realized simultaneous light stimulation and electrophysiological recording in the brains of freely moving rats. Additionally, Zhou et al. utilized the thermal drawing process to controllably embed and distribute metal electrodes in a biocompatible polymer fiber with a double-clad optical waveguide, achieving long-term (>10 weeks) simultaneous light stimulation and neural recording at the single-cell level in behavioral mice (Figure 5.10) (Du et al., 2020).

5.5.3 Soft Electronics for MRI-Compatible Electrodes

Simultaneous monitoring of neural electrophysiology and MRI holds significant promise for advancing the diagnosis and treatment of various neurodegenerative diseases (Oribe et al., 2019). However, metal electrodes can introduce artifacts in MRI images due to their magnetic susceptibility mismatch with brain tissue and water. Additionally, radiofrequency fields in MRI may heat probe, potentially causing brain damage, and gradient fields from coils can generate eddy currents in conductive materials. To address these challenges, Fallegger et al. employed stretchable gold thin films and Pt-silicone composite as electrode coatings. They designed ECoG electrode arrays of varied sizes (250 μm to 5 mm diameter) and layouts (0.2 to 10 mm electrode spacing) on 150 μm-thick silicone membranes (Fallegger et al., 2021). In the presence of a 3T MRI scanner, as depicted in Figure 5.11a–h, this array displayed no imaging artifacts (less than 1 mm, in contrast to clinical grids that exhibit nearly 1 cm length), and no local tissue heating, thereby enabling an accurate diagnosis.

Certain MRI-compatible materials were introduced into the neural electrodes to mitigate geometric signal distortion caused by the magnetic field during MRI. The magnetic susceptibility of copper is close to that of brain tissue and water. Zhao et al. deposited graphene on a 100-μm diameter copper wire and encapsulated it with parylene-C, preventing direct contact between copper and brain tissue while averting corrosion (Zhao et al., 2020). Comparative analysis with Pt microwire of the same size revealed negligible artifacts in the electrode at a high magnetic field of 7-Tesla (7T), signifying superior MRI compatibility. In

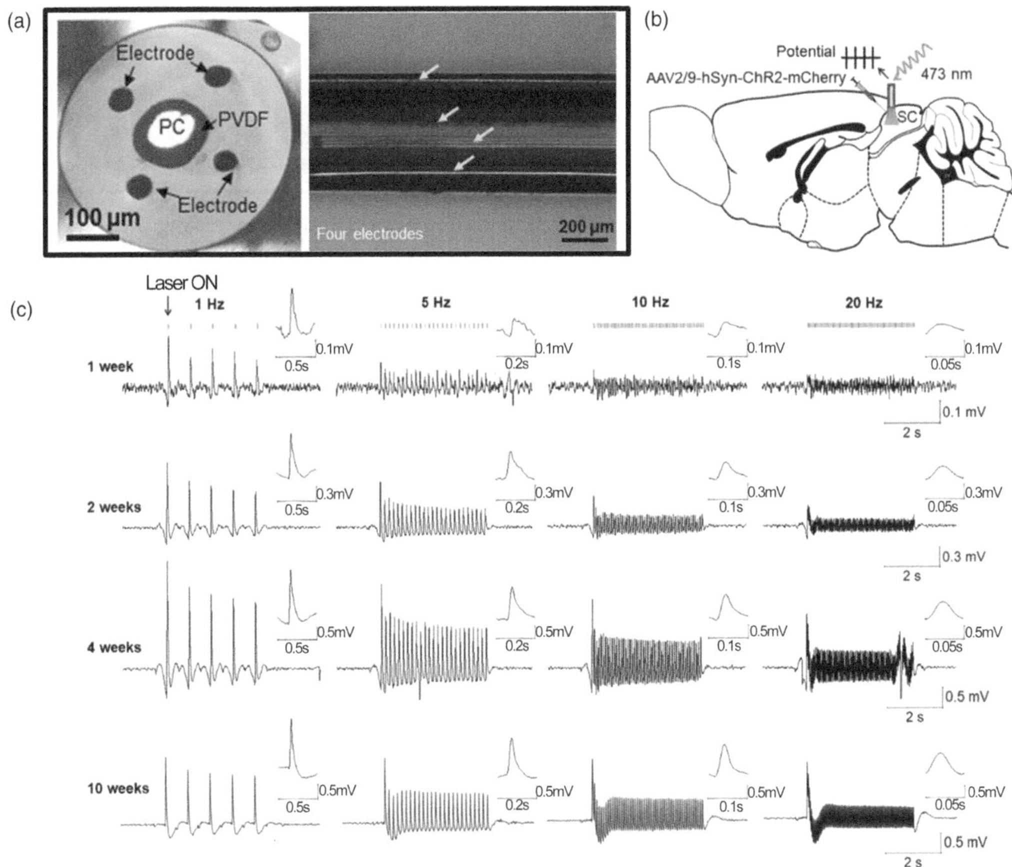

FIGURE 5.10 Flexible fiber probe for optogenetics. (a) Polymer fiber with four metal electrodes. (b, c) Simultaneous light stimulation and neural recording (lasting from 1 to 10 weeks). (Adapted with permission. (Du et al., 2020) Copyright 2020, Wiley-VCH.)

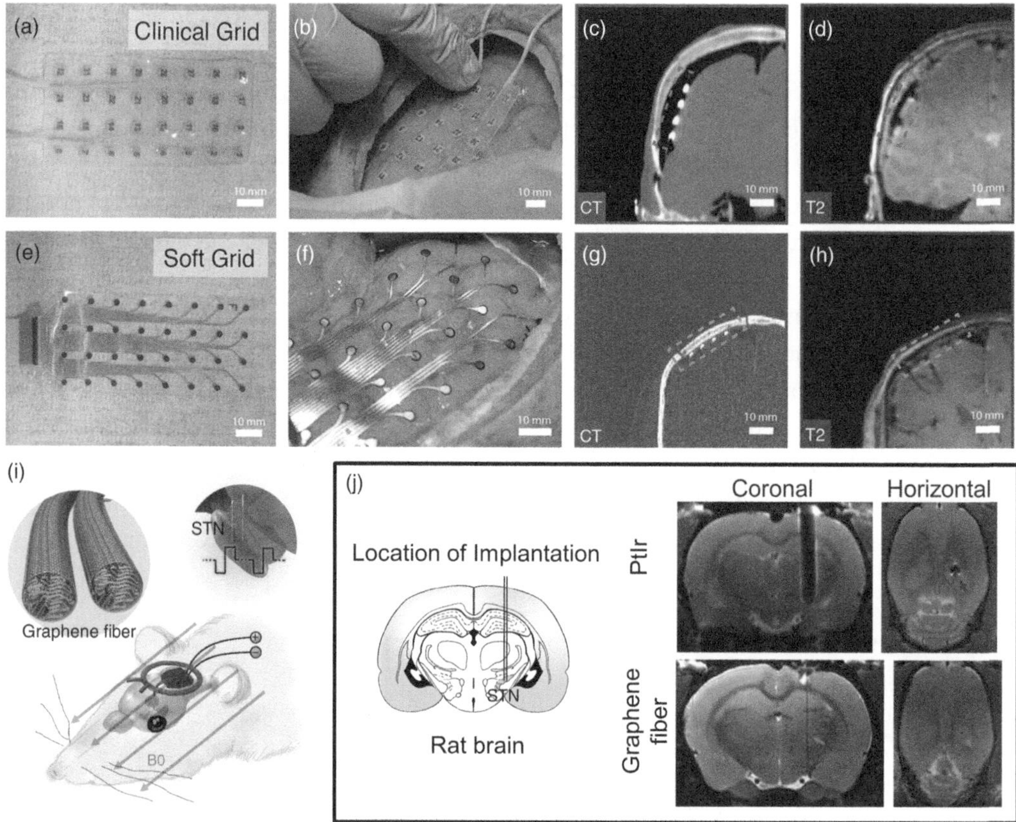

FIGURE 5.11   MRI-compatible electrodes. A clinical ECoG grid (a, b) and a soft ECoG grid (e, f) were implanted and placed on the surface of the cadaveric specimen. CT and T2-weighted MRI scans of the clinical ECoG grid (c, d) and the soft ECoG grid (g, h) The dashed line boxes indicate the position of two grids, respectively. (i) Graphene fiber for neural stimulation and MRI scanning. (j) MRI artifact size of graphene fiber and PtIr wires implanted to the subthalamic nucleus (STN). ([a–h] Adapted with permission. (Fallegger et al., 2021) Copyright 2021, Wiley-VCH; [i, j] Adapted with permission. (Zhao et al., 2020) Copyright 2023, Springer Nature.)

another study shown in Figure 5.11i and j, Zhao et al. developed graphene fiber electrodes with high CIC and no MRI artifact at 9.4T for DBS-fMRI (Zhao et al., 2020). Furthermore, Lu et al. demonstrated minimal artifacts in 7T magnetic resonance scans with CNT fiber electrodes (20-μm diameter), considerably smaller than PtIr microwire, allowing for the visualization of brain tissue near the electrodes (Lu et al., 2019). Furthermore, Cho et al. developed a flexible transparent electrode based on PEDOT:PSS and successfully applied it in 9.4T high magnetic fields, showcasing its artifact-free properties (2023).

5.6 RECENT ADVANCES IN SOFT ELECTRONICS FOR NEURAL INTERFACES

High-resolution and multichannel neural electrode arrays are at the forefront of advancements in implantable neural interfaces. The primary goal is to enhance the spatial coverage provided by soft electronics while maintaining the resolution of individual cells.

One approach involves reducing the dimensions of electrodes and interconnects to a few microns using micro–nanoprocessing techniques such as lithography and electron-beam lithography. However, this approach poses the risk of increasing electrode impedance.

For example, the nanoelectronic thread (NET) series electrodes, developed by Xie et al. using specialized photolithography, feature interconnect wires measuring only 2–3 μm. These electrodes integrate 16 electrodes on a single array with a width of 30 μm and the most densely implanted arrays achieve approximately 1000 recording sites per cubic mm of cortical volume. In Musk et al.'s Neuralink, individual threads created through lithography consist of 48 or 96 threads, each hosting 32 electrodes with contacts spaced at 50 μm or 75 μm. Each thread also exhibits a small geometric surface area of $14 \times 24 \ \mu m^2$.

An alternative method involves active matrix addressing technology, incorporating active devices in the electrode front end to multiplex the electrode interconnection lines. This method reduces the interconnection line area, enhancing electrode resolution. The Neural Matrix integrates an active matrix based on flexible silicon transistors, featuring a kilo-scale 28×36 electrode neural matrix array in $9 \times 9.24 \ mm^2$ for brain mapping in non-human primates.

In addition to multiplexing, various transistors, such as organic electrochemical transistors (OECTs), graphene solution–gated transistors, and zinc oxide thin-film transistors (ZnO-TFTs), can serve as preamplifiers for the electrodes. Noise is inevitably introduced during the transmission of electrophysiological signals from the interconnect to the amplifier. Placing the preamplifiers at the front end can mitigate the impact of noise on neural signals during the transmission process, thereby enhancing the SNR. OECTs, embedded in ultrathin organic films, demonstrate superior performance in recording electrophysiological signals from the brain surface, achieving a high SNR through local amplification. In a study by Zhang et al., a fully transparent active electrode array using ZnO-TFTs as front-end amplifiers was fabricated (Figure 5.12). This array was employed for simultaneous cortical electrophysiological recordings and optical stimulation, resulting in neuro-electrical signals with a notably high SNR.

Soft neural implants can be designed to be transient or bioresorbable, allowing them to be naturally absorbed by the body after a certain period. This feature eliminates the need for surgical removal, reducing the invasiveness of the implantation procedure and minimizing potential long-term risks. Luo et al. developed a bioabsorbable device using poly(l-lactide) and polycaprolactone (PLLA/PCL) composites with a transient metal, molybdenum. This device functioned for electrophysiological recording and intracranial pressure sensing, remaining functional in vivo for approximately five days before complete absorption within 100 days. Rogers et al. engineered a biodegradable device comprising Si photodetectors, poly(lactic-co-glycolic acid) (PLGA) fibers, Zn electrodes, SiO_2 insulating layers, and PLGA substrates. This device continuously monitors brain temperature, oxygenation, and neural activity in freely moving mice and is entirely absorbed by the human body after a controlled service life.

The convergence of soft electronic technology with wireless transmission allows for real-time data transmission, making these devices more practical for long-term monitoring and modulation of the brain in freely moving animals. The integration of flexible probes

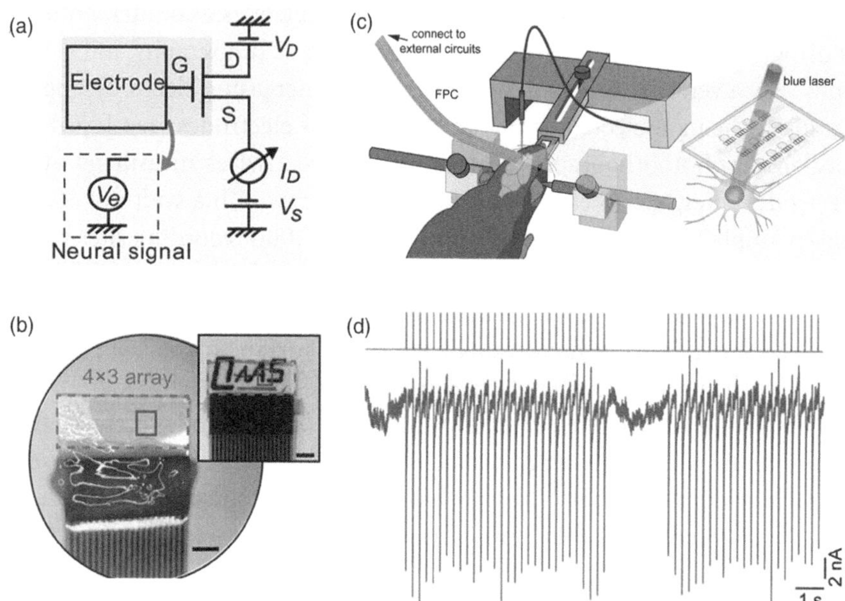

FIGURE 5.12   Multimodal ECoG active electrode array based on ZnO-TFTs. (a) Circuit diagram of ZnO-TFT electrode array. Ve represents the neural signals captured by the gate electrode and the transistors are biased by voltage sources at the drain and source. A colored square indicates the brain tissue. (b) An image of the ZnO-TFT array. Scale bar: 2.5 mm. The inset showcases its high transparency. Scale bar: 2 mm. The dashed frames outline the edge of the electrode array, while the dark red frames indicate the electrode region. (c, d) The transparent ZnO-TFT array is used for optogenetics. (Adapted with permission. (Zhang et al., 2023) Copyright 2022, Wiley-VCH.)

with electronic systems is crucial in advancing implantable systems that are biocompatible, fully-integrated, and equipped with high spatiotemporal resolution and multimodal capabilities.

In conclusion, soft neural electronics contribute significantly to the evolution of neural engineering and brain–computer interfaces by addressing critical aspects such as biocompatibility, flexibility, multimodal integration, and high-resolution recording. These innovations pave the way for safer, more effective, and longer-term neural interfaces, bringing us closer to unlocking the full potential of brain–machine communication and interaction.

REFERENCES

Abdulkader, S. N., Atia, A., Mostafa, M.-S. M. (2015). Brain computer interfacing: Applications and challenges. *Egyptian Informatics Journal*, 16(2), 213–230.

Abgrall, P., Conedera, V., Camon, H., Gue, A. M., Nguyen, N. T. (2007). SU-8 as a structural material for labs-on-chips and microelectromechanical systems. *Electrophoresis*, 28(24), 4539–4551.

Alahi, M. E. E., Liu, Y., Xu, Z., Wang, H., Wu, T., Mukhopadhyay, S. C. (2021). Recent advancement of electrocorticography (ECoG) electrodes for chronic neural recording/stimulation. *Materials Today Communications*, 29, 102853.

Altuna, A., Bellistri, E., Cid, E., Aivar, P., Gal, B., Berganzo, J., Fernández, L. J. (2013). SU-8 based microprobes for simultaneous neural depth recording and drug delivery in the brain. *Lab on a Chip*, 13(7), 1422–1430.

Alvarez, N. T., Buschbeck, E., Miller, S., Le, A. D., Gupta, V. K., Ruhunage, C., Ma, Y. (2020). Carbon nanotube fibers for neural recording and stimulation. *ACS Applied BioMaterials*, 3(9), 6478–6487.

Apollo, N. V., Murphy, B., Prezelski, K., Driscoll, N., Richardson, A. G., Lucas, T. H., Vitale, F. (2020). Gels, jets, mosquitoes, and magnets: a review of implantation strategies for soft neural probes. *Journal of Neural Engineering*, 17(4), 041002.

Aqrawe, Z., Montgomery, J., Travas-Sejdic, J., Svirskis, D. (2018). Conducting polymers for neuronal microelectrode array recording and stimulation. *Sensors and Actuators B: Chemical*, 257, 753–765.

Aqrawe, Z., Wright, B., Patel, N., Vyas, Y., Malmstrom, J., Montgomery, J. M., Svirskis, D. (2019). The influence of macropores on PEDOT/PSS microelectrode coatings for neuronal recording and stimulation. *Sensors and Actuators B: Chemical*, 281, 549–560.

Arcot Desai, S., Rolston, J. D., Guo, L., Potter, S. M. (2010). Improving impedance of implantable microwire multi-electrode arrays by ultrasonic electroplating of durable platinum black. *Frontiers in Neuroengineering*, 3, 1303.

Ariati, R., Sales, F., Souza, A., Lima, R. A., Ribeiro, J. (2021). Polydimethylsiloxane composites characterization and its applications: a review. *Polymers*, 13(23), 4258.

Bakhshaee Babaroud, N., Palmar, M., Velea, A. I., Coletti, C., Weingärtner, S., Vos, F., Giagka, V. (2022). Multilayer CVD graphene electrodes using a transfer-free process for the next generation of optically transparent and MRI-compatible neural interfaces. *Microsystems & Nanoengineering*, 8(1), 107.

Baranauskas, G., Maggiolini, E., Castagnola, E., Ansaldo, A., Mazzoni, A., Angotzi, G. N., Fadiga, L. (2011). Carbon nanotube composite coating of neural microelectrodes preferentially improves the multiunit signal-to-noise ratio. *Journal of Neural Engineering*, 8(6), 066013.

Birbaumer, N. (2006). Breaking the silence: brain–computer interfaces (BCI) for communication and motor control. *Psychophysiology*, 43(6), 517–532.

Bobacka, J., Lewenstam, A., Ivaska, A. (2000). Electrochemical impedance spectroscopy of oxidized poly (3, 4-ethylenedioxythiophene) film electrodes in aqueous solutions. *Journal of Electroanalytical Chemistry*, 489(1–2), 17–27.

Boehler, C., Carli, S., Fadiga, L., Stieglitz, T., Asplund, M. (2020). Tutorial: guidelines for standardized performance tests for electrodes intended for neural interfaces and bioelectronics. *Nature Protocols*, 15(11), 3557–3578.

Bourrier, A., Shkorbatova, P., Bonizzato, M., Rey, E., Barraud, Q., Courtine, G., Delacour, C. (2019). Monolayer graphene coating of intracortical probes for long-lasting neural activity monitoring. *Advanced Healthcare Materials*, 8(18), 1801331.

Brocker, D. T., Grill, W. M. (2013). Principles of electrical stimulation of neural tissue. *Handbook of Clinical Neurology*, 116, 3–18.

Brummer, S., Turner, M. (1975). Electrical stimulation of the nervous system: the principle of safe charge injection with noble metal electrodes. *Bioelectrochemistry and Bioenergetics*, 2(1), 13–25.

Brummer, S., Turner, M. (1977a). Electrical stimulation with Pt electrodes: II-estimation of maximum surface redox (theoretical non-gassing) limits. *IEEE Transactions on Biomedical Engineering*, 5, 440–443.

Brummer, S. B., Turner, M. (1977b). Electrochemical considerations for safe electrical stimulation of the nervous system with platinum electrodes. *IEEE Transactions on Biomedical Engineering*, 1, 59–63.

Buzsáki, G., Anastassiou, C. A., Koch, C. (2012). The origin of extracellular fields and currents — EEG, ECoG, LFP and spikes. *Nature Reviews Neuroscience*, 13(6), 407–420.

Campbell, A., Wu, C. (2018). Chronically implanted intracranial electrodes: tissue reaction and electrical changes. *Micromachines*, 9(9), 430.

Campbell, P. K., Jones, K. E., Huber, R. J., Horch, K. W., Normann, R. A. (1991). A silicon-based, three-dimensional neural interface: manufacturing processes for an intracortical electrode array. *IEEE Transactions on Biomedical Engineering*, 38(8), 758–768.

Chakraborty, B., Joshi-Imre, A., Cogan, S. F. (2022). Charge injection characteristics of sputtered ruthenium oxide electrodes for neural stimulation and recording. *Journal of Biomedical Materials Research Part B: Applied Biomaterials*, 110(1), 229–238.

Chen, C.-H., Lin, C.-T., Hsu, W.-L., Chang, Y.-C., Yeh, S.-R., Li, L.-J., Yao, D.-J. (2013). A flexible hydrophilic-modified graphene microprobe for neural and cardiac recording. *Nanomedicine: Nanotechnology, Biology and Medicine*, 9(5), 600–604.

Chen, R., Canales, A., Anikeeva, P. (2017). Neural recording and modulation technologies. *Nature Reviews Materials*, 2(2), 1–16.

Chen, Z., Yin, R. T., Obaid, S. N., Tian, J., Chen, S. W., Miniovich, A. N., Lu, L. (2020). Flexible and transparent metal oxide/metal grid hybrid interfaces for electrophysiology and optogenetics. *Advanced Materials Technologies*, 5(8), 2000322.

Cho, Y. U., Kim, K., Dutta, A., Park, S. H., Lee, J. Y., Kim, H. W., Won, C. (2023). MRI-Compatible, Transparent PEDOT: PSS Neural Implants for the Alleviation of Neuropathic Pain with Motor Cortex Stimulation. *Advanced Functional Materials*, 34, 2310908.

Cho, Y. U., Lee, J. Y., Jeong, U. J., Park, S. H., Lim, S. L., Kim, K. Y., Shin, H. (2022a). Ultra-low cost, facile fabrication of transparent neural electrode array for electrocorticography with photoelectric artifact-free optogenetics. *Advanced Functional Materials*, 32(10), 2105568.

Cho, Y. U., Lim, S. L., Hong, J.-H., Yu, K. J. (2022b). Transparent neural implantable devices: a comprehensive review of challenges and progress. *NPJ Flexible Electronics*, 6(1), 1–18.

Cogan, S. F. (2008). Neural stimulation and recording electrodes. *Annu. Rev. Biomed. Eng.*, 10, 275–309.

Cogan, S. F., Ehrlich, J., Plante, T. D., Smirnov, A., Shire, D. B., Gingerich, M., Rizzo, J. F. (2009). Sputtered iridium oxide films for neural stimulation electrodes. *Journal of Biomedical Materials Research Part B: Applied Biomaterials*, 89B(2), 353–361.

Cogan, S. F., Peramunage, D., Smirnov, A., Ehrlich, J., McCreery, D. B., Manoonkitiwongsa, P. S. (2007). Polyethylenedioxythiophene (PEDOT) coatings for neural stimulation and recording electrodes. *Materials Research Society Meetings*, 2007, 26–30.

Cogan, S. F., Plante, T., Ehrlich, J. (2004). Sputtered iridium oxide films (SIROFs) for low-impedance neural stimulation and recording electrodes. *The 26th Annual International Conference of the IEEE Engineering in Medicine and Biology Society*,

Cogan, S. F., Troyk, P. R., Ehrlich, J., Plante, T. D., Detlefsen, D. E. (2006). Potential-biased, asymmetric waveforms for charge-injection with activated iridium oxide (AIROF) neural stimulation electrodes. *IEEE Transactions on Biomedical Engineering*, 53(2), 327–332.

Constantin, C. P., Aflori, M., Damian, R. F., Rusu, R. D. (2019). Biocompatibility of polyimides: A mini-review. *Materials*, 12(19), 3166.

Cui, Y., Zhang, F., Chen, G., Yao, L., Zhang, N., Liu, Z., Chen, X. (2021). A stretchable and transparent electrode based on PEGylated silk fibroin for in vivo dual-modal neural-vascular activity probing. *Advanced Materials*, 33(34), 2100221.

Dalrymple, A. N., Huynh, M., Nayagam, B. A., Lee, C. D., Weiland, G. R., Petrossians, A., Shepherd, R. K. (2020). Electrochemical and biological characterization of thin-film platinum-iridium alloy electrode coatings: a chronic in vivo study. *Journal of Neural Engineering*, 17(3), 036012.

Degenhart, A. D., Eles, J., Dum, R., Mischel, J. L., Smalianchuk, I., Endler, B., Wang, W. (2016). Histological evaluation of a chronically-implanted electrocorticographic electrode grid in a non-human primate. *Journal of Neural Engineering*, 13(4), 046019.

Deslouis, C., El Moustafid, T., Musiani, M., Tribollet, B. (1996). Mixed ionic-electronic conduction of a conducting polymer film. Ac impedance study of polypyrrole. *Electrochimica Acta*, 41(7–8), 1343–1349.

Devi, M., Vomero, M., Fuhrer, E., Castagnola, E., Gueli, C., Nimbalkar, S., Sharma, S. (2021). Carbon-based neural electrodes: Promises and challenges. *Journal of Neural Engineering*, 18(4), 041007.

Dong, S., Chen, W., Wang, X., Zhang, S., Xu, K., Zheng, X. (2017). Flexible ECoG electrode for implantation and neural signal recording applications. *Vacuum*, 140, 96–100.

Du, M., Huang, L., Zheng, J., Xi, Y., Dai, Y., Zhang, W., So, K. F. (2020). Flexible fiber probe for efficient neural stimulation and detection. *Advanced Science*, 7(15), 2001410.

Fallegger, F., Schiavone, G., Pirondini, E., Wagner, F. B., Vachicouras, N., Serex, L., Palma, M. (2021). MRI-Compatible and conformal electrocorticography grids for translational research. *Advanced Science*, 8(9), 2003761.

Feig, V. R., Tran, H., Lee, M., Liu, K., Huang, Z., Beker, L., Bao, Z. (2019). An electrochemical gelation method for patterning conductive PEDOT: PSS hydrogels. *Advanced Materials*, 31(39), 1902869.

Fekete, Z., Pongrácz, A. (2017). Multifunctional soft implants to monitor and control neural activity in the central and peripheral nervous system: a review. *Sensors and Actuators B: Chemical*, 243, 1214–1223.

Fertonani, A., Miniussi, C. (2017). Transcranial electrical stimulation: what we know and do not know about mechanisms. *The Neuroscientist*, 23(2), 109–123.

Fouad, M. M., Amin, K. M., El-Bendary, N., Hassanien, A. E. (2015). Brain computer interface: a review. *Brain-Computer Interfaces: Current Trends and Applications*, 3–30. https://doi.org/10.1007/978-3-319-10978-7_1

Ganji, M., Tanaka, A., Gilja, V., Halgren, E., Dayeh, S. A. (2017). Scaling effects on the electrochemical stimulation performance of Au, Pt, and PEDOT: PSS electrocorticography arrays. *Advanced Functional Materials*, 27(42), 1703019.

Garma, L. D., Ferrari, L. M., Scognamiglio, P., Greco, F., Santoro, F. (2019). Inkjet-printed PEDOT: PSS multi-electrode arrays for low-cost in vitro electrophysiology. *Lab on a Chip*, 19(22), 3776–3786.

Gnadt, J. W., Echols, S. D., Yildirim, A., Zhang, H., Paul, K. (2003). Spectral cancellation of microstimulation artifact for simultaneous neural recording in situ. *IEEE Transactions on Biomedical Engineering*, 50(10), 1129–1135.

Gordon, B., Lesser, R. P., Rance, N. E., Hart Jr, J., Webber, R., Uematsu, S., Fisher, R. S. (1990). Parameters for direct cortical electrical stimulation in the human: histopathologic confirmation. *Electroencephalography and Clinical Neurophysiology*, 75(5), 371–377.

Green, R. A., Lovell, N. H., Wallace, G. G., Poole-Warren, L. A. (2008). Conducting polymers for neural interfaces: challenges in developing an effective long-term implant. *Biomaterials*, 29(24–25), 3393–3399.

Grill, W. M., Bhadra, N., Wang, B. (1999). Bladder and urethral pressures evoked by microstimulation of the sacral spinal cord in cats. *Brain Research*, 836(1–2), 19–30.

Guo, B., Ma, P. X. (2018). Conducting polymers for tissue engineering. *Biomacromolecules*, 19(6), 1764–1782.

Guo, Z., Wang, F., Wang, L., Tu, K., Jiang, C., Xi, Y., Yang, B. (2022). A flexible neural implant with ultrathin substrate for low-invasive brain–computer interface applications. *Microsystems & Nanoengineering*, 8(1), 133.

Gupta, S., Dixit, M., Sharma, K., Saxena, N. (2009). Mechanical study of metallized polyethylene terephthalate (PET) films. *Surface and Coatings Technology*, 204(5), 661–666.

Guyton, D. L., Terry Hambrecht, F. (1974). Theory and design of capacitor electrodes for chronic stimulation. *Medical and biological engineering*, 12, 613–620.

Hassler, C., von Metzen, R. P., Ruther, P., Stieglitz, T. (2010). Characterization of parylene C as an encapsulation material for implanted neural prostheses. *Journal of Biomedical Materials Research Part B: Applied Biomaterials*, 93B(1), 266–274.

He, F., Lycke, R., Ganji, M., Xie, C., Luan, L. (2020). Ultraflexible neural electrodes for long-lasting intracortical recording. *IScience*, 23(8). https://doi.org/10.1016/j.isci. 2020.101387

Heeger, A. J. (2001). Semiconducting and metallic polymers: the fourth generation of polymeric materials (Nobel lecture). *Angewandte Chemie International Edition*, 40(14), 2591–2611.

Hejazi, M., Tong, W., Ibbotson, M. R., Prawer, S., Garrett, D. J. (2021). Advances in carbon-based microfiber electrodes for neural interfacing. *Frontiers in Neuroscience*, 15, 658703.

Herculano-Houzel, S. (2009). The human brain in numbers: a linearly scaled-up primate brain. *Frontiers in Human Neuroscience*, 3, 857.

Herculano-Houzel, S. (2012). The remarkable, yet not extraordinary, human brain as a scaled-up primate brain and its associated cost. *Proceedings of the National Academy of Sciences*, 109, 10661–10668.

Hong, G., Lieber, C. M. (2019). Novel electrode technologies for neural recordings. *Nature Reviews Neuroscience*, 20(6), 330–345.

Hong, G., Yang, X., Zhou, T., Lieber, C. M. (2018). Mesh electronics: a new paradigm for tissue-like brain probes. *Current Opinion in Neurobiology*, 50, 33–41.

Huang, W. C., Ong, X. C., Kwon, I. S., Gopinath, C., Fisher, L. E., Wu, H., Bettinger, C. J. (2018). Ultracompliant hydrogel-based neural interfaces fabricated by aqueous-phase microtransfer printing. *Advanced Functional Materials*, 28(29), 1801059.

Hughes, C., Herrera, A., Gaunt, R., Collinger, J. (2020). Bidirectional brain-computer interfaces. *Handbook of Clinical Neurology*, 168, 163–181.

Hwang, E., Sarma, S. D. (2008). Acoustic phonon scattering limited carrier mobility in two-dimensional extrinsic graphene. *Physical Review B*, 77(11), 115449.

Iijima, S. (1991). Helical microtubules of graphitic carbon. *Nature*, 354(6348), 56–58.

Iijima, S., Brabec, C., Maiti, A., Bernholc, J. (1996). Structural flexibility of carbon nanotubes. *The Journal of Chemical Physics*, 104(5), 2089–2092.

Im, C., Seo, J.-M. (2016). A review of electrodes for the electrical brain signal recording. *Biomedical Engineering Letters*, 6(3), 104–112.

Imai, A., Takahashi, S., Furubayashi, S., Mizuno, Y., Sonoda, M., Miyazaki, T., Fujie, T. (2023). Flexible Thin-Film Neural Electrodes with Improved Conformability for ECoG Measurements and Electrical Stimulation. *Advanced Materials Technologies*, 8(21), 2300300.

Janders, M., Egert, U., Stelzle, M., Nisch, W. (1996). Novel thin film titanium nitride micro-electrodes with excellent charge transfer capability for cell stimulation and sensing applications. *Proceedings of 18th Annual International Conference of the IEEE Engineering in Medicine and Biology Society*,

Jeong, J.-W., Shin, G., Park, S. I., Yu, K. J., Xu, L., Rogers, J. A. (2015). Soft materials in neuroengineering for hard problems in neuroscience. *Neuron*, 86(1), 175–186.

Ji, B., Ge, C., Guo, Z., Wang, L., Wang, M., Xie, Z., Wang, X. (2020). Flexible and stretchable optoelectric neural interface for low-noise electrocorticogram recordings and neuromodulation in vivo. *Biosensors and Bioelectronics*, 153, 112009.

Jimbo, Y., Matsuhisa, N., Lee, W., Zalar, P., Jinno, H., Yokota, T., Someya, T. (2017). Ultraflexible transparent oxide/metal/oxide stack electrode with low sheet resistance for electrophysiological measurements. *ACS applied materials & interfaces*, 9(40), 34744–34750.

Johnston, I. D., McCluskey, D. K., Tan, C. K., Tracey, M. C. (2014). Mechanical characterization of bulk Sylgard 184 for microfluidics and microengineering. *Journal of Micromechanics and Microengineering*, 24(3), 035017.

Kaiju, T., Doi, K., Yokota, M., Watanabe, K., Inoue, M., Ando, H., Suzuki, T. (2017). High spatiotemporal resolution ECoG recording of somatosensory evoked potentials with flexible microelectrode arrays. *Frontiers in Neural Circuits*, 11, 20.

Khodagholy, D., Gelinas, J. N., Thesen, T., Doyle, W., Devinsky, O., Malliaras, G. G., Buzsáki, G. (2015). NeuroGrid: recording action potentials from the surface of the brain. *Nature Neuroscience*, 18(2), 310–315.

Kim, D.-H., Viventi, J., Amsden, J. J., Xiao, J., Vigeland, L., Kim, Y.-S., Contreras, D. (2010a). Dissolvable films of silk fibroin for ultrathin conformal bio-integrated electronics. *Nature Materials*, 9(6), 511–517.

Kim, D.-H., Wiler, J. A., Anderson, D. J., Kipke, D. R., Martin, D. C. (2010b). Conducting polymers on hydrogel-coated neural electrode provide sensitive neural recordings in auditory cortex. *Acta Biomaterialia*, 6(1), 57–62.

Kim, T., Cho, M., Yu, K. J. (2018). Flexible and stretchable bio-integrated electronics based on carbon nanotube and graphene. *Materials*, 11(7), 1163.

Kim, T.-I., McCall, J. G., Jung, Y. H., Huang, X., Siuda, E. R., Li, Y., Kim, R.-H. (2013). Injectable, cellular-scale optoelectronics with applications for wireless optogenetics. *Science*, 340(6129), 211–216.

Kostarelos, K., Vincent, M., Hebert, C., Garrido, J. A. (2017). Graphene in the design and engineering of next-generation neural interfaces. *Advanced Materials*, 29(42), 1700909.

Kozai, T. D., Gugel, Z., Li, X., Gilgunn, P. J., Khilwani, R., Ozdoganlar, O. B., Cui, X. T. (2014). Chronic tissue response to carboxymethyl cellulose based dissolvable insertion needle for ultra-small neural probes. *Biomaterials*, 35(34), 9255–9268.

Kozai, T. D., Jaquins-Gerstl, A. S., Vazquez, A. L., Michael, A. C., Cui, X. T. (2015). Brain tissue responses to neural implants impact signal sensitivity and intervention strategies. *ACS Chemical Neuroscience*, 6(1), 48–67.

Kumar, R., Ranwa, S., Kumar, G. (2019). Biodegradable flexible substrate based on chitosan/PVP blend polymer for disposable electronics device applications. *The Journal of Physical Chemistry B*, 124(1), 149–155.

Kumar, R., Rauti, R., Scaini, D., Antman-Passig, M., Meshulam, O., Naveh, D., Shefi, O. (2021). Graphene-based nanomaterials for neuroengineering: recent advances and future prospective. *Advanced Functional Materials*, 31(46), 2104887.

Kunori, N., Takashima, I. (2015). A transparent epidural electrode array for use in conjunction with optical imaging. *Journal of Neuroscience Methods*, 251, 130–137.

Kunugi, T., Ichinose, C., Suzuki, A. (1986). Preparation of high-modulus and high-strength poly (ethylene terephthalate) film by zone-annealing method. *Journal of Applied Polymer Science*, 31(2), 429–439.

Kuzum, D., Takano, H., Shim, E., Reed, J. C., Juul, H., Richardson, A. G., Lucas, T. H. (2014). Transparent and flexible low noise graphene electrodes for simultaneous electrophysiology and neuroimaging. *Nature Communications*, 5(1), 5259.

Lacour, S. P., Benmerah, S., Tarte, E., FitzGerald, J., Serra, J., McMahon, S., Morrison, B. (2010). Flexible and stretchable micro-electrodes for in vitro and in vivo neural interfaces. *Medical & Biological Engineering & Computing*, 48, 945–954.

Lacour, S. P., Wagner, S., Huang, Z., Suo, Z. (2003). Stretchable gold conductors on elastomeric substrates. *Applied Physics Letters*, 82(15), 2404–2406.

Leber, M., Körner, J., Reiche, C. F., Yin, M., Bhandari, R., Franklin, R., Solzbacher, F. (2019). Advances in penetrating multichannel microelectrodes based on the utah array platform. *Neural Interface: Frontiers and Applications*, 1–40. https://doi.org/10.1007/978-981-13-2050-7_1

Lecomte, A., Castagnola, V., Descamps, E., Dahan, L., Blatché, M. C., Dinis, T. M., Bergaud, C. (2015). Silk and PEG as means to stiffen a parylene probe for insertion in the brain: toward a double time-scale tool for local drug delivery. *Journal of Micromechanics and Microengineering*, 25(12), 125003.

Ledochowitsch, P., Yazdan-Shahmorad, A., Bouchard, K., Diaz-Botia, C., Hanson, T., He, J.-W., Blanche, T. (2015). Strategies for optical control and simultaneous electrical readout of extended cortical circuits. *Journal of Neuroscience Methods*, 256, 220–231.

Lee, C., Wei, X., Kysar, J. W., Hone, J. (2008). Measurement of the elastic properties and intrinsic strength of monolayer graphene. *Science*, 321(5887), 385–388.

Lee, K. Y., Moon, H., Kim, B., Kang, Y. N., Jang, J. W., Choe, H. K., Kim, S. (2020). Development of a polydimethylsiloxane-based electrode array for electrocorticography. *Advanced Materials Interfaces*, 7(24), 2001152.

Lee, W., Kim, D., Matsuhisa, N., Nagase, M., Sekino, M., Malliaras, G. G., Someya, T. (2017). Transparent, conformable, active multielectrode array using organic electrochemical transistors. *Proceedings of the National Academy of Sciences*, 114(40), 10554–10559.

Liang, Q., Shen, Z., Sun, X., Yu, D., Liu, K., Mugo, S. M., Zhang, Q. (2023). Electron Conductive and Transparent Hydrogels for Recording Brain Neural Signals and Neuromodulation. *Advanced Materials*, 35(9), 2211159.

Liang, Q., Xia, X., Sun, X., Yu, D., Huang, X., Han, G., Zhang, Q. (2022). Highly stretchable hydrogels as wearable and implantable sensors for recording physiological and brain neural signals. *Advanced Science*, 9(16), 2201059.

Liang, Y., Offenhäusser, A., Ingebrandt, S., Mayer, D. (2021). PEDOT: PSS-based bioelectronic devices for recording and modulation of electrophysiological and biochemical cell signals. *Advanced Healthcare Materials*, 10(11), 2100061.

Lin, C.-M., Lee, Y.-T., Yeh, S.-R., Fang, W. (2009). Flexible carbon nanotubes electrode for neural recording. *Biosensors and Bioelectronics*, 24(9), 2791–2797.

Liu, J., Fu, T.-M., Cheng, Z., Hong, G., Zhou, T., Jin, L., Xie, C. (2015). Syringe-injectable electronics. *Nature Nanotechnology*, 10(7), 629–636.

Liu, X.-J., Zheng, M.-S., Chen, G., Dang, Z.-M., Zha, J.-W. (2022). High-temperature polyimide dielectric materials for energy storage: theory, design, preparation and properties. *Energy & Environmental Science*, 15(1), 56–81.

López-Larraz, E., Sarasola-Sanz, A., Irastorza-Landa, N., Birbaumer, N., Ramos-Murguialday, A. (2018). Brain-machine interfaces for rehabilitation in stroke: a review. *NeuroRehabilitation*, 43(1), 77–97.

Lu, L., Fu, X., Liew, Y., Zhang, Y., Zhao, S., Xu, Z., Stanley, G. B. (2019). Soft and MRI compatible neural electrodes from carbon nanotube fibers. *Nano Letters*, 19(3), 1577–1586.

Lu, Y., Liu, X., Kuzum, D. (2018). Graphene-based neurotechnologies for advanced neural interfaces. *Current Opinion in Biomedical Engineering*, 6, 138–147.

Lu, Y., Lyu, H., Richardson, A. G., Lucas, T. H., Kuzum, D. (2016). Flexible neural electrode array based-on porous graphene for cortical microstimulation and sensing. *Scientific Reports*, 6(1), 33526.

Luan, L., Wei, X., Zhao, Z., Siegel, J. J., Potnis, O., Tuppen, C. A., Holloway, S. (2017). Ultraflexible nanoelectronic probes form reliable, glial scar–free neural integration. *Science Advances*, 3(2), 1601966.

Marin, C., Fernández, E. (2010). Biocompatibility of intracortical microelectrodes: current status and future prospects. *Frontiers in Neuroengineering*, 3, 1212.

Maynard, E. M., Nordhausen, C. T., Normann, R. A. (1997). The utah intracortical electrode array: a recording structure for potential brain-computer interfaces. *Electroencephalography and Clinical Neurophysiology*, 102(3), 228–239.

McClain, M. A., Clements, I. P., Shafer, R. H., Bellamkonda, R. V., LaPlaca, M. C., Allen, M. G. (2011). Highly-compliant, microcable neuroelectrodes fabricated from thin-film gold and PDMS. *Biomedical Microdevices*, 13, 361–373.

McConnell, G. C., Rees, H. D., Levey, A. I., Gutekunst, C.-A., Gross, R. E., Bellamkonda, R. V. (2009). Implanted neural electrodes cause chronic, local inflammation that is correlated with local neurodegeneration. *Journal of Neural Engineering*, 6(5), 056003.

McCreery, D., Bullara, L., Agnew, W. (1986). Neuronal activity evoked by chronically implanted intracortical microelectrodes. *Experimental Neurology*, 92(1), 147–161.

McCreery, D. B., Agnew, W. F., Bullara, L. A. (2002). The effects of prolonged intracortical microstimulation on the excitability of pyramidal tract neurons in the cat. *Annals of Biomedical Engineering*, 30, 107–119.

Morikawa, Y., Yamagiwa, S., Sawahata, H., Numano, R., Koida, K., Ishida, M., Kawano, T. (2018). Ultrastretchable kirigami bioprobes. *Advanced Healthcare Materials*, 7(3), 1701100.

Mozota, J., Conway, B. (1983). Surface and bulk processes at oxidized iridium electrodes—I. Monolayer stage and transition to reversible multilayer oxide film behaviour. *Electrochimica Acta*, 28(1), 1–8.

Musk, E., Neuralink. (2019). An Integrated Brain-achine Interface Platform With Thousands of Channels. *J Med Internet Res*, 21(10), e16194.

Nair, R. R., Blake, P., Grigorenko, A. N., Novoselov, K. S., Booth, T. J., Stauber, T., Geim, A. K. (2008). Fine structure constant defines visual transparency of graphene. *Science*, 320(5881), 1308–1308.

Negi, S., Bhandari, R., Rieth, L., Solzbacher, F. (2010a). In vitro comparison of sputtered iridium oxide and platinum-coated neural implantable microelectrode arrays. *Biomedical Materials*, 5(1), 015007.

Negi, S., Bhandari, R., Rieth, L., Van Wagenen, R., Solzbacher, F. (2010b). Neural electrode degradation from continuous electrical stimulation: comparison of sputtered and activated iridium oxide. *Journal of Neuroscience Methods*, 186(1), 8–17.

Nemani, K. V., Moodie, K. L., Brennick, J. B., Su, A., Gimi, B. (2013). In vitro and in vivo evaluation of SU-8 biocompatibility. *Materials Science and Engineering: C*, 33(7), 4453–4459.

Neto, J. P., Costa, A., Vaz Pinto, J., Marques-Smith, A., Costa, J. C., Martins, R., Barquinha, P. (2021). Transparent and flexible electrocorticography electrode arrays based on silver nanowire networks for neural recordings. *ACS Applied Nano Materials*, 4(6), 5737–5747.

Nguyen, J. K., Park, D. J., Skousen, J. L., Hess-Dunning, A. E., Tyler, D. J., Rowan, S. J., Capadona, J. R. (2014). Mechanically-compliant intracortical implants reduce the neuroinflammatory response. *Journal of Neural Engineering*, 11(5), 056014.

Nordhausen, C. T., Rousche, P. J., Normann, R. A. (1994). Optimizing recording capabilities of the Utah Intracortical Electrode Array. *Brain Research*, 637(1), 27–36.

Nordström, M., Keller, S., Lillemose, M., Johansson, A., Dohn, S., Haefliger, D., Boisen, A. (2008). SU-8 cantilevers for bio/chemical sensing; fabrication, characterisation and development of novel read-out methods. *Sensors*, 8(3), 1595–1612.

Oribe, S., Yoshida, S., Kusama, S., Osawa, S.-i., Nakagawa, A., Iwasaki, M., Nishizawa, M. (2019). Hydrogel-based organic subdural electrode with high conformability to brain surface. *Scientific Reports*, 9(1), 13379.

Ouyang, S., Xie, Y., Wang, D., Zhu, D., Xu, X., Tan, T., Fong, H. H. (2015). Surface patterning of PEDOT: PSS by photolithography for organic electronic devices. *Journal of Nanomaterials*, 2015, 4–4.

Pan, J., Xia, J., Zhang, F., Zhang, L., Zhang, S., Pan, G., Dong, S. (2023). 7T Magnetic Compatible Multimodality Electrophysiological Signal Recording System. *Electronics*, 12(17), 3648.

Park, D.-W., Brodnick, S. K., Ness, J. P., Atry, F., Krugner-Higby, L., Sandberg, A., Kim, H. (2016). Fabrication and utility of a transparent graphene neural electrode array for electrophysiology, in vivo imaging, and optogenetics. *Nature Protocols*, 11(11), 2201–2222.

Park, D.-W., Ness, J. P., Brodnick, S. K., Esquibel, C., Novello, J., Atry, F., Swanson, K. I. (2018). Electrical neural stimulation and simultaneous in vivo monitoring with transparent graphene electrode arrays implanted in GCaMP6f mice. *ACS Nano*, 12(1), 148–157.

Park, D.-W., Schendel, A. A., Mikael, S., Brodnick, S. K., Richner, T. J., Ness, J. P., Williams, J. C. (2014). Graphene-based carbon-layered electrode array technology for neural imaging and optogenetic applications. *Nature Communications*, 5(1), 5258.

Park, S., Yuk, H., Zhao, R., Yim, Y. S., Woldeghebriel, E. W., Kang, J., Zhao, X. (2021). Adaptive and multifunctional hydrogel hybrid probes for long-term sensing and modulation of neural activity. *Nature Communications*, 12(1), 3435.

Patel, P. R., Na, K., Zhang, H., Kozai, T. D., Kotov, N. A., Yoon, E., Chestek, C. A. (2015). Insertion of linear 8.4 μm diameter 16 channel carbon fiber electrode arrays for single unit recordings. *Journal of Neural Engineering*, 12(4), 046009.

Peigney, A., Laurent, C., Flahaut, E., Bacsa, R., Rousset, A. (2001). Specific surface area of carbon nanotubes and bundles of carbon nanotubes. *Carbon*, 39(4), 507–514.

Peng, Q., Chen, J., Wang, T., Peng, X., Liu, J., Wang, X., Zeng, H. (2020). Recent advances in designing conductive hydrogels for flexible electronics. *InfoMat*, 2(5), 843–865.

Petersen, K. E. (1982). Silicon as a mechanical material. *Proceedings of the IEEE*, 70(5), 420–457.

Polikov, V. S., Tresco, P. A., Reichert, W. M. (2005). Response of brain tissue to chronically implanted neural electrodes. *Journal of Neuroscience Methods*, 148(1), 1–18.

Pranti, A. S., Schander, A., Bödecker, A., Lang, W. (2017). Highly stable PEDOT: PSS coating on gold microelectrodes with improved charge injection capacity for chronic neural stimulation. *Proceedings, Proceedings*, 1, 492.

Qiang, Y., Seo, K. J., Zhao, X., Artoni, P., Golshan, N. H., Culaclii, S., Fagiolini, M. (2017). Bilayer nanomesh structures for transparent recording and stimulating microelectrodes. *Advanced Functional Materials*, 27(48), 1704117.

Renz, A. F., Reichmuth, A. M., Stauffer, F., Thompson-Steckel, G., Vörös, J. (2018). A guide towards long-term functional electrodes interfacing neuronal tissue. *Journal of Neural Engineering*, 15(6), 061001.

Rivnay, J., Wang, H., Fenno, L., Deisseroth, K., Malliaras, G. G. (2017). Next-generation probes, particles, and proteins for neural interfacing. *Science Advances*, 3(6), 1601649.

Robblee, L., McHardy, J., Agnew, W., Bullara, L. (1983). Electrical stimulation with Pt electrodes. VII. Dissolution of Pt electrodes during electrical stimulation of the cat cerebral cortex. *Journal of Neuroscience Methods*, 9(4), 301–308.

Rose, T., Kelliher, E., Robblee, L. (1985). Assessment of capacitor electrodes for intracortical neural stimulation. *Journal of Neuroscience Methods*, 12(3), 181–193.

Rose, T. L., Robblee, L. S. (1990). Electrical stimulation with Pt electrodes. VIII. Electrochemically safe charge injection limits with 0.2 ms pulses (neuronal application). *IEEE Transactions on Biomedical Engineering*, 37(11), 1118–1120.

Rousche, P. J., Normann, R. A. (1998). Chronic recording capability of the Utah Intracortical Electrode Array in cat sensory cortex. *Journal of Neuroscience Methods*, 82(1), 1–15.

Salvetat, J.-P., Bonard, J.-M., Thomson, N., Kulik, A., Forro, L., Benoit, W., Zuppiroli, L. (1999). Mechanical properties of carbon nanotubes. *Applied Physics A*, 69, 255–260.

Scharf, R., Tsunematsu, T., McAlinden, N., Dawson, M. D., Sakata, S., Mathieson, K. (2016). Depth-specific optogenetic control in vivo with a scalable, high-density μLED neural probe. *Scientific Reports*, 6(1), 28381.

Seo, J. W., Kim, K., Seo, K. W., Kim, M. K., Jeong, S., Kim, H., Lee, J. Y. (2020). Artifact-free 2D mapping of neural activity in vivo through transparent gold nanonetwork array. *Advanced Functional Materials*, 30(34), 2000896.

Shannon, R. V. (1992). A model of safe levels for electrical stimulation. *IEEE Transactions on Biomedical Engineering*, 39(4), 424–426.

Sharafkhani, N., Kouzani, A. Z., Adams, S. D., Long, J. M., Lissorgues, G., Rousseau, L., Orwa, J. O. (2022). Neural tissue-microelectrode interaction: Brain micromotion, electrical impedance, and flexible microelectrode insertion. *Journal of Neuroscience Methods*, 365, 109388.

Shepherd, R. K., Carter, P. M., Dalrymple, A. N., Enke, Y. L., Wise, A. K., Nguyen, T., Fallon, J. B. (2021). Platinum dissolution and tissue response following long-term electrical stimulation at high charge densities. *Journal of Neural Engineering*, 18(3), 036021.

Sin, L. T., Tueen, B. S. (2022). *Plastics and Sustainability: Practical Approaches*. Elsevier.

Sinha, S. K., Noh, Y., Reljin, N., Treich, G. M., Hajeb-Mohammadalipour, S., Guo, Y., Sotzing, G. A. (2017). Screen-printed PEDOT: PSS electrodes on commercial finished textiles for electrocardiography. *ACS Applied Materials & Interfaces*, 9(43), 37524–37528.

Sironi, V. A. (2011). Origin and evolution of deep brain stimulation. *Frontiers in Integrative Neuroscience*, 5, 42.

Slavcheva, E., Vitushinsky, R., Mokwa, W., Schnakenberg, U. (2004). Sputtered iridium oxide films as charge injection material for functional electrostimulation. *Journal of the Electrochemical Society*, 151(7), E226.

Smart, S., Cassady, A., Lu, G., Martin, D. (2006). The biocompatibility of carbon nanotubes. *Carbon*, 44(6), 1034–1047.

Soldano, C., Mahmood, A., Dujardin, E. (2010). Production, properties and potential of graphene. *Carbon*, 48(8), 2127–2150.

Stieglitz, T., Beutel, H.R., Schuettler, M., Meyer, J.-U. (2000). Micromachined, polyimide-based devices for flexible neural interfaces. *Biomedical Microdevices*, 2, 283–294.

Stiller, A. M., Black, B. J., Kung, C., Ashok, A., Cogan, S. F., Varner, V. D., Pancrazio, J. J. (2018). A meta-analysis of intracortical device stiffness and its correlation with histological outcomes. *Micromachines*, 9(9), 443.

Tang, X., Shen, H., Zhao, S., Li, N., Liu, J. (2023). Flexible brain–computer interfaces. *Nature Electronics*, 6(2), 109–118.

Thompson, B., Yoon, H.-S. (2013). Aerosol-printed strain sensor using PEDOT: PSS. *IEEE Sensors Journal*, 13(11), 4256–4263.

Thunemann, M., Lu, Y., Liu, X., Kılıç, K., Desjardins, M., Vandenberghe, M., Kuzum, D. (2018). Deep 2-photon imaging and artifact-free optogenetics through transparent graphene microelectrode arrays. *Nature Communications*, 9(1), 2035.

Tian, H., Xu, K., Zou, L., Fang, Y. (2022). Multimodal neural probes for combined optogenetics and electrophysiology. *IScience*, 25(1). https://doi.org/10.1016/j.isci.2021.103612

Tian, J., Lin, Z., Chen, Z., Obaid, S. N., Efimov, I. R., Lu, L. (2021). Stretchable and transparent metal nanowire microelectrodes for simultaneous electrophysiology and optogenetics applications. *Photonics. Photonics*, 8, 220.

Tien, L. W., Wu, F., Tang-Schomer, M. D., Yoon, E., Omenetto, F. G., Kaplan, D. L. (2013). Silk as a multifunctional biomaterial substrate for reduced glial scarring around brain-penetrating electrodes. *Advanced Functional Materials*, 23(25), 3185–3193.

Vitale, F., Summerson, S. R., Aazhang, B., Kemere, C., Pasquali, M. (2015). Neural stimulation and recording with bidirectional, soft carbon nanotube fiber microelectrodes. *ACS Nano*, 9(4), 4465–4474.

Vomero, M., Oliveira, A., Ashouri, D., Eickenscheidt, M., Stieglitz, T. (2018). Graphitic carbon electrodes on flexible substrate for neural applications entirely fabricated using infrared nanosecond laser technology. *Scientific Reports*, 8(1), 14749.

Von Metzen, R. P., Stieglitz, T. (2013). The effects of annealing on mechanical, chemical, and physical properties and structural stability of Parylene C. *Biomedical Microdevices*, 15, 727–735.

Wang, K., Fishman, H. A., Dai, H., Harris, J. S. (2006). Neural stimulation with a carbon nanotube microelectrode array. *Nano Letters*, 6(9), 2043–2048.

Wang, K., Frewin, C. L., Esrafilzadeh, D., Yu, C., Wang, C., Pancrazio, J. J., Wallace, G. (2019). High-performance graphene-fiber-based neural recording microelectrodes. *Advanced Materials*, 31(15), 1805867.

Weatherup, R. S., Dlubak, B., Hofmann, S. (2012). Kinetic control of catalytic CVD for high-quality graphene at low temperatures. *ACS Nano*, 6(11), 9996–10003.

Wei, X., Luan, L., Zhao, Z., Li, X., Zhu, H., Potnis, O., Xie, C. (2018). Nanofabricated ultraflexible electrode arrays for high-density intracortical recording. *Advanced Science*, 5(6), 1700625.

Weiland, J. D., Anderson, D. J., Humayun, M. S. (2002). In vitro electrical properties for iridium oxide versus titanium nitride stimulating electrodes. *IEEE Transactions on Biomedical Engineering*, 49(12), 1574–1579.

Widge, A. S., Malone Jr, D. A., Dougherty, D. D. (2018). Closing the loop on deep brain stimulation for treatment-resistant depression. *Frontiers in Neuroscience*, 12, 175.

Woeppel, K., Yang, Q., Cui, X. T. (2017). Recent advances in neural electrode–tissue interfaces. *Current O pinion in Biomedical Engineering*, 4, 21–31.

Wolf, M. P., Salieb-Beugelaar, G. B., Hunziker, P. (2018). PDMS with designer functionalities—Properties, modifications strategies, and applications. *Progress in Polymer Science*, 83, 97–134.

Xiang, Z., Yen, S.-C., Xue, N., Sun, T., Tsang, W. M., Zhang, S., Lee, C. (2014). Ultra-thin flexible polyimide neural probe embedded in a dissolvable maltose-coated microneedle. *Journal of Micromechanics and Microengineering*, 24(6), 065015.

Xie, C., Liu, J., Fu, T.-M., Dai, X., Zhou, W., Lieber, C. M. (2015). Three-dimensional macroporous nanoelectronic networks as minimally invasive brain probes. *Nature Materials*, 14(12), 1286–1292.

Xie, K., Zhang, S., Dong, S., Li, S., Yu, C., Xu, K., Wu, Z. (2017). Portable wireless electrocorticography system with a flexible microelectrodes array for epilepsy treatment. *Scientific Reports*, 7(1), 7808.

Yang, C., Suo, Z. (2018). Hydrogel ionotronics. *Nature Reviews Materials*, 3(6), 125–142.

Yang, M., Chen, P., Qu, X., Zhang, F., Ning, S., Ma, L., Jiang, W. (2023). Robust neural interfaces with photopatternable, bioadhesive, and highly conductive hydrogels for stable chronic neuromodulation. *ACS Nano*, 17(2), 885–895.

Yang, W., Gong, Y., Yao, C.-Y., Shrestha, M., Jia, Y., Qiu, Z., Li, W. (2021). A fully transparent, flexible PEDOT: PSS–ITO–Ag–ITO based microelectrode array for ECoG recording. *Lab on a Chip*, 21(6), 1096–1108.

Yu, J., Ling, W., Li, Y., Ma, N., Wu, Z., Liang, R., Wang, K. (2021). A multichannel flexible optoelectronic fiber device for distributed implantable neurological stimulation and monitoring. *Small*, 17(4), 2005925.

Yuk, H., Lu, B., Lin, S., Qu, K., Xu, J., Luo, J., Zhao, X. (2020). 3D printing of conducting polymers. *Nature Communications*, 11(1), 1604.

Zhang, F., Zhang, L., Xia, J., Zhao, W., Dong, S., Ye, Z., Zhang, S. (2023). Multimodal electrocorticogram active electrode array based on zinc oxide-thin film transistors. *Advanced Science*, 10(2), 2204467.

Zhang, J., Liu, X., Xu, W., Luo, W., Li, M., Chu, F., Duan, X. (2018). Stretchable transparent electrode arrays for simultaneous electrical and optical interrogation of neural circuits in vivo. *Nano Letters*, 18(5), 2903–2911.

Zhang, P., Travas-Sejdic, J. (2021). Fabrication of conducting polymer microelectrodes and microstructures for bioelectronics. *Journal of Materials Chemistry C*, 9(31), 9730–9760.

Zhao, S., Li, G., Tong, C., Chen, W., Wang, P., Dai, J., Duan, X. (2020). Full activation pattern mapping by simultaneous deep brain stimulation and fMRI with graphene fiber electrodes. *Nature Communications*, 11(1), 1788.

Zhao, Z., Gong, R., Zheng, L., Wang, J. (2016). In vivo neural recording and electrochemical performance of microelectrode arrays modified by rough-surfaced AuPt alloy nanoparticles with nanoporosity. *Sensors*, 16(11), 1851.

Zhao, Z., Li, X., He, F., Wei, X., Lin, S., Xie, C. (2019). Parallel, minimally-invasive implantation of ultra-flexible neural electrode arrays. *Journal of Neural Engineering*, 16(3), 035001.

Zhao, Z., Zhu, H., Li, X., Sun, L., He, F., Chung, J. E., Xie, C. (2023). Ultraflexible electrode arrays for months-long high-density electrophysiological mapping of thousands of neurons in rodents. *Nature Biomedical Engineering*, 7(4), 520–532.

Zheng, X. S., Tan, C., Castagnola, E., Cui, X. T. (2021a). Electrode materials for chronic electrical microstimulation. *Advanced Healthcare Materials*, 10(12), 2100119.

Zheng, X. S., Yang, Q., Vazquez, A. L., Tracy Cui, X. (2021b). Imaging the efficiency of poly (3, 4-ethylenedioxythiophene) doped with acid-functionalized carbon nanotube and iridium oxide electrode coatings for microstimulation. *Advanced NanoBiomed Research*, 1(7), 2000092.

Zheng, Y., Wang, Y., Zhang, F., Zhang, S., Piatkevich, K. D., Zhou, N., Pokorski, J. K. (2022). Coagulation bath-sssisted 3D printing of PEDOT: PSS with high resolution and strong substrate adhesion for bioelectronic devices. *Advanced Materials Technologies*, 7(7), 2101514.

Zhou, H., Cheng, X., Rao, L., Li, T., Duan, Y. Y. (2013). Poly (3, 4-ethylenedioxythiophene)/multiwall carbon nanotube composite coatings for improving the stability of microelectrodes in neural prostheses applications. *Acta Biomaterialia*, 9(5), 6439–6449.

CHAPTER 6

Soft Electronics for Wearable and Implantable Systems

Zhe Wang, Xiahua Cui, Kaiwei Li, and Lei Ren

6.1 INTRODUCTION

In recent years, the field of wearable and implantable systems has experienced explosive growth, driven by advances in materials science, microfabrication, and microelectronics technologies. The key to realizing the full potential of wearable and implantable systems lies in developing soft and biocompatible devices through soft materials or structures that can seamlessly integrate with the human body or clothes. Soft electronics, featuring materials or structures with high deformability or stretchability, offer a comfortable and conformal interface with the skin and underlying tissues. These wearable and implantable systems have revolutionized healthcare, allowing for continuous monitoring of vital signs, personalized interventions, and real-time data analysis. Moreover, these systems hold immense promise for a wide range of applications beyond the healthcare sector, including fitness tracking, human–computer interaction, and augmented reality (Hassan et al., 2021).

Soft electronic skins (e-skins), with their unparalleled ability to conform to the complex contours of the body, represent a significant leap forward in wearable technology. These e-skins mimic the structure and functionality of human skin, enabling them to sense various physiological parameters such as pressure, temperature, strain, and even biochemical signals (Yang et al., 2019). This opens doors to a wide range of applications in healthcare, motion detection, environmental monitoring, etc. Underneath the surface, soft implantable sensors offer a minimally invasive approach to monitoring internal physiological activities. These sensors are flexible and biocompatible and can be implanted directly into organs and tissues, providing real-time data on temperature, pressure, pH, and even tissue oxygenation (Koydemir & Ozcan, 2018). This allows for early detection and treatment of diseases, personalized drug delivery, and improved understanding of disease progression.

However, the functionality and implementation of these innovative systems are contingent upon the development of efficient and compliant energy storage strategies. Traditional batteries are often bulky and rigid, posing challenges for integration into soft and flexible systems. Therefore, efforts are directed toward developing novel energy storage solutions

DOI: 10.1201/9781003493631-6

such as biocompatible and stretchable supercapacitors and batteries (Gong & Cheng, 2017). These advancements are crucial for ensuring the long-term operation of soft wearable and implantable systems without the need for frequent recharging or replacement, maximizing their potential impact in healthcare and beyond.

In this chapter, we will introduce the latest research advancements in soft wearable and implantable systems. We will delve into the working principles and structure designs of disparate soft e-skins, explore the diverse applications of soft implantable sensors, and discuss the development of innovative energy storage strategies for soft electronics. Finally, we will address the remaining challenges and future directions for this rapidly evolving field, highlighting its potential for real-world applications, ultimately improving healthcare, human–computer interaction, and our understanding of human behavior.

6.2 SOFT ELECTRONIC SKINS

The skin, the body's largest organ, contains a network of receptors distributed at different depths within the soft tissues that are sensitive to energy (Soni & Dahiya, 2020). It allows us to perceive temperature, distinguish texture, recognize shapes, provide haptic feedback, and facilitate communication. The design of flexible e-skins aims to emulate the tactile and other perceptual capabilities of human skin, enabling the detection, perception, and responsive behavior to external stimuli (W. Wang et al., 2023b). Here we focus on describing the sensing mechanism of e-skin and the performance improvement method based on structural design.

6.2.1 Sensing Mechanisms of e-skins

For tactile sensing e-skin, according to the sensing mechanism, it can be divided into piezoresistive sensor skin, capacitive sensor skin, piezoelectric sensor skin, and electrostatic sensor skin (Lee et al., 2021; Wang et al., 2015).

6.2.1.1 Piezoresistive Sensor Skin

A piezoresistive sensor consists of an active layer in contact with two electrodes, which can be either an elastic conductor or a semiconductor. Its resistance changes when external pressure is applied. The overall resistance of the sensor comprises two parts: electrode resistance and active layer resistance. In specific piezoresistive sensors, the electrode resistance is typically a constant value. Therefore, the variation of the sensor resistance signal is primarily influenced by changes in the resistance of the active layer. A conductor's resistance can be calculated from the following equation:

$$R = \frac{\rho L}{A}$$

where ρ is material resistivity, L is the length of the conductor, and A is the cross-sectional area. The applied pressure induces changes in the length or cross-sectional area of the active layer, leading to a systematic variation in resistance. Typically, the relative resistance change is described by $\Delta R/R$ to characterize the relationship between resistance and pressure. The advantages of piezoresistive sensors include a simple device structure, a broad pressure-detecting range, high sensitivity, and fast response (Kumar, 2022). However, its drawbacks include pronounced hysteresis effects and relatively poor cyclic stability.

As pressure is applied, the material undergoes compression, altering the resistance between overlapped electrodes. Flexible piezoresistive sensor skins are primarily composed of supporting materials and active materials (Pierre Claver & Zhao, 2021). The most commonly used active materials include metal-based materials, carbon-based materials, conductive polymers, and other materials. These active materials have excellent mechanical properties, outstanding electrical conductivity, and long-term stability. The choice of supporting material is an important factor affecting the performance of piezoresistive sensor skins. At present, a variety of supporting materials have been studied, including silicone, hydrogels, and biomaterials. Chen et al. prepared a double-layer piezoresistive sensor skin using MXene and polydimethylsiloxane (PDMS). It exhibits a wide sensing range, high sensitivity, short response/recovery time, and excellent repeatability as shown in Figure 6.1a (2022). Gao et al. selected thin paper coated with silver nanowires (AgNWs) and nanocellulose paper (NCP) as materials to prepare an all-paper-based piezoresistive (APBP) pressure sensor. Figure 6.1b shows that the proposed sensor shows a high sensitivity of 1.5 kPa^{-1} in the range of 0.03–30.2 kPa (Gao et al., 2019). Qiao et al. developed a multifunctional e-skin based on substrate-free laser-scribed graphene (SFG). It could be used to detect respiration, human motion, and electrocardiogram (ECG), as presented in Figure 6.1c (2020).

6.2.1.2 Capacitive Sensor Skin

A flexible capacitive pressure sensor is a crucial type of sensor for detecting loads. Capacitive sensing is commonly accomplished by assessing the changes in capacitance between two electrodes that overlap, with their separation maintained by a dielectric elastomer (Roberts et al., 2013) or an air gap (Weigel et al., 2015). A typical flexible capacitive sensor takes the form of a sandwich structure (Li et al., 2021). Ensuring superior flexibility involves fabricating the electrodes from flexible substrates and choosing conductive materials based on the sensor's intended performance. The applied pressure predominantly alters the distance between the two electrodes or the sensing area of the capacitor, leading to a corresponding capacitance change described by the following equation:

$$C = \frac{\varepsilon_r \varepsilon_0 A}{d}$$

C is the sensor capacitance, ε_0 is the vacuum permittivity, ε_r is the relative permittivity of the dielectric, A is the overlapping area, and d is the distance between the two electrodes. The sensor comprises four layers, namely the contact layer, upper plate with its electrode, dielectric layer, and lower plate with its electrode (Ye et al., 2021), as illustrated in Figure 6.2. Sputtered onto the surfaces of the upper and lower plates, the upper and lower electrodes are separated by an intermediate dielectric layer. The application of

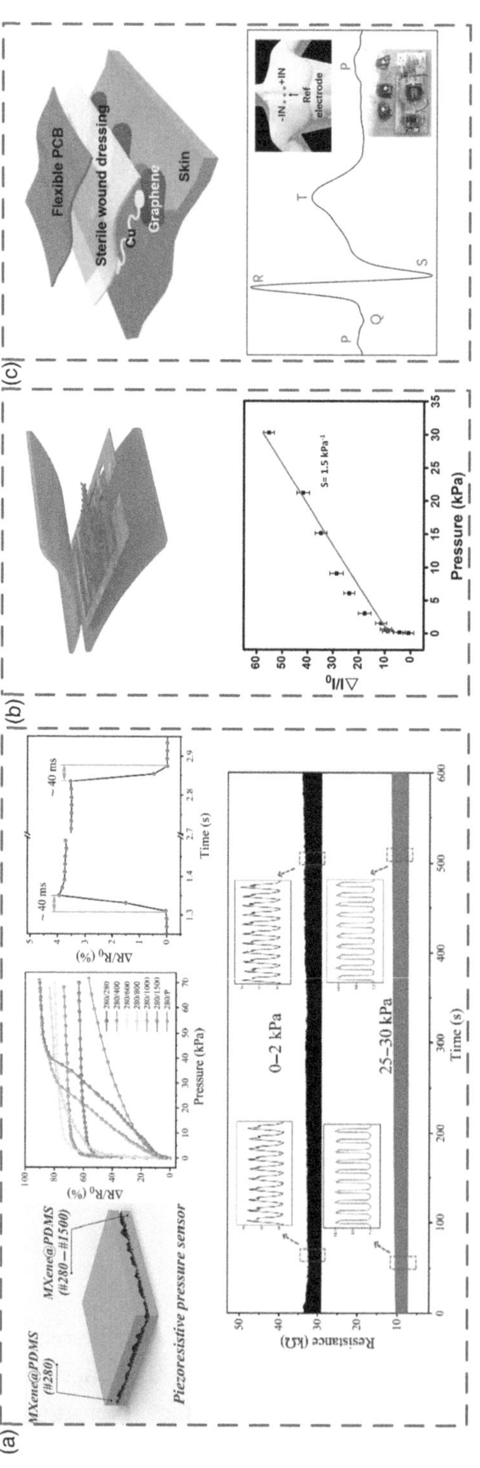

FIGURE 6.1 (a) A double-layer piezoresistive sensor skin with good performance. (b) An all-paper-based piezoresistive (APBP) pressure sensor. (c) A multifunctional e-skin. ([a] Adapted with permission. (Chen et al., 2022) Copyright 2022, Elsevier Inc.; [b] Adapted with permission. (Gao et al., 2019) Copyright 2019, American Chemical Society; [c] Adapted with permission. (Qiao et al., 2020) Copyright 2020, American Chemical Society.)

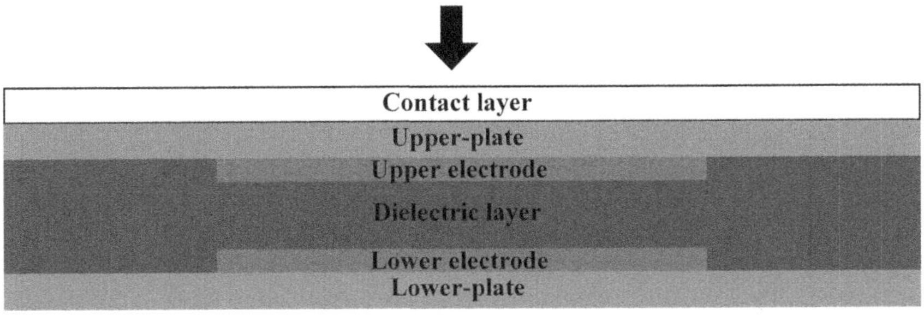

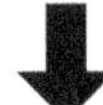

Contact layer
Upper-plate
Upper electrode
Dielectric layer
Lower electrode
Lower-plate

FIGURE 6.2 The composition of the capacitive sensor. (Adapted with permission.)

pressure above the electrodes induces a change in distance between them, causing a corresponding variation in capacitance for pressure measurement.

The sensitivity of a capacitive pressure sensor is defined as:

$$S = \frac{\left(\dfrac{C}{C_0}\right)-1}{\Delta P}$$

Combined with the capacitance equation, it can be obtained:

$$S = \frac{\left(\dfrac{A}{A_0}\times\dfrac{d_0}{d}\times\dfrac{\varepsilon_r}{\varepsilon_{r0}}\right)-1}{\Delta P}$$

S represents sensitivity, C_0 is the initial capacitance of the capacitive pressure sensor, C is the capacitance after applying the load, ΔP is the pressure change. A_0 and A, d_0 and d, as well as ε_{r0} and ε_r, respectively, represent the relative areas, distances, and relative permittivities of the two electrode layers before and after loading. The improvement of capacitive sensor performance involves several aspects, including geometric structures, materials, compressive modulus, and permittivity. The stretchability, linearity, and response time of the device are influenced by both the geometric structure and materials. Permittivity governs the capacitance both before and after sensing. Simultaneously, modulus may impact the deformation and recovery time of the dielectric material under identical pressure conditions.

Compared to the traditional pressure sensors that utilize rigid metals and semiconductor materials, flexible substrates in pressure sensors are more suitable for a broader range of applications. Used polymer films for flexible substrates commonly include PDMS, polyethylene terephthalate (PET), Ecoflex, polyurethane (PU), polyimide (PI), and polyvinyl alcohol (PVA) (Li et al., 2021). Furthermore, fabrics that have more gaps and superior flexibility are commonly utilized as flexible substrates. Yu et al. proposed a full-fabric capacitive sensor (AFCS) based on a nanofiber dielectric layer. Figure 6.3a shows that the sensor has a high sensitivity of 8.31 kPa^{-1} under 1 kPa (2021). Chen et al. prepared a capacitive sensor using a microstructured PDMS film as the microstructured conductive electrode

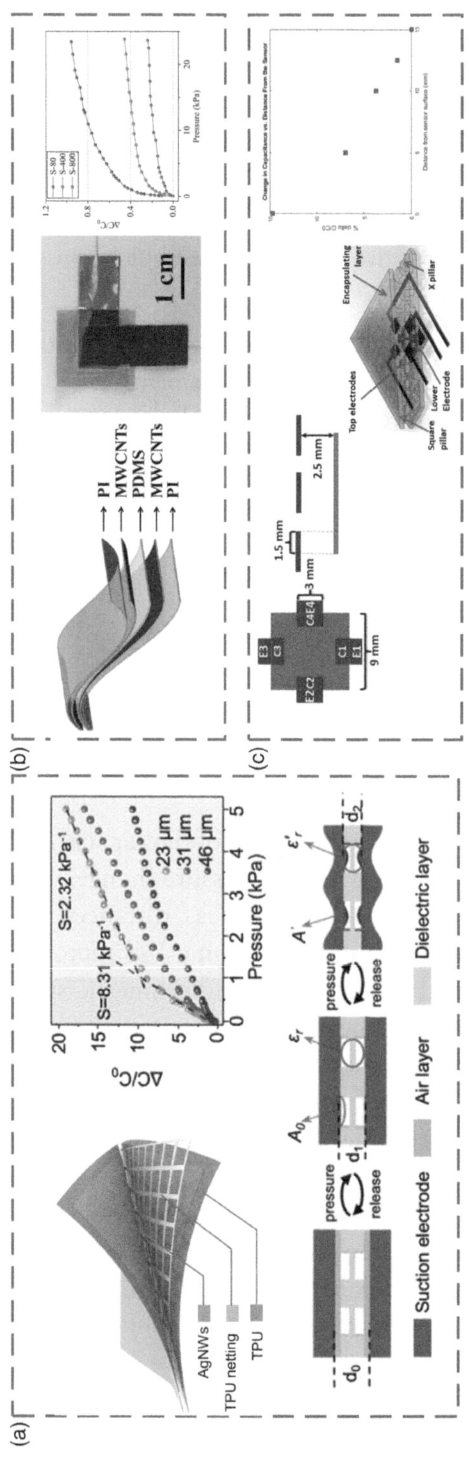

FIGURE 6.3 (a) A full-fabric capacitive sensor. (b) Capacitive pressure sensor with multi-walled carbon nanotube microstructure electrodes. (c) Schematic scenario in touchless mode. ([a] Adapted with permission. (Yu et al., 2021) Copyright 2021, American Chemical Society; [b] Adapted with permission. (Chen et al., 2021) Copyright 2021, IOP Publishing Ltd.; [c] Adapted with permission. (Sarwar et al., 2023) Copyright 2023, Springer Nature.)

and a smooth PDMS film as a dielectric layer. And multi-walled carbon nanotubes (MWCNTs) are embedded on microstructured PDMS film. After optimizing the size of the electrode microstructure, the sensitivity of the proposed sensor can reach 1.3 kPa^{-1} as shown in Figures 6.3b (Chen et al., 2021). In addition to detecting contact force and surface pressure, capacitive sensors can also sense proximity. When detecting proximity, the sensor relies on the conductivity of a non-contact object, such as a human finger, to act as the capacitor electrode. A capacitive sensor consisting of five electrodes is investigated. Four sense electrodes (E1–E4) are capacitively coupled to one ground electrode, and four sense electrodes are on top of the ground electrode. Figure 6.3c illustrates the average taxel capacitive response to an approaching finger with a baseline capacitance distance of 15 mm (Sarwar et al., 2023).

6.2.1.3 Piezoelectric Sensor Skin

A piezoelectric sensor is a type of sensor that utilizes the piezoelectric effect to detect and measure changes in pressure. Most piezoelectric sensors make use of the positive piezoelectric effect, allowing piezoelectric materials to convert mechanical energy into electrical energy (Wu et al., 2021). When an external force acts on the piezoelectric material, it can generate polarized charges on its surface, resulting in a piezoelectric potential due to the piezoelectric effect. The pressure/strain is detected by detecting the strain-induced polarization charge in the piezoelectric material.

A piezoelectric nanogenerator (PENG) is a device that utilizes the piezoelectric effect. The piezoelectric materials used in nanogenerators commonly include lead zirconate titanate (PZT), zinc oxide (ZnO), polyvinylidene fluoride (PVDF), and other materials with strong piezoelectric properties. PVDF and poly(vinylidene fluoride-trifluoroethylene) (P(VDF-TrFE)) are the most researched piezoelectric polymers in nanogenerators. Due to their structural flexibility, biocompatibility, chemical stability, and piezoelectric performance, they hold tremendous potential in the field of electronic skin.

PENGs have been employed as sensing devices for biomechanical stimuli, such as heart rate, heart rate variability, respiration, and body movements. The use of flexible PENGs enables the easy monitoring of movements in limbs, joints, hands, and feet. During squatting, PENGs generate electrical signals due to the periodic compression and release of the device. While walking or running, the output signals of PENGs can indicate step frequency and the intensity of force applied during body movement. Different intensities and frequencies allow real-time monitoring of human movement conditions. As shown in Figure 6.4a and b, the motion of joints can provide bending forces for flexible PENGs, and PENGs generate electrical signals to detect the movement of human joints (Guan et al., 2020; Khan et al., 2020). The different bending positions of joints result in varying bending forces, leading to changes in signal strength. In addition, a self-powered electronic skin (SPES) based on PENG is investigated and used for robot sensing. As presented in Figure 6.4c, the test results show that the bending sensitivity of SPES is 0.44 mV/° and the pressing sensitivity is 2.5 mV/N (M. Zhang et al., 2023a). Therefore, sensors based on piezoelectric sensing

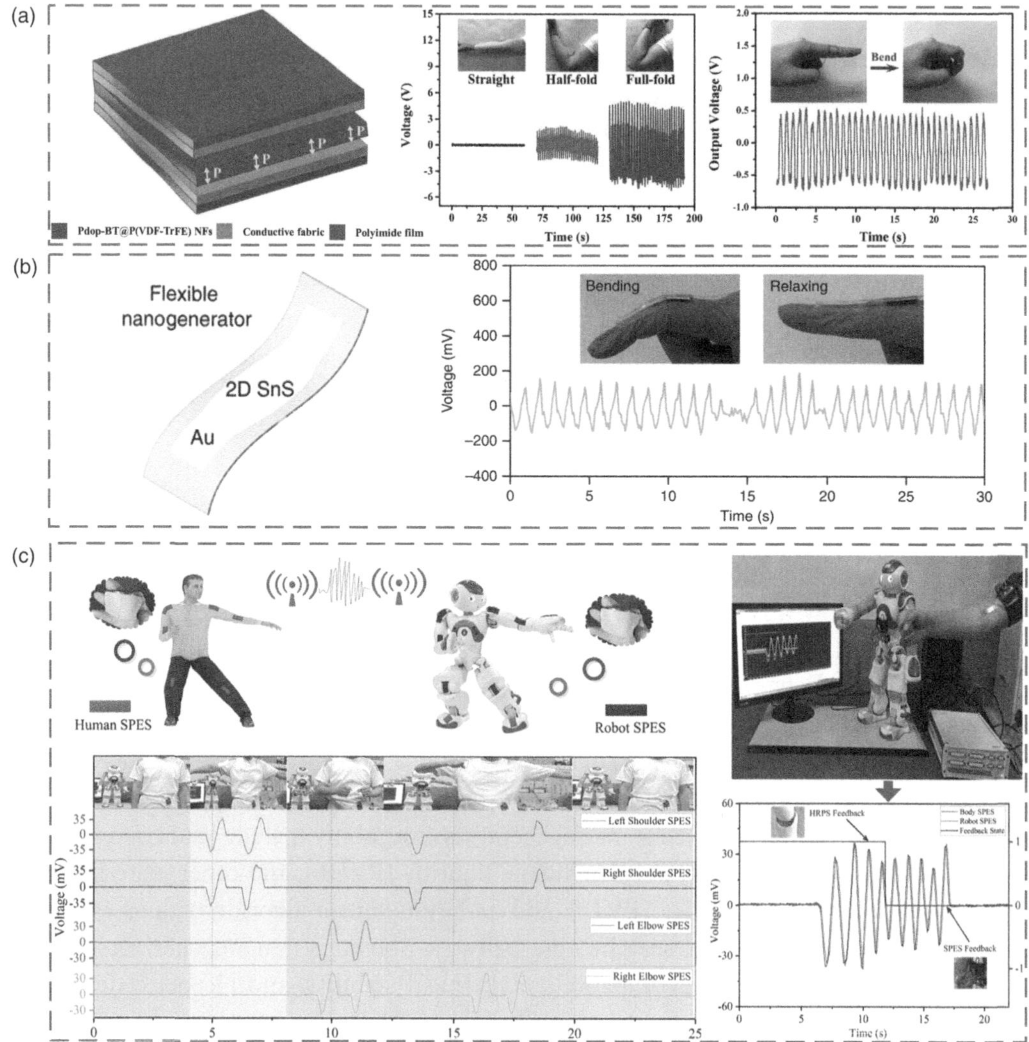

FIGURE 6.4   (a) The flexible Pdop-BT@P(VDF-TrFE) nanocomposite PENG. (b) The flexible nanogenerator PENG. (c) Self-powered e-skin for remote human–machine. ([a] Adapted with permission. (Guan et al., 2020) Copyright 2020, Elsevier Ltd.; [b] Adapted with permission. (Khan et al., 2020) Copyright 2020, Springer Nature; [c] Adapted with permission. (M. Zhang et al., 2023a) Copyright 2023, American Chemical Society.)

demonstrate potential application value in real-time controlling mechanical hands or arms in human–machine interaction systems.

6.2.1.4 Triboelectric Sensor Skin

Triboelectric nanogenerators (TENGs) leverage the coupled effects of contact electrification and electrostatic induction, effectively converting mechanical energy into electrical energy. Typically, TENGs are composed of two materials with distinct frictional electrical properties. When the two materials come into contact, contact electrification occurs, resulting in opposite static charges on the surfaces. Additionally, electrodes are present on the back of the materials. The charges flow between the two electrodes through an external circuit, generating a potential difference as the materials separate.

Two typical structures of TENG sensors are single-fiber-shaped and flat-plate-shaped. Silver nanowire/carbon nanotube conductive materials and encapsulated PDMS are deposited in an ordered manner onto stretchable nylon fibers onto stretchable nylon fibers, forming a coaxial structure fiber-shaped friction nanogenerator (F-TENG) with a diameter of 0.63 mm. The preparation process of the F-TENG is shown in Figure 6.5a. It can be stretched by over 140% and folded into various shapes, as shown in Figure 6.5b. As a self-powered tactile sensor, the F-TENGs can be applied to human organs for monitoring various human motions. Output measurement of fingers and wrist movements with the photograph of motion states is presented in Figure 6.5c–e (Ning et al., 2021).

A soft skin-like TENG (STENG) is developed. PAAm-LiCl hydrogel wrapped with PDMS was used as a single-electrode TENG to detect pressure, and its structure is presented in Figure 6.6a. The sensor has a transmittance of 96.2% and a maximum elongation of 1160%. These STENGs can generate an open-circuit voltage of up to 145 V and an instantaneous areal power density of 35 mWm^{-2}. Simultaneously, the e-skin based on STENG can detect pressures as low as 1.3 kPa (Pu et al., 2017). A completely transparent and highly stretchable contact-separation TENG is prepared based on PDMS and applied to self-powered tactile sensing, its structure is presented in Figure 6.6b. Under different stretching ratios (0%, 10%, 50%, and 80% strain), the frictional electrical signal maintains a good

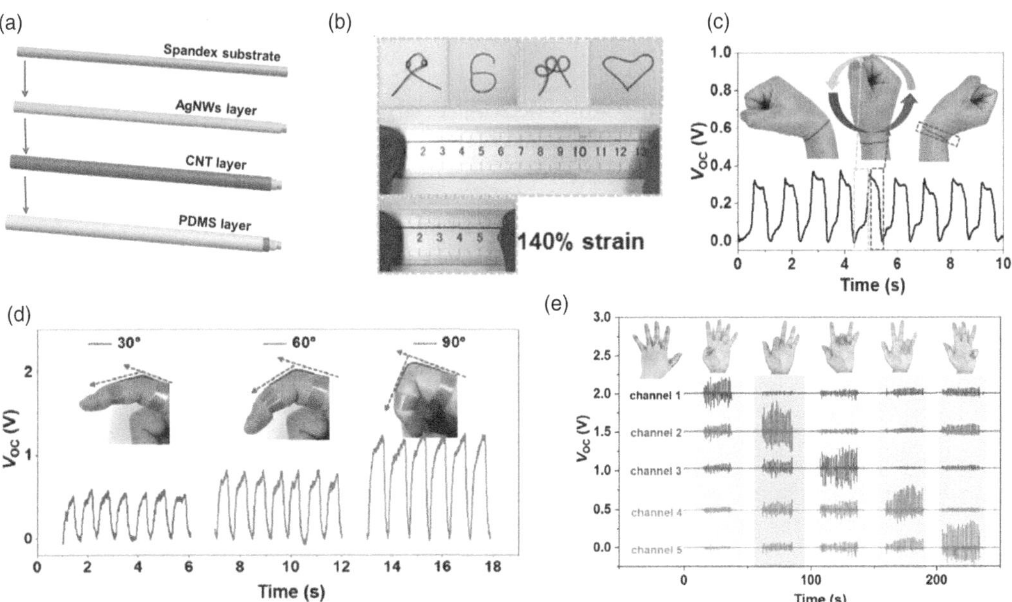

FIGURE 6.5   (a) The process of obtaining F-TENGs. (b) Photographs of the stretchable F-TENG. (c) The voltage of an F-TENG for different wrist states. (d) The peak value of an F-TENG under varying finger bending angles. (e) Voltage readings from the five F-TENGs fixed on the fingers. (Adapted with permission. (Ning et al., 2021) Copyright 2021, Wiley.)

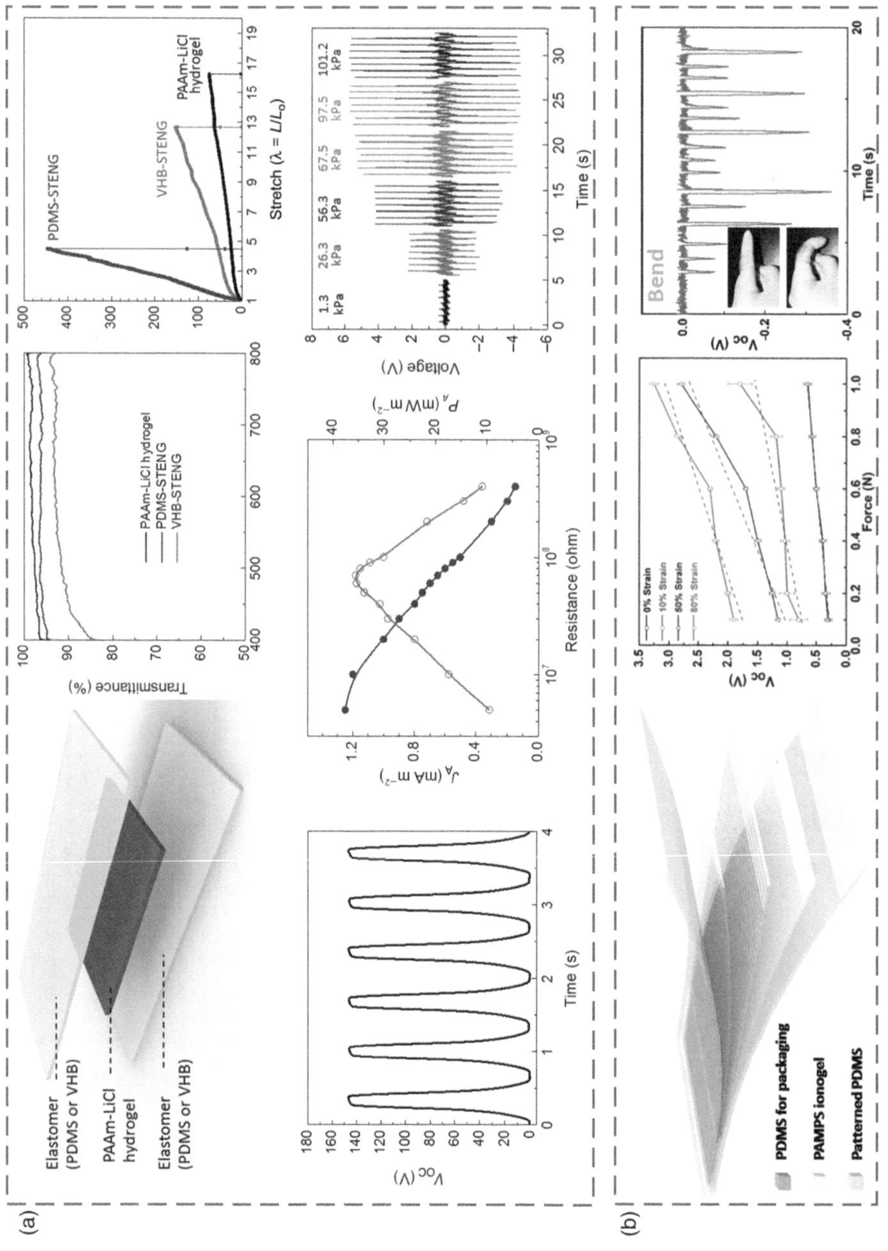

FIGURE 6.6 (a) Structure scheme and output measurement of the STENG. (b) The contact-separation TENG. ([a] Adapted with permission. (Pu et al., 2017) Copyright 2017, AAAS; [b] Adapted with permission. (Zhao et al., 2019) Copyright 2019, Elsevier Ltd.)

linear correlation. So that the sensor could be used to detect various human activities, such as the bend of a finger (Zhao et al., 2019).

6.2.2 Structural Design of E-skins

With the development of e-skin, high needs for flexible pressure sensors are placed on. Microengineering efficiently tunes the mechanical properties of active layers, enhancing sensor performance (Ruth et al., 2020). The sensor's sensitivity can be significantly improved by designing microscopic patterns on the surface of the sensitive layer. Various micropatterned designs were compared with a flat frictional electric surface of the same material, including lines, cubes, and pyramid structures, as shown in Figure 6.7a (Fan et al., 2012). The output trend is consistent with the increase in effective contact area caused by the surface structure (pyramid > cube > line > flat), leading to enhanced output. As shown in Figure 6.7b, microstructures such as microcolumns, hemispheres, and sponges have also been studied (Cheng et al., 2020; Lee et al., 2016; S. Wang et al., 2023a). The patterns provide different mechanical characteristics, resulting in diverse pressure sensor performances. The uneven stress distribution at the top of pyramid structures leads to small initial induction values but significant resistance changes can occur at relatively low pressures. Microspheres and laterally semi-circular shapes exhibit a more uniformly changing contact area, maintaining sensitivity at a given pressure.

As shown in Figure 6.8a, natural leaf patterns are utilized as molds to obtain micro-structured PDMS films (Jian et al., 2017). Aligned carbon nanotubes/graphene (ACNT/G) is used as the active material and microstructured PDMS is used as the flexible matrix. The obtained pressure sensors demonstrate high sensitivity (19.8 kPa^{-1}, <0.3 kPa), low detection limit (0.6 Pa), fast response time (<16.7 ms), low operating voltage (0.03 V), and excellent stability for more than 35,000 loading–unloading cycles. All the performance and devices were obtained at 0.03 V, proving the feasibility of working at low voltage. Inspired by the morphology of natural plant surfaces, a biomimetic self-powered TENG e-skin is developed. Figure 6.8b illustrates interlocking microstructures that have been incorporated into the friction layer to enhance the frictional electric effect (Yao et al., 2020).

Furthermore, the implementation of porous designs and multilayer stacking structures is also an effective strategy for improving the performance of pressure sensors. When the conductive material within the sensor exhibits unique micro and nanostructures, the deformation in the polymer matrix caused by external pressure creates additional permeation pathways for electrons, thereby increasing conductivity. The size and density of micropores play a crucial role in modifying Young's modulus of the active layer, influencing the sensitivity of the sensors. Larger pore sizes and increased porosity in the active layer help to improve sensor deformability, and thus sensitivity, although the detection range may decrease. An e-skin with a uniform-size micropore structure is proposed. The micropores are self-assembled in an orderly and uniform close-packed manner over a large area. As shown in Figure 6.9a, the sensitivity and dynamic range of the e-skin were controlled to be as high as 0.86 kPa^{-1} and up to 100 kPa through micropores ranging in size from 100 to 500 μm (Kim et al., 2019). Multilayer stacking structures provide another avenue for constructing the active layer, amplifying sensitivity through interactions

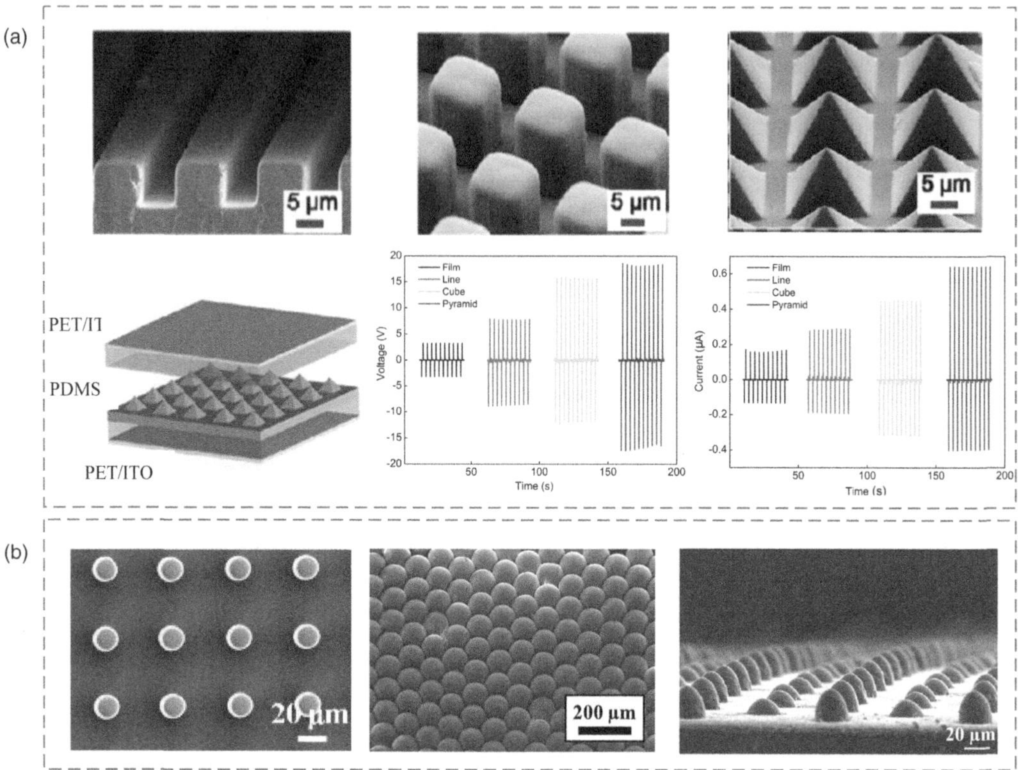

FIGURE 6.7   (a) The schematic and output measurement of pressure sensors made with different micropatterns. (b) Microstructures, namely microcolumns, hemispheres, and sponges. ([a] Adapted with permission. (Fan et al., 2012) Copyright 2012, American Chemical Society; [b] Adapted with permission. (Cheng et al., 2020; Lee et al., 2016; S. Wang et al., 2023a) Copyright 2020, Royal Society of Chemistry. Adapted with permission. Copyright 2016, Wiley. Adapted with permission. Copyright 2023, Wiley.)

between layers. An e-skin is developed that mimics mushrooms with a "stipe–pileus–papillary groove" architecture. The e-skin possesses high sensitivity (up to 600 kPa⁻¹), a broad pressure sensing range (up to 150 kPa), a short response time (<20 ms), and excellent durability (15,000 cycles) (Y. J. Zhang et al., 2023b) (Figure 6.9b).

6.3   SOFT IMPLANTABLE SENSORS

The field of medicine and biomedicine has continuously pursued more accurate and real-time data to enhance the effectiveness of diagnosis, treatment, and monitoring. The rapid development of flexible and stretchable electronic devices has provided the possibility to integrate sensors into implants for real-time physiological monitoring and optimization of implant functionality (Veletic et al., 2022). As a crucial branch of sensing technology, implantable sensors have gained widespread attention in the medical field. Their significance lies in the real-time collection, monitoring, and transmission of various physiological parameters, enabling healthcare professionals to get comprehensive and detailed data

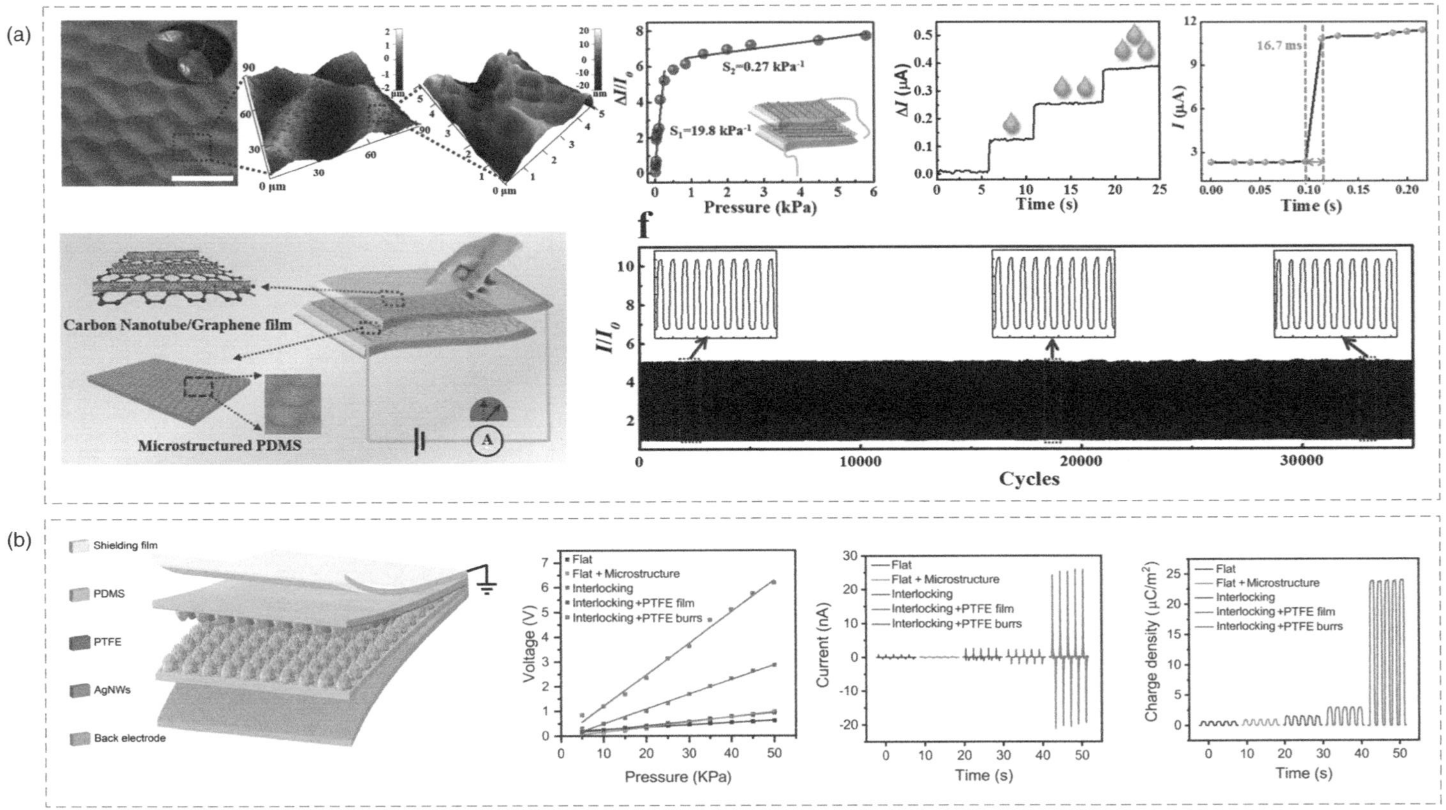

FIGURE 6.8 (a) The schematic and output measurement of pressure sensors made with micropatterns of a leaf (Jian et al., 2017). (b) The schematic and output measurement of a biomimetic self-powered TENG e-skin (Yao et al., 2020). ([a] Adapted with permission. Copyright 2017, Wiley; [b] Adapted with permission. Copyright 2020, Wiley.)

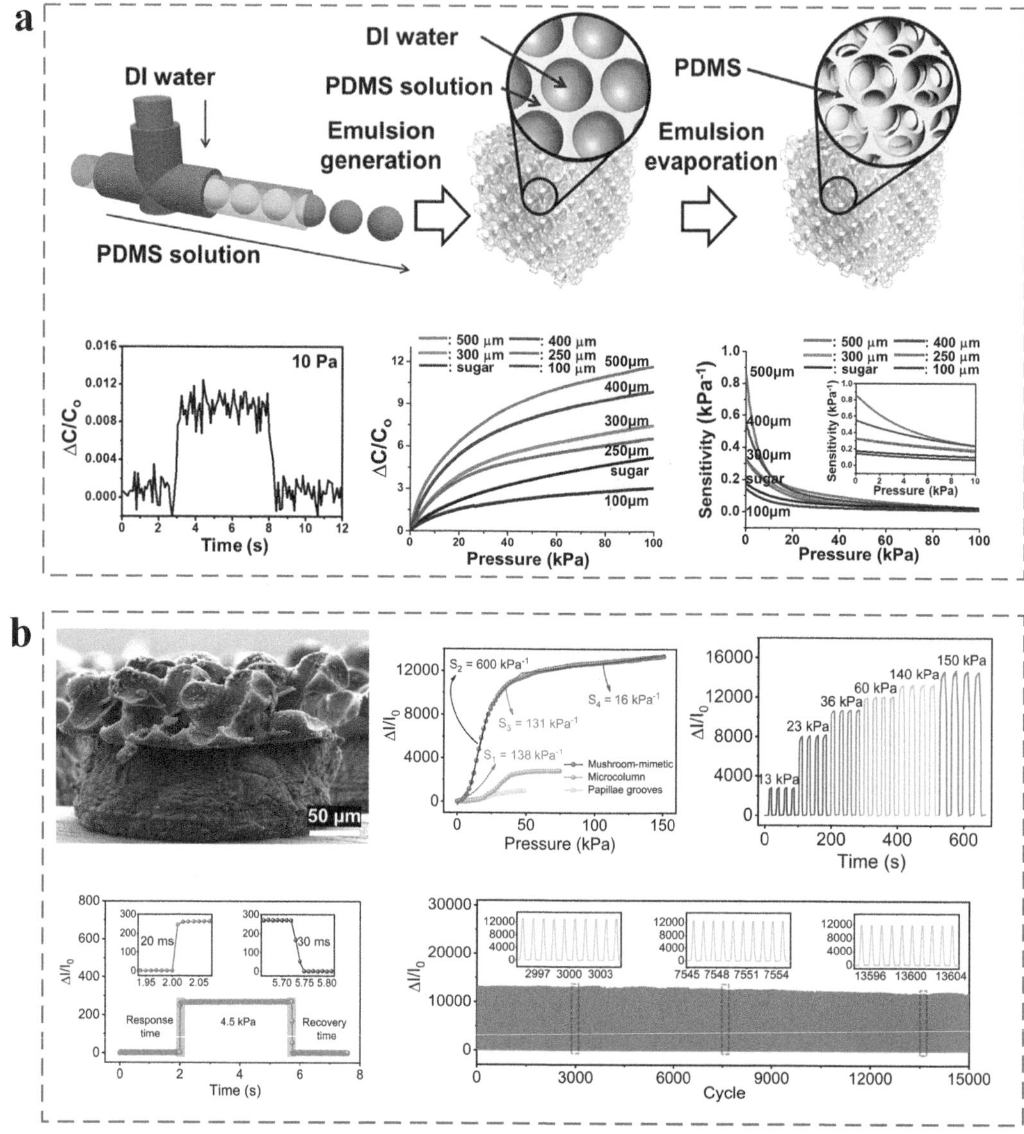

FIGURE 6.9 (a) The implementation of porous design on the e-skins. (b) The implementation of multilayer stacking structure designs on e-skins. ([a] Adapted with permission. (Kim et al., 2019) Copyright 2019, Wiley; [b] Adapted with permission. (Y. J. Zhang et al., 2023b) Copyright 2023, Royal Society of Chemistry.)

without causing harm. The sensors can monitor, track, and record vital signs (e.g., tissue deformation, electrical signals, and concentrations of molecular biomarkers). It empowers medical practitioners with detailed data while allowing patients to actively engage in their health management without adverse effects.

In the human body, soft and complex tissues necessitate that implantable sensors exhibit excellent compatibility in both mechanics and biology. Materials employed for implantable sensors must ensure that the sensors make soft and conformal contact with tissues while minimizing damage to the tissues during the sensing process (Hong et al., 2019), thereby achieving high sensitivity and stability. Concerning the *in vivo* environment, sensor implantation sites can be categorized into subcutaneous tissues, the digestive tract, visceral organs, and the brain as shown in Figure 6.10. Different implantation sites impose distinct design requirements on sensors. Sensors intended for ingestion into the digestive tract should maintain stability in highly acidic environments. Sensors adhered to visceral organs require high flexibility and tensile strength. Devices implanted in the brain not only need to exhibit high mechanical similarity to the brain but also require high biocompatibility to avoid interference with the central nervous system (Mei et al., 2022). Therefore, the customization of suitable materials is necessary for constructing implantable sensors with different mechanical, chemical, and electrical properties.

Generally, implantable devices are primarily prepared from three types of materials: polymers, hydrogels, and carbon-based materials. Polymers are organic macromolecules composed of repeating monomers. Its materials are often utilized as flexible substrates and coating materials to enhance the performance of sensors during the manufacturing process (Biswas et al., 2022). Benefiting from monomer synthesis and chain engineering, polymers can be designed as insulators, semiconductors, and conductors with rich electrical and mechanical properties. Synthetic polymers exhibit significant advantages in terms of implantability, biodegradability, catalysis, energy storage, and energy conversion. The polymer materials can also adapt to different specifications of sensors and their high designability promotes the development of implantable sensors. Hydrogels have excellent

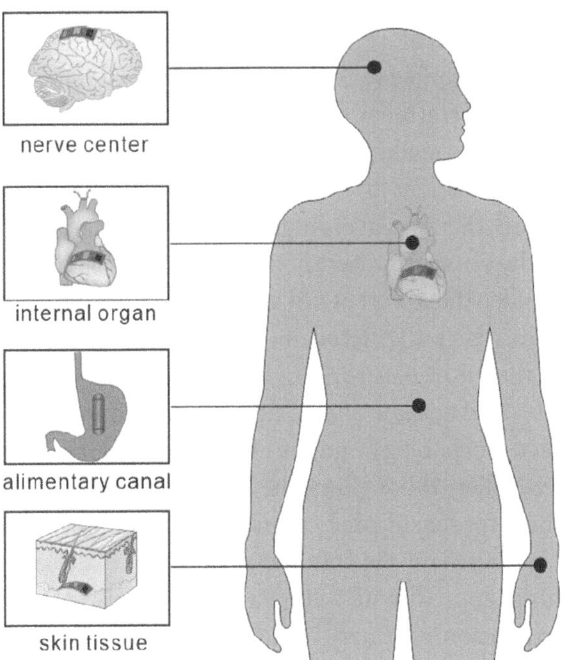

FIGURE 6.10   Schematic diagram of the distribution of implantable sensors in the human body. (Adapted with permission. (Mei et al., 2022) Copyright 2022, Wiley.)

biocompatibility due to their solubility, reactivity, and modification properties (Nishat et al., 2022). Carbon nanomaterials possess outstanding conductivity, performance metrics, and unique nanostructures, thereby exhibiting excellent biocompatibility and various biological effects, garnering widespread attention (Gaihre et al., 2022; Verma et al., 2022).

Non-degradable implantable sensors may interfere with imaging and become foci for bacterial infections or encounter displacement issues (Ribeiro et al., 2012). Therefore, a new generation of implantable sensors made from biodegradable materials is being explored. Firstly, sensors manufactured from biodegradable materials exhibit better biocompatibility, seamlessly integrating with the biological system and minimizing physiological impact on patients. In comparison to traditional implantable sensors that may trigger allergy or rejection, biodegradable sensors can alleviate tissue inflammation, enhancing the stability of implants within the biological system. Secondly, traditional implantable sensors often require secondary surgeries for removal, adding to patient discomfort and introducing risks of infection and other complications. Biodegradable sensors can naturally decompose after completing monitoring tasks, eliminating the need for additional surgeries and reducing the burden on patients. Additionally, due to the use of degradable materials, the shape and structure of the sensor can better adapt to the needs of the implantation site, providing more flexibility in design. It provides possibilities for monitoring within complex biological environments while minimizing interference with surrounding tissues during sensor implantation. Lastly, the development of biodegradable sensors is also to solve the power supply problem of traditional sensors. As the sensors degrade after completing tasks, they may no longer rely on conventional batteries for power. It offers a more flexible solution for wireless communication and data transmission, providing greater freedom in sensor design. The advancement of biodegradable sensors is expected to facilitate the broader application of implantable sensor technology. It can not only be used for monitoring vital signs and disease treatment but also has wider application and development in neuroscience research, sports medicine, and other fields.

The most stringent requirement for implant materials is biocompatibility; it ensures biomaterial effectiveness in therapy, avoiding harm and optimizing response (Williams, 2008). In addition to biocompatibility, the selection of biological materials for sensing devices must also consider the different physical/mechanical characteristics and dynamic features of various organs/tissues. Different mechanical properties and micro-environments of various tissues are shown in Figure 6.11. The elastic modulus should be similar to the surrounding tissues to avoid adverse effects such as tissue damage. The human brain has a complex curved surface morphology and the elastic modulus of brain tissue is between 0.5 and 1.0 kPa (Taylor & Miller, 2004). Since the brain undergoes minimal volume changes, the primary requirement for sensing devices in direct contact with the brain is a conformal covering with low impedance on the soft and folded brain surface. In contrast, the heart has an elastic modulus of approximately 20 kPa, significantly higher than the brain. And it undergoes periodic expansion/contraction movements, with a volume expansion/contraction ratio of about 10% (Carlsson et al., 2004). Cardiovascular diseases can increase the hardness of heart tissue by 2–3 times (Hiesinger et al., 2012). Therefore, cardiac devices need to exhibit stretchability that adapts to the movement and microenvironment changes

Tissue	Young's modulus Indentation (tensile)	Dynamics/Microenvironment	Sample Devices
(a) Brain	~1 kPa	- Highly convoluted surface topography - Neural activities occurring in submillimeter scale	
(b) Peripheral nerve	~10 kPa (~2 MPa)	- Surrounded by multiple layers of connective tissues - Constantly experiences non-uniform deformations	
(c) Heart	~20 kPa	- Periodic volumetric expansion/shrinkage (10%) - Shift in stiffness during different pathological conditions	
(d) Skin (abrasion)	-	- Change in mechanical and biochemical properties with respect to time (healing)	
(e) Blood Vessel	~125 kPa (~2 MPa)	- Significant noises from peripheral tissues - Lies deep inside the dermis	
(f) Skin	~85 kPa (~30 MPa)	- Stiffness varying by location, age, ethnicity - Complicated surface topography with nano-/micro-hierarchical structures	

FIGURE 6.11 Different mechanical properties and micro-environments of various tissues. (Adapted with permission. (Koo et al., 2020) Copyright 2020, Wiley.)

in the heart. Additionally, due to the surrounding muscle movements, nerves undergo continuous uneven deformation. Devices applied to these nerves should be manufactured using materials with extremely high toughness, durability, and sufficient stretchability.

All components of biodegradable sensors should be fabricated from degradable materials. Currently, degradable materials mainly include biodegradable metals, polymers, silicon, and their composites (Ashammakhi et al., 2021). The most commonly used metals in biodegradable sensors are magnesium (Mg), iron (Fe), tungsten (W), molybdenum (Mo), and zinc (Zn) (Li et al., 2018). Mg is suitable for sensor fabrication because of its high conductivity, ease of processing, and rapid degradation (Sezer et al., 2018). Fe has been extensively used in medical implants due to its excellent mechanical properties, while Mo is often employed in the communication components of implantable sensors (Curry et al., 2018). Biodegradable polymers are another crucial material for manufacturing biodegradable sensors. They can be used not only as substrates and sensor encapsulation materials but also as adhesives and dielectric layers for sensors (Hwang et al., 2014). Additionally, conductive polymers offer a range of advantages applicable in medical settings, including biocompatibility, biodegradability, and flexibility. They also support electronic and ionic transport, allowing for the easy presentation of specific chemical affinities and sensing characteristics (Balint et al., 2014). Silicon nanofilms (Si-NMs), porous and nanostructured variants and films, and SiO_2 are the most popular silicon-based materials. Generally, silicon-based materials are rigid and unsuitable for implantable devices. Hence, they are often prepared as flexible and elastic thin films (Ashammakhi et al., 2021).

Although biodegradable implantable sensors with proven biocompatibility and biodegradability in both *in vitro* and *in vivo* experiments have been developed, there is still a lack of published reports on clinical applications. However, an increasing number of reports are emerging regarding application in experimental animals. One such example is a fully biodegradable cuff-like pressure sensor made entirely of biodegradable materials; the illustration of a biodegradable and flexible arterial-pulse sensor is shown in Figure 6.12a (Boutry et al., 2019). It can be wrapped around blood vessels to measure arterial blood flow in both contact and non-contact modes. The sensor operates wirelessly through inductive coupling, where arterial pulsation causes changes in the capacitance of the sensor, subsequently altering the resonant frequency detected by the externally coupled coil. The artificial artery model *in vitro* and the rat model *in vivo* are tested. The set-up used in *in vitro* experiments is presented in Figure 6.12b and the test results of wired and wireless sensors are, respectively, shown in Figure 6.12c and d. The implantation site with the wired

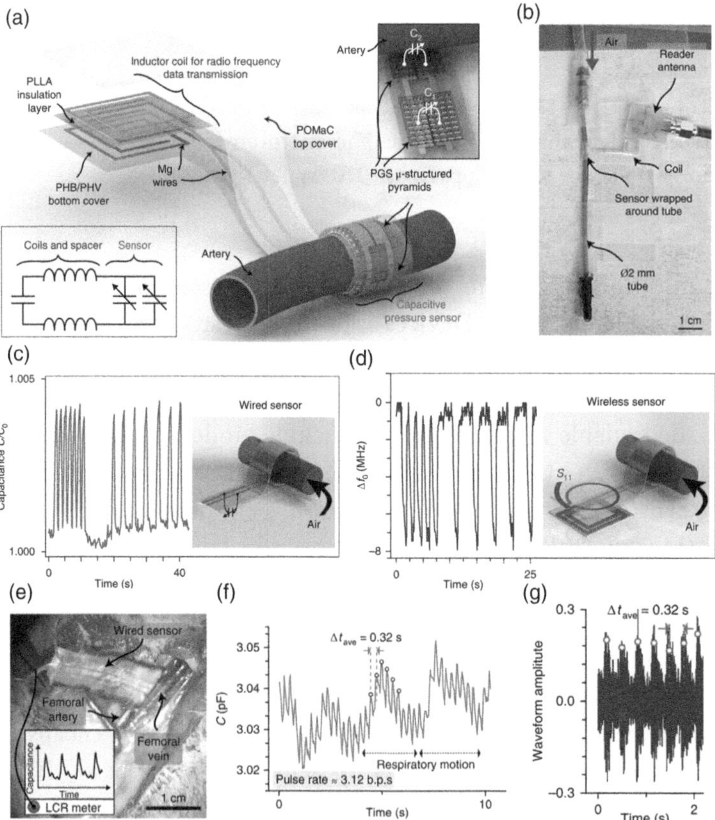

FIGURE 6.12　(a) Illustration of the sensor with an exposed view. The top-right portion provides a close-up of the pressure-sensitive region of the sensor, featuring the two variable capacitors, C_1 and C_2, before being encased around the artery. In the lower-left section, the equivalent electrical circuit is illustrated, with the two variable capacitors corresponding to C_1 and C_2. (b) Corresponding photograph of the sensor *in vitro* experiment. (c) The measured capacitance for a wired sensor. (d) Measured Δf_0 for a wireless sensor under various applied pressure patterns. (e) Image of the implantation site. (f) Measured capacitance of implanted wired sensor during *in vivo* tests. (g) Measured sound waveform of the external Doppler ultrasound.

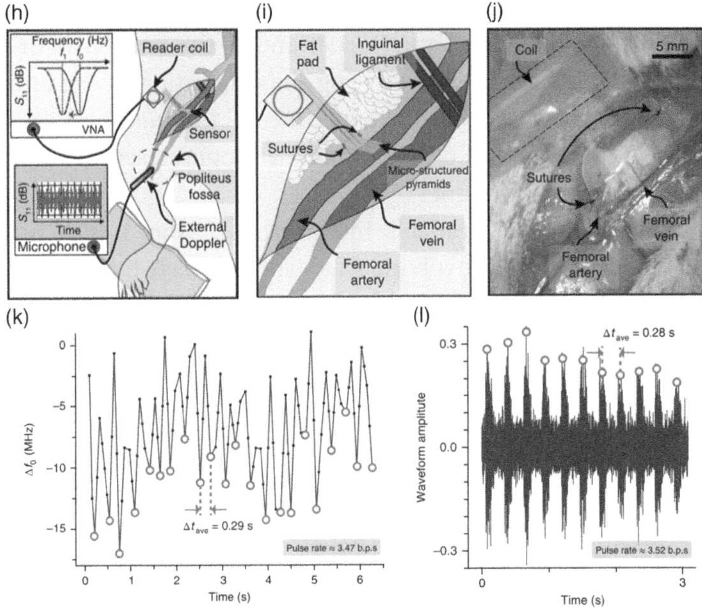

FIGURE 6.12 (Cont.) (h) Schematic of the measurement sensor. (i) Close-up view of the implantation site. (j) Image of an implant site. (k) Plot of measured Δf_0 versus time. (l) Sound waveform of the external Doppler ultrasound. (Adapted with permission. (Boutry et al., 2019) Copyright 2019, Spring Nature.)

sensor wrapped around the femoral artery and fixed with sutures is shown in Figure 6.12e. The measured capacitance and measured sound waveform of the external Doppler ultrasound of the implanted wired sensor are presented in Figure 6.12f and g, respectively. Figure 6.12h and i show the schematic and the placement of the measurement set-up. The image after the sensor is implanted and the skin is sutured is shown in Figure 6.12j. The measured capacitance and measured sound waveform of the external Doppler ultrasound of the implanted wireless sensor are presented in Figure 6.12k and l, respectively. The results show that both wired and wireless sensor configurations demonstrated excellent biocompatibility and pulse monitoring functionality.

Another proposed device is a fully biodegradable implantable pressure and strain sensor made entirely of biodegradable materials (Boutry et al., 2018). It distinguishes between strain and pressure by employing two vertically stacked sensors. The concepts of strain and pressure sensing are respectively shown in Figure 6.13a and b. When strain is applied, two thin film comb-like electrodes slide relative to each other, resulting in a change in capacitance. When pressure is applied, changes in the distance between the electrodes lead to variations in capacitance. The thin-film capacitor features a microstructured elastic dielectric based on poly (glycerol sebacate) (PGS). It is positioned between high-sensitivity plates made of Mg. Materials and structure of the sensor can be obtained from Figure 6.13c. The results of *in vitro* experiments (Figure 6.13d) compared with the reference microtester signal are shown in Figure 6.13e. Figure 6.13f and g depict the implanted position of the sensor and the method of signal application in *in vivo* experiments. Pressure and strain signals are respectively shown in Figure 6.13h and i. The bottom figures in both cases depict the corresponding baseline, illustrating the respiration of the animal as recorded with the pressure and strain sensors. The experimental findings, both *in vitro* and *in vivo*, clearly demonstrate the successful utilization of the proposed sensor for measuring physiological strain signals on the tendon.

Currently, research on biodegradable implantable sensors is still in its early stages. Several proof-of-concept studies involving small animals have demonstrated the potential for clinical applications. However, before biodegradable implantable sensors can be practically applied in clinical settings, numerous challenges still need to be addressed (Ashammakhi et al., 2021; Koo et al., 2020, 2021).

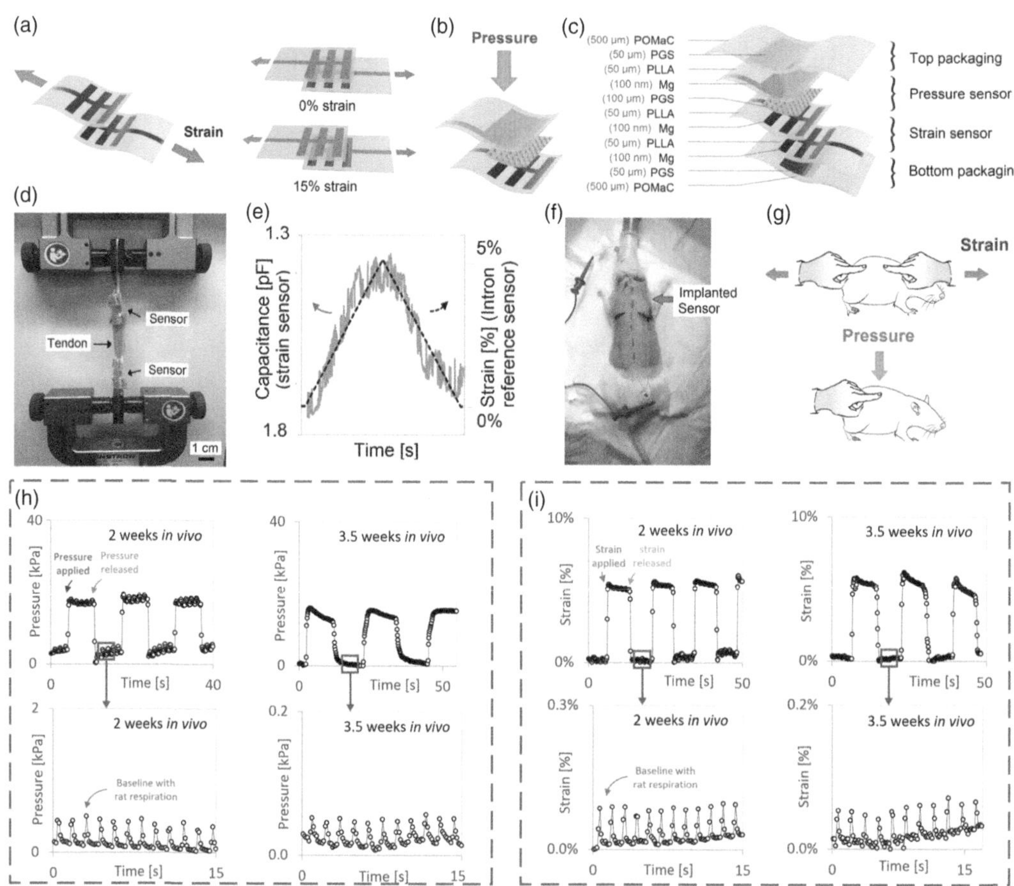

FIGURE 6.13 (a) Concepts used for strain sensing. (b) Concepts used for pressure sensing. (c) Materials and overall assembly of the full sensor. (d) *In vitro* study of the biodegradable strain and pressure sensor. (e) The signal was measured with the strain sensor and the reference microtester signal. (f) The sensors tested *in vivo* were implanted into the back of a Sprague–Dawley rat. (g) In the *in vivo* study, the implanted sensor registers signals of both strain and pressure. (h) Pressure signal recorded after 2 weeks and 3.5 weeks. (i) Strain signal recorded after 2 weeks and 3.5 weeks. (Adapted with permission. (Boutry et al., 2018) Copyright 2018, Spring Nature.)

Firstly, considering the degradation rate of implant devices in the body and their compatibility with existing manufacturing technologies, the material options for biodegradable sensors become more limited. There is a need for further exploration of new materials for semiconductors, conductors, dielectrics, and encapsulation, especially biodegradable semiconductor materials with high conductivity and flexibility. However, the degradation rate of the material determines the operational lifespan of the sensor. Once a biodegradable sensor comes into contact with bodily fluids, its components start to degrade, altering the characteristics and functionality of the sensor, and thereby affecting the accuracy and reliability of the measured signals. Therefore, encapsulating the sensor to protect it from the influence of bodily fluids is crucial. The development of novel materials and advancements in manufacturing technologies are necessary to enhance the performance and durability of sensor encapsulation.

Secondly, for compatibility with the soft and irregular contours of surrounding tissues, biodegradable sensors should have high flexibility. Most biodegradable materials are prone to dissolution at high temperatures, making them unsuitable for traditional microfabrication techniques. Although photolithography and printing technologies have been developed for manufacturing biodegradable sensors, photolithography struggles to create sensor components small enough for intricate interconnections and fine microstructures, while printing technologies are costly and time-consuming. Therefore, there is still a need to explore manufacturing technologies that integrate different biodegradable materials to prepare sensors effectively.

Lastly, power supply and battery life are significant challenges for implantable sensors. Power sources and sensor communication are among the most challenging components made from biodegradable materials. Traditional batteries have limited lifespans, requiring regular replacement or recharging, which is impractical for sensors intended for long-term implantation. Additionally, battery recharging may require the support of external devices, causing inconvenience for patients and increasing the risk of infection and mechanical failures. The development of nanogenerators and self-powering technologies is expected to improve power supply and endurance issues.

6.4 ENERGY STORAGE STRATEGIES FOR SOFT WEARABLE SYSTEMS

6.4.1 Structural Stretchability

As mentioned before, energy storage devices are essential for most wearable and implantable systems to provide a reliable and efficient source of power and enable long-term operation. To ensure conformity to the human body and improve comfort and wearability, stretchable and deformable materials and structures are crucial for the energy storage devices of wearable and implantable systems.

Although researchers have developed numerous intrinsically stretchable materials for electrodes and electrolytes including silicon-based composite materials and hydrogels (Song et al., 2019), their stretchability and performance are usually limited. Moreover, utilizing traditional non-stretchable materials and components is often inevitable in some cases where high electrode conductivity or different functionalities are required.

Therefore, in addition to intrinsically stretchable materials, realizing stretchability through structure design has been widely studied in wearable and implantable energy storage devices.

Researchers have explored various approaches to achieve structural stretchability, including wrinkle, serpentine, kirigami, and origami structures. Wrinkled structures have attracted significant attention in recent years due to their remarkable properties, including high stretchability, tunable surface area, and improved mechanical stability. Wrinkled structures are formed by pre-straining a thin film and then releasing it. This creates a network of wrinkles that can accommodate strain without breaking the film, as shown in Figure 6.14a, b (Yu et al., 2009). Yu et al. presented a stretchable supercapacitor using buckled single-walled carbon nanotube (SWNT) macrofilms. These supercapacitors can be stretched up to 130% without compromising their electrochemical performance. For better stretchability, Huang et al. reported a novel electrolyte comprised of polyacrylic acid cross-linked by hydrogen bonds and vinyl hybrid silica nanoparticles, which endows the supercapacitor with high stretchability, reaching 600% strain with enhanced performance (2015) (Figure 6.14c, d).

Serpentine structures are created by winding a thin film or wire into a snake-like pattern. This design allows the device to stretch by uncoiling the serpentine structure. John A. Rogers' group introduced soft network composite materials with serpentine metal mesh structures (Jang et al., 2015) as shown in Figure 6.14e, f. This low-modulus matrix exhibits a range of desired mechanical responses and can be stretched up to 57%, showing promising applications in skin-mounted electrophysiological sensors. Also, Figure 6.14g, h illustrates a "self-similar" serpentine geometry used for developing a rechargeable lithium-ion battery (Xu et al., 2013). Such a battery could be reversibly stretched up to 300% while maintaining a capacity density of 1.1 mAh cm^{-2}.

Kirigami structures are created by cutting a thin film into certain patterns. These cuts allow the film to stretch and deform without tearing. Figure 6.14i shows three kirigami patterns, that is, zigzag-cut pattern, cut-N-twist pattern, and cut-N-shear pattern (Song et al., 2015) (from left to right). Among these patterns, the cut-N-shear pattern achieves the highest package density without out-of-plane deformation under stretching. Therefore, Song et al. developed a stretchable lithium-ion battery based on this kirigami pattern which can be stretched over 150% while maintaining its functionality, which shows its application perspective in powering wearable electronics. Origami structures are created by folding a thin film into complex three-dimensional shapes. These shapes can be designed to expand and collapse, allowing the device to stretch and compress. Figure 6.14j sketched two examples of origami lithium-ion batteries using Miura folding (Song et al., 2014). These batteries are highly twistable and bendable without sacrificing their electrochemical performance, opening up exciting possibilities for diverse applications in wearable and implantable devices. Additionally, there are many other options to achieve structural stretchability, such as woven structures based on the interconnected nature of textiles and porous structures benefiting from the presence of internal voids in porous structures, which we will not discuss in detail here.

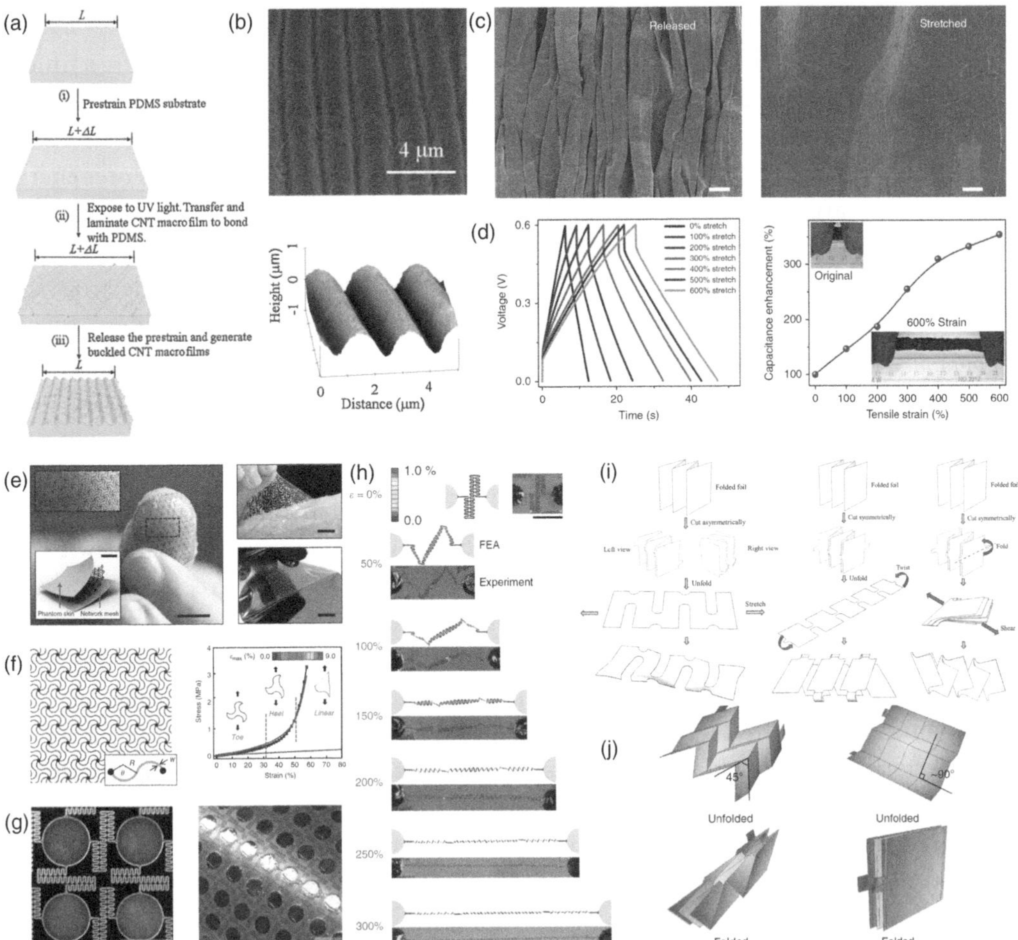

FIGURE 6.14 (a) Fabrication of wrinkled SWNT macrofilms on an elastomeric substrate. (b) Optical image and AFM image of the surface morphology. (c) SEM images of released and stretched PPy@CNT paper electrode after pre-stretching. (d) Galvanostatic charge/discharge curves and capacitance enhancement under different stretch ratios. (e) Optical images of skin-like composite elastomer wrapped on a thumb. (f) The design of the serpentine line. (g) Optical images of the Al electrode pads and serpentine layouts on a Si wafer (left) and silicone (right). (h) Simulation and experiment results of serpentine layouts under different stretch ratios. (i) Sketch of three kirigami patterns. (j) Two examples of origami batteries using Miura folding. ([a, b] Adapted with permission. (Yu et al., 2009) Copyright 2009, Wiley; [c, d] Adapted with permission. (Huang et al., 2015) Copyright 2015, Spring Nature; [e, f] Adapted with permission. (Jang et al., 2015) Copyright 2015, Spring Nature; [g, h] Adapted with permission. (Xu et al., 2013) Copyright 2013, Spring Nature; [i] Adapted with permission. (Song et al., 2015) Copyright 2015, AAAS; [j] Adapted with permission. (Song et al., 2014) Copyright 2014, Spring Nature.)

6.4.2 Wearable and Implantable Supercapacitors

Supercapacitors, also known as electrochemical capacitors or ultracapacitors, are a unique class of energy storage devices. A supercapacitor usually consists of two electrodes separated by an electrolyte. When a voltage is applied, positive and negative charges accumulate on the surface of the electrodes. The electric field between the electrodes stores energy. Based on the charge storage mechanism, there are two main types of supercapacitors (Gong & Cheng, 2017). One is electrochemical double-layer capacitors (EDLCs), where energy is stored in the electrostatic double layer formed at the interface between the electrode and the electrolyte. This double layer acts like a capacitor plate, storing charge without involving any chemical reactions. The other one is pseudocapacitors. These supercapacitors store energy through Faradaic reactions, where charge transfer occurs between the electrode and the electrolyte. This results in a higher energy density compared to EDLCs, while the charging and discharging rate is usually lower than EDLCs.

To accommodate the requirements of wearable and implantable systems, such as biocompatibility, flexibility, stretchability, and long lifespan, various supercapacitors with different materials and structures ranging from 1D to 3D have been reported. He et al. introduced biocompatible hydrophilic carbon nanotube (CNT) fibers for implantable supercapacitors (2017) (Figure 6.15a). Such supercapacitors can work in physiological fluids directly and their good biocompatibility is proved. As a result, this supercapacitor shows good flexibility and its specific capacitance reaches 10.4 F/cm^3 or 20.8 F/g. Also, the cyclic performance test demonstrates that its capacitance only dropped by 1.7% after 10,000 working cycles, as shown in Figure 6.15b. However, an *in vivo* test is required to fully confirm the biocompatibility and long-term safety. Another work from Hanyang University in South Korea developed a novel biosupercapacitor based on NAD/BQ/CNT yarn electrodes inspired by the cellular redox system (Jang et al., 2021). This biosupercapacitor has a maximum area capacitance of 55.73 mF/cm^2. The *in vivo* test is conducted under a rat's skin, showing good biocompatibility. As shown in Figure 6.15c, the performance of the supercapacitor *in vivo* is similar to that in PBS buffer solution. It is stable for two weeks of continuous testing, holding promise for powering implantable medical devices without the need for batteries.

As an example of film-based supercapacitors, Tian et al. demonstrated an implantable and biodegradable transient supercapacitor, which can be fully dissolved and broken down into environmentally friendly byproducts after fulfilling its function (Tian et al., 2021). As illustrated in Figure 6.15d, patterned Zn@PPy hybrid is an electrode prepared by screen printing and electrochemical deposition, while NaCl/agarose is selected as the electrolyte. Such a supercapacitor possesses a maximum energy density of 0.394 mWh/cm^2 and an *in vivo* biodegrading test is conducted as shown in Figure 6.15e. After being implanted in the subcutaneous region of rats, the supercapacitor was dissolved after 30 days, providing a feasible way for transient electronics in diverse implantable applications. For better stretchability, Bingqing Wei's group produced all-solid-state asymmetric stretchable supercapacitors based on the wrinkle structure design (Figure 6.15f), reaching a tensile strain of up to 100% (Gu & Wei, 2016). The wrinkled structure offers a large surface area

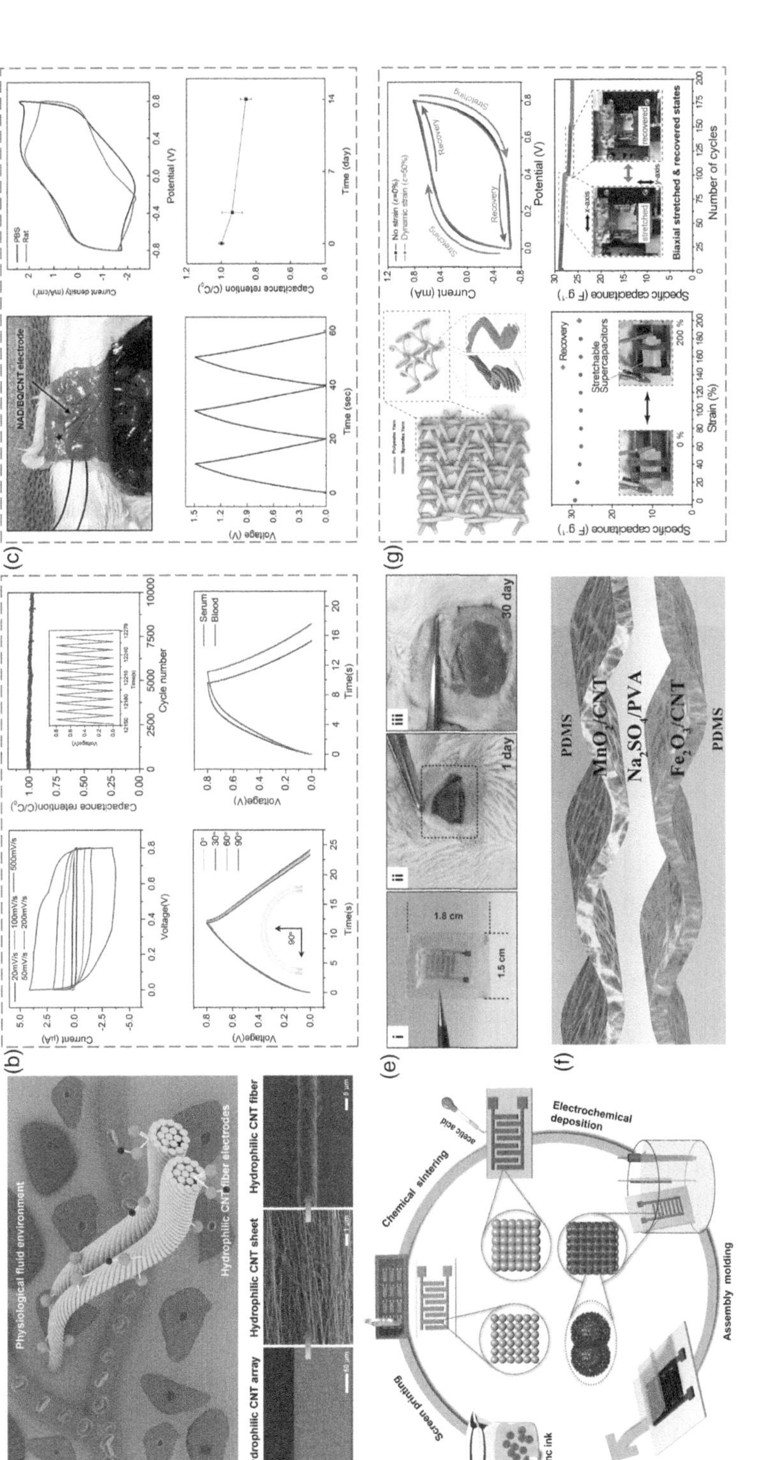

FIGURE 6.15 (a) Biocompatible fiber-based supercapacitor in the physiological fluids. (b) Performance of the biocompatible fiber-based supercapacitor. (c) Biosupercapacitor based on NAD/BQ/CNT yarn electrodes and their performance. (d) Fabrication of an implantable and biodegradable transient supercapacitor. (e) *In vivo* tests for the biodegradable transient supercapacitor. (f) A stretchable supercapacitor based on the wrinkle structure. (g) A stretchable supercapacitor based on an engineered tricot woven structure. ([a, b] Adapted with permission. (He et al., 2017) Copyright 2017, Elsevier Ltd.; [c] Adapted with permission. (Jang et al., 2021) Copyright 2021, Wiley; [d, e] Adapted with permission. (Tian et al., 2021) Copyright 2021, American Chemical Society; [f] Adapted with permission. (Gu & Wei, 2016) Copyright 2016, Royal Society of Chemistry; [g] Adapted with permission. (Lee et al., 2015) Copyright 2015, American Chemical Society.)

for efficient charge storage and a highly conductive network for rapid electron transport, achieving a high energy density of 45.8 Wh/kg and great cycling stability and durability. Woven structure can also be employed for supercapacitor applications. As shown in Figure 6.15g, Lee et al. demonstrated an engineered tricot weave that exhibits anomalous stretchable conductivity, which can maintain its exceptional electrical performance even when subjected to significant stretching (2015) (200 tensile strain). Both its CV curve and specific capacitance remained unchanged under dynamic strain. The capacitance of the textile-based supercapacitors could be well retained under repeated biaxial stretching, indicating a promising approach to wearable applications.

6.4.3 Wearable and Implantable Batteries

One great advantage of batteries compared to supercapacitors is the high energy density, which is crucial for device usage time, especially for implantable devices. In general, a battery is an electrochemical device that converts chemical energy directly into electrical energy. It consists of two or more connected electrochemical cells, each with a positive electrode (anode) and a negative electrode (cathode) separated by an electrolyte. To date, various batteries have been developed based on different materials and mechanisms, such as lithium-ion batteries utilizing lithium ions as the charge carriers, multivalent-based batteries utilizing multivalent ions, such as Mg^{2+}, Ca^{2+}, and Al^{3+}, as charge carriers instead of single-charged lithium ions, and metal–air batteries utilizing oxygen from the surrounding air as the oxidant, offering potentially high energy density. For wearable and implantable systems, there are additional requirements for batteries, including stretchability, biocompatibility, and safety even under leakage.

Figure 6.16a shows an all-solid-state fiber-shaped aluminum–air battery with exceptional flexibility, stretchability, and high electrochemical performance (Xu et al., 2016). This fiber battery was fabricated layer-by-layer around the aluminum spring anode using a coating and wrapping process, which enabled its stretchability (up to 30%). The energy density reached 935 mAh/g and its power density reached 1168 Wh/kg. After being woven into textiles, it was further applied to powering a commercial LED watch. For a larger scale integration, Huisheng Peng's group developed a continuous production line of fiber lithium-ion fiber batteries (FLIBs), including coating electrode slurry, wrapping separator, twisting fibers, and winding processes (He et al., 2021) (Figure 6.16b). Hundreds of meters of uniform FLIB were produced and the energy density exceeded 80 Wh/kg, which is comparable to commercial pouch cells. Such fiber batteries were subsequently woven into textiles using conventional industrial looms. Furthermore, a series of applications of the textile battery were exhibited, such as charging a cell phone wirelessly and powering textile displays and fiber sensors. For implanting purposes, Zhao et al. reported an injectable fiber battery which offers a promising solution for powering implantable medical devices throughout the body (Zhao et al., 2021). Such biocompatible and injectable fiber batteries use two twisted CNT-based fibers, CNT/NMO hybrid fiber and CNT/MoO$_3$/PPy hybrid fiber, as the cathode and anode, respectively (Figure 6.16c). Encapsulation isn't required as body fluid can be used as the electrolyte, which makes it quite soft and deliver a power

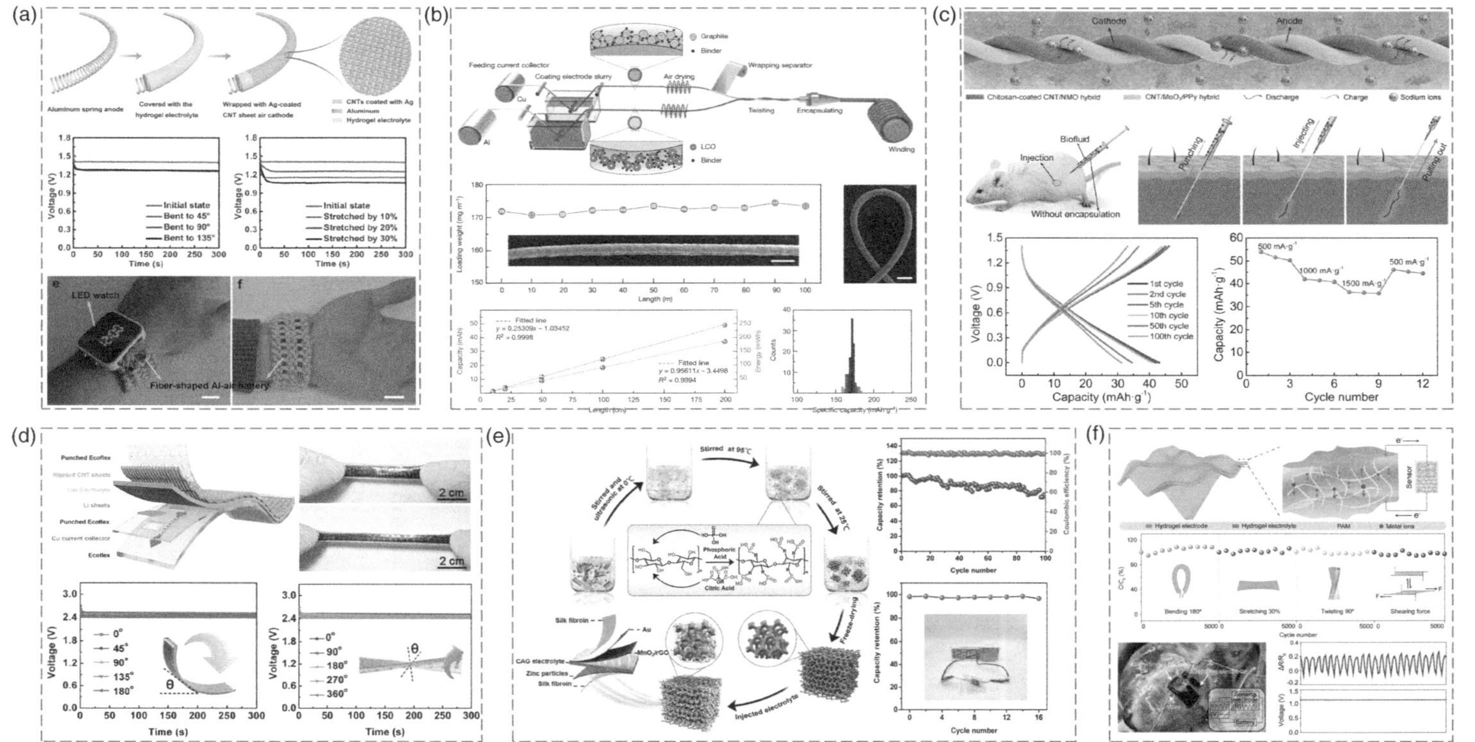

FIGURE 6.16   (a) An all-solid-state fiber-shaped aluminum–air battery with good bendability and stretchability. (b) Fiber lithium-ion fiber batteries and their scalable production. (c) Biocompatible and injectable fiber batteries and their durability. (d) A stretchable lithium–air battery based on Ecoflex substrate. (e) A biodegradable transient multivalent-based battery. [e] Adapted with permission. (Zhou et al., 2022) Copyright 2022, Wiley. (f) An all-hydrogel tissue-like battery. ([a] Adapted with permission. (Xu et al., 2016) Copyright 2016, Wiley; [b] Adapted with permission. (He et al., 2021) Copyright 2021, Spring Nature; [c] Adapted with permission. (Zhao et al., 2021) Copyright 2021, Royal Society of Chemistry; [d] Adapted with permission. (Wang et al., 2016) Copyright 2016, Royal Society of Chemistry; [f] Adapted with permission. (Ye et al., 2021) Copyright 2021, Wiley.)

density of 78.9 mW/cm³ *in vivo*. And the mini-invasive implanting methods also decrease the health risks of pain and morbidity for patients.

Film-based batteries were also extensively studied. Figure 6.16d displays a stretchable lithium–air battery based on Ecoflex substrate (Wang et al., 2016). The unique micro-structured design allows the battery to maintain its performance even when stretched up to 100%. The discharge capacity achieved 7111 mAh/g. And dynamic bending or twisting won't affect the discharging process obviously, providing a stable power supply for wearable applications. Moreover, Biao Kong's group developed a transient multivalent-based battery that is implantable and biodegradable (Zhou et al., 2022). The key to this device is its unique three-dimensional electrode structure (Figure 6.16e), which combines zinc and polypyrrole (PPy) in a super-assembled network. The specific capacity achieves 211.5 mAh/g, and this device can be completely degraded in 30 days, suggesting its potential in clinical applications. Hydrogel is also a popular material for wearable and implantable applications because of its merits in biocompatibility and tunable properties. Ye et al. developed an all-hydrogel battery that replicates the softness and flexibility of human tissue as shown in Figure 6.16f (2021). The interconnected hydrogel network enables efficient ion transport, resulting in high energy density (370 mAh/g at a current density of 0.5 A/g), which is comparable to conventional batteries. Furthermore, heart beating monitoring is realized by implanting this battery as well as a sensing electrode on the surface of the heart, indicating its future applications in powering wearable and implantable bioelectronics.

Additionally, it is worth mentioning that energy storage devices are not indispensable in all wearable and implantable systems. Some systems may only use energy conversion devices such as photovoltaic devices, thermoelectric devices, or generators to generate electricity and power the system in real time (Gong & Cheng, 2017). Also, wireless power has been widely studied as a power supply (Ho et al., 2014). These strategies offer wider choices for powering wearable and implantable systems under different circumstances.

6.5 CONCLUSION

The continuous advancements in materials science, microfabrication, and microelectronics technologies are propelling the field of soft wearable and implantable systems forward at an unprecedented pace. In this chapter, we have discussed different kinds of e-skins, presented the materials and configurations of implantable sensors, and introduced energy storage devices for wearable and implantable systems. Despite the remarkable progress, several challenges remain to be addressed. For example, the integration of various functionalities within a single platform requires seamless bonding of sensors, energy storage components, etc. Also, the biocompatibility and long-term stability of soft materials need further improvement to ensure the safety and efficacy of implantable systems. Further efforts should be made to address these challenges. And the combination between these systems and artificial intelligence could be an effective way to boost its future applications. We expect to see even more exciting developments in this field and believe it would change our lives in countless ways, improving health, enhancing well-being, and reshaping human–machine interactions.

REFERENCES

Ashammakhi, N., Hernandez, A. L., Unluturk, B. D., Quintero, S. A., De Barros, N. R., Apu, E. H., Holgado, M. (2021). Biodegradable implantable sensors: Materials design, fabrication, and applications. *Advanced Functional Materials*, 31(49), 2104149.

Balint, R., Cassidy, N. J., Cartmell, S. H. (2014). Conductive polymers: Towards a smart biomaterial for tissue engineering. *Acta Biomaterialia*, 10(6), 2341–2353.

Biswas, S., Kim, Hyeok, Lee, Y., Hyojeong, C. (2022). Current development in bio-implantable sensors. *Journal of Sensor Science and Technology*, 31(6), 403–410.

Boutry, C. M., Beker, L., Kaizawa, Y., Vassos, C., Tran, H., Hinckley, A. C., Bao, Z. N. (2019). Biodegradable and flexible arterial-pulse sensor for the wireless monitoring of blood flow. *Nature Biomedical Engineering*, 3(1), 47–57.

Boutry, C. M., Kaizawa, Y., Schroeder, B. C., Chortos, A., Legrand, A., Wang, Z., Bao, Z. N. (2018). A stretchable and biodegradable strain and pressure sensor for orthopaedic application. *Nature Electronics*, 1(5), 314–321.

Carlsson, M., Cain, P., Holmqvist, C., Stahlberg, F., Lundback, S., Arheden, H. (2004). Total heart volume variation throughout the cardiac cycle in humans. *American Journal of Physiology-Heart and Circulatory Physiology*, 287(1), H243–H250.

Chen, B. D., Zhang, L., Li, H. Q., Lai, X. J., Zeng, X. R. (2022). Skin-inspired flexible and high-performance MXene@polydimethylsiloxane piezoresistive pressure sensor for human motion detection. *Journal of Colloid and Interface Science*, 617, 478–488.

Chen, Y. C., Zhang, P., Li, Y. X., Zhang, K., Su, J. P., Huang, L. S. (2021). Flexible capacitive pressure sensor based on multi-walled carbon nanotubes microstructure electrodes. *Journal of Physics D-Applied Physics*, 54(15), 155101.

Cheng, L., Qian, W., Wei, L., Zhang, H., Zhao, T., Li, M., Wu, H. (2020). A highly sensitive piezoresistive sensor with interlocked graphene microarrays for meticulous monitoring of human motions. *Journal of Materials Chemistry C*, 8(33), 11525–11531.

Curry, E. J., Ke, K., Chorsi, M. T., Wrobel, K. S., Miller, A. N., Patel, A., Nguyen, T. D. (2018). Biodegradable piezoelectric force sensor. *Proceedings of the National Academy of Sciences of the United States of America*, 115(5), 909–914.

Fan, F. R., Lin, L., Zhu, G., Wu, W. Z., Zhang, R., Wang, Z. L. (2012). Transparent triboelectric nanogenerators and self-powered pressure sensors based on micropatterned plastic films. *Nano Letters*, 12(6), 3109–3114.

Gaihre, B., Potes, M. A., Serdiuk, V., Tilton, M., Liu, X. F., Lu, L. C. (2022). Two-dimensional nanomaterials-added dynamism in 3D printing and bioprinting of biomedical platforms: Unique opportunities and challenges. *Biomaterials*, 284, 121507.

Gao, L., Zhu, C. X., Li, L., Zhang, C. W., Liu, J. H., Yu, H. D., Huang, W. (2019). All paper-based flexible and wearable piezoresistive pressure sensor. *Acs Applied Materials & Interfaces*, 11(28), 25034–25042.

Gong, S., Cheng, W. (2017). Toward soft skin-like wearable and implantable energy devices. *Advanced Energy Materials*, 7(23), 1700648.

Gu, T., Wei, B. (2016). High-performance all-solid-state asymmetric stretchable supercapacitors based on wrinkled MnO2/CNT and Fe2O3/CNT macrofilms. *Journal of Materials Chemistry A*, 4(31), 12289–12295.

Guan, X. Y., Xu, B. G., Gong, J. L. (2020). Hierarchically architected polydopamine modified BaTiO3@P(VDF-TrFE) nanocomposite fiber mats for flexible piezoelectric nanogenerators and self-powered sensors. *Nano Energy*, 70, 104516.

Hassan, M., Abbas, G., Li, N., Afzal, A., Haider, Z., Ahmed, S., Peng, Z. (2021). Significance of flexible substrates for wearable and implantable devices: Recent advances and perspectives. *Advanced Materials Technologies*, 7(3).

He, J., Lu, C., Jiang, H., Han, F., Shi, X., Wu, J., Peng, H. (2021). Scalable production of high-performing woven lithium-ion fibre batteries. *Nature*, 597(7874), 57–63.

He, S., Hu, Y., Wan, J., Gao, Q., Wang, Y., Xie, S., Peng, H. (2017). Biocompatible carbon nanotube fibers for implantable supercapacitors. *Carbon*, 122, 162–167.

Hiesinger, W., Brukman, M. J., McCormick, R. C., Fitzpatrick, J. R., Frederick, J. R., Yang, E. C., Woo, Y. J. (2012). Myocardial tissue elastic properties determined by atomic force microscopy after stromal cell-derived factor 1α angiogenic therapy for acute myocardial infarction in a murine model. *Journal of Thoracic and Cardiovascular Surgery*, 143(4), 962–966.

Ho, J. S., Yeh, A. J., Neofytou, E., Kim, S., Tanabe, Y., Patolla, B., Poon, A. S. Y. (2014). Wireless power transfer to deep-tissue microimplants. *Proceedings of the National Academy of Sciences*, 111(22), 7974–7979.

Hong, Y. J., Jeong, H., Cho, K. W., Lu, N., Kim, D. H. (2019). Wearable and implantable devices for cardiovascular healthcare: from monitoring to therapy based on flexible and stretchable electronics. *Advanced Functional Materials*, 29(19), 1808247.

Huang, Y., Zhong, M., Huang, Y., Zhu, M., Pei, Z., Wang, Z., Zhi, C. (2015). A self-healable and highly stretchable supercapacitor based on a dual crosslinked polyelectrolyte. *Nature Communications*, 6(1), 1–8.

Hwang, S. W., Song, J. K., Huang, X., Cheng, H. Y., Kang, S. K., Kim, B. H., Rogers, J. A. (2014). High-performance biodegradable/transient electronics on biodegradable polymers. *Advanced Materials*, 26(23), 3905–3911.

Jang, K.-I., Chung, H. U., Xu, S., Lee, C. H., Luan, H., Jeong, J., Rogers, J. A. (2015). Soft network composite materials with deterministic and bio-inspired designs. *Nature Communications*, 6(1), 6566.

Jang, Y., Park, T., Kim, E., Park, J. W., Lee, D. Y., Kim, S. J. (2021). Implantable biosupercapacitor inspired by the cellular redox system. *Angewandte Chemie International Edition*, 60(19), 10563–10567.

Jian, M. Q., Xia, K. L., Wang, Q., Yin, Z., Wang, H. M., Wang, C. Y., Zhang, Y. Y. (2017). Flexible and highly sensitive pressure sensors based on bionic hierarchical structures. *Advanced Functional Materials*, 27(9), 1606066.

Khan, H., Mahmood, N., Zavabeti, A., Elbourne, A., Rahman, M. A., Zhang, B. Y., Kalantar-Zadeh, K. (2020). Liquid metal-based synthesis of high performance monolayer SnS piezoelectric nanogenerators. *Nature Communications*, 11(1), 3449.

Kim, J. O., Kwon, S. Y., Kim, Y., Choi, H. B., Yang, J. C., Oh, J., Park, S. (2019). Highly ordered 3D microstructure-based electronic skin capable of differentiating pressure, temperature, and proximity. *ACS Applied Materials & Interfaces*, 11(1), 1503–1511.

Koo, J. H., Song, J. K., Kim, D. H., Son, D. (2021). Soft implantable bioelectronics. *Acs Materials Letters*, 3(11), 1528–1540.

Koo, J. H., Song, J. K., Yoo, S., Sunwoo, S. H., Son, D., Kim, D. H. (2020). Unconventional device and material approaches for monolithic biointegration of implantable sensors and wearable electronics. *Advanced Materials Technologies*, 5(10), 2000407.

Koydemir, H. C., Ozcan, A. (2018). wearable and implantable sensors for biomedical applications. *Annual Review of Analytical Chemistry*, 11(1), 127–146.

Kumar, A. (2022). Recent progress in the fabrication and applications of flexible capacitive and resistive pressure sensors. *Sensors and Actuators A: Physical*, 344, 113770.

Lee, K. Y., Yoon, H. J., Jiang, T., Wen, X., Seung, W., Kim, S. W., Wang, Z. L. (2016). Fully packaged self-powered triboelectric pressure sensor using hemispheres-array. *Advanced Energy Materials*, 6(11), 1502566.

Lee, Y., Myoung, J., Cho, S., Park, J., Kim, J., Lee, H., Ko, H. (2021). Bioinspired Gradient Conductivity and Stiffness for Ultrasensitive Electronic Skins. *Acs Nano*, 15(1), 1795–1804.

Lee, Y. H., Kim, Y., Lee, T. I., Lee, I., Shin, J., Lee, H. S., Choi, J. W. (2015). Anomalous stretchable conductivity using an engineered tricot weave. *Acs Nano*, 9(12), 12214–12223.

Li, R., Wang, L., Kong, D., Yin, L. (2018). Recent progress on biodegradable materials and transient electronics. *Bioactive Materials*, 3(3), 322–333.

Li, R. Q., Zhou, Q., Bi, Y., Cao, S. J., Xia, X., Yang, A. L., Xiao, X. L. (2021). Research progress of flexible capacitive pressure sensor for sensitivity enhancement approaches. *Sensors and Actuators a-Physical*, 321, 112425.

Mei, X. Y., Ye, D. K., Zhang, F. J., Di, C. A. (2022). Implantable application of polymer-based biosensors. *Journal of Polymer Science*, 60(3), 328–347.

Ning, C., Dong, K., Cheng, R. W., Yi, J., Ye, C. Y., Peng, X., Wang, Z. L. (2021). Flexible and stretchable fiber-shaped triboelectric nanogenerators for biomechanical monitoring and human-interactive sensing. *Advanced Functional Materials*, 31(4), 2006679.

Nishat, Z. S., Hossain, T., Islam, M. N., Phan, H. P., Wahab, M. A., Moni, M. A., Masud, M. K. (2022). Hydrogel nanoarchitectonics: An evolving paradigm for ultrasensitive biosensing. *Small*, 18(26), 2107571.

Pierre Claver, U., Zhao, G. (2021). Recent progress in flexible pressure sensors based electronic skin. *Advanced Engineering Materials*, 23(5), 2001187.

Pu, X., Liu, M. M., Chen, X. Y., Sun, J. M., Du, C. H., Zhang, Y., Wang, Z. L. (2017). Ultrastretchable, transparent triboelectric nanogenerator as electronic skin for biomechanical energy harvesting and tactile sensing. *Science Advances*, 3(5), 1700015.

Qiao, Y. C., Li, X. S., Jian, J. M., Wu, Q., Wei, Y. H., Shuai, H., Ren, T. L. (2020). Substrate-free multilayer graphene electronic skin for intelligent diagnosis. *Acs Applied Materials & Interfaces*, 12(44), 49945–49956.

Ribeiro, M., Monteiro, F. J., Ferraz, M. P. (2012). Infection of orthopedic implants with emphasis on bacterial adhesion process and techniques used in studying bacterial-material interactions. *Biomatter*, 2(4), 176–194.

Roberts, P., Damian, D. D., Shan, W. L., Lu, T., Majidi, C., IEEE. (2013). Soft-Matter Capacitive Sensor for Measuring Shear and Pressure Deformation. *IEEE International Conference on Robotics and Automation ICRA*.

Ruth, S. R. A., Feig, V. R., Tran, H., Bao, Z. (2020). Microengineering pressure sensor active layers for improved performance. *Advanced Functional Materials*, 30(39), 2003491.

Sarwar, M. S., Ishizaki, R., Morton, K., Preston, C., Nguyen, T., Fan, X., Madden, J. D. W. (2023). Touch, press and stroke: a soft capacitive sensor skin. *Scientific Reports*, 13(1), 17390.

Sezer, N., Evis, Z., Kayhan, S. M., Tahmasebifar, A., Koç, M. (2018). Review of magnesium-based biomaterials and their applications. *Journal of Magnesium and Alloys*, 6(1), 23–43.

Song, W. J., Yoo, S., Song, G., Lee, S., Kong, M., Rim, J., Park, S. (2019). Recent progress in stretchable batteries for wearable electronics. *Batteries & Supercaps*, 2(3), 181–199.

Song, Z., Ma, T., Tang, R., Cheng, Q., Wang, X., Krishnaraju, D., Jiang, H. (2014). Origami lithium-ion batteries. *Nature Communications*, 5(1), 3140.

Song, Z., Wang, X., Lv, C., An, Y., Liang, M., Ma, T., Jiang, H. (2015). Kirigami-based stretchable lithium-ion batteries. *Scientific Reports*, 5(1), 10988.

Soni, M., Dahiya, R. (2020). Soft eSkin: distributed touch sensing with harmonized energy and computing. *Philosophical Transactions of the Royal Society A*, 378(2164), 20190156.

Taylor, Z., Miller, K. (2004). Reassessment of brain elasticity for analysis of biomechanisms of hydrocephalus. *Journal of Biomechanics*, 37(8), 1263–1269.

Tian, W., Li, Y., Zhou, J., Wang, T., Zhang, R., Cao, J., Kong, B. (2021). Implantable and biodegradable micro-supercapacitor based on a superassembled three-dimensional network Zn@PPy hybrid electrode. *Acs Applied Materials & Interfaces*, 13(7), 8285–8293.

Veletic, M., Apu, E. H., Simic, M., Bergsland, J., Balasingham, I., Contag, C. H., Ashammakhi, N. (2022). Implants with sensing capabilitie. *Chemical Reviews*, 122(21), 16329–16363.

Verma, M. L., Sukriti, D. B. S., Saini, R., Das, A., Varma, R. S. (2022). Synthesis and application of graphene-based sensors in biology: a review. *Environmental Chemistry Letters*, 20(3), 2189–2212.

Wang, L., Zhang, Y., Pan, J., Peng, H. (2016). Stretchable lithium-air batteries for wearable electronics. *Journal of Materials Chemistry A*, 4(35), 13419–13424.

Wang, S., Deng, W., Yang, T., Ao, Y., Zhang, H., Tian, G., Lan, B. (2023a). Bioinspired MXene-based piezoresistive sensor with two-stage enhancement for motion capture. *Advanced Functional Materials*, 2214503.

Wang, W., Jiang, Y., Zhong, D., Zhang, Z., Choudhury, S., Lai, J. C., Bao, Z. (2023b). Neuromorphic sensorimotor loop embodied by monolithically integrated, low-voltage, soft e-skin. *Science*, 380(6646), 735–742.

Wang, X. D., Dong, L., Zhang, H. L., Yu, R. M., Pan, C. F., Wang, Z. L. (2015). Recent progress in electronic skin. *Advanced Science*, 2(10), 1500169.

Weigel, M., Lu, T., Bailly, G., Oulasvirta, A., Majidi, C., Steimle, J., Assoc Comp, M. (2015, Apr 18–23). iSkin: Flexible, stretchable and visually customizable on-body touch sensors for mobile computing. *33rd Annual CHI Conference on Human Factors in Computing Systems (CHI)*.

Williams, D. F. (2008). On the mechanisms of biocompatibility. *Biomaterials*, 29(20), 2941–2953.

Wu, Y. L., Ma, Y. L., Zheng, H. Y., Ramakrishna, S. (2021). Piezoelectric materials for flexible and wearable electronics: A review. *Materials & Design*, 211, 110164.

Xu, S., Zhang, Y., Cho, J., Lee, J., Huang, X., Jia, L., Rogers, J. A. (2013). Stretchable batteries with self-similar serpentine interconnects and integrated wireless recharging systems. *Nature Communications*, 4(1), 1543.

Xu, Y., Zhao, Y., Ren, J., Zhang, Y., Peng, H. (2016). An all-solid-state fiber-shaped aluminum–air battery with flexibility, stretchability, and high electrochemical performance. *Angewandte Chemie*, 128(28), 8111–8114.

Yang, J. C., Mun, J., Kwon, S. Y., Park, S., Bao, Z. N., Park, S. (2019). Electronic skin: Recent progress and future prospects for skin-attachable devices for health monitoring, robotics, and prosthetics. *Advanced Materials*, 31(48), 1904765.

Yao, G., Xu, L., Cheng, X. W., Li, Y. Y., Huang, X., Guo, W., Wu, H. (2020). Bioinspired triboelectric nanogenerators as self-powered electronic skin for robotic tactile sensing. *Advanced Functional Materials*, 30(6), 1907312.

Ye, T., Wang, J., Jiao, Y., Li, L., He, E., Wang, L., Zhang, Y. (2021). A tissue-like soft all-hydrogel battery. *Advanced Materials*, 34(4), 2105120.

Yu, C., Masarapu, C., Rong, J., Wei, B., Jiang, H. (2009). Stretchable supercapacitors based on buckled single-walled carbon-nanotube macrofilms. *Advanced Materials*, 21(47), 4793–4797.

Yu, P. T., Li, X., Li, H. Y., Fan, Y. J., Cao, J. W., Wang, H. L., Zhu, G. (2021). All-fabric ultrathin capacitive sensor with high pressure sensitivity and broad detection range for electronic skin. *Acs Applied Materials & Interfaces*, 13(20), 24062–24069.

Zhang, M., Wang, W. L., Xia, G. T., Wang, L. C., Wang, K. (2023a). Self-powered electronic skin for remote human-machine synchronization. *Acs Applied Electronic Materials*, 5(1), 498–508.

Zhang, Y. J., Zhang, X. Y., Ning, C., Dai, K., Zheng, G. Q., Liu, C. T., Shen, C. Y. (2023b). Mushroom-mimetic 3D hierarchical architecture-based e-skin with high sensitivity and a wide sensing range for intelligent perception. *Materials Horizons*, 10, 5666–5676.

Zhao, G. R., Zhang, Y. W., Shi, N., Liu, Z. R., Zhang, X. D., Wu, M. Q., Wang, Z. L. (2019). Transparent and stretchable triboelectric nanogenerator for self-powered tactile sensing. *Nano Energy*, 59, 302–310.

Zhao, Y., Mei, T., Ye, L., Li, Y., Wang, L., Zhang, Y., Peng, H. (2021). Injectable fiber batteries for all-region power supply in vivo. *Journal of Materials Chemistry A*, 9(3), 1463–1470.

Zhou, J., Zhang, R., Xu, R., Li, Y., Tian, W., Gao, M., Kong, B. (2022). Super-assembled hierarchical cellulose aerogel-gelatin solid electrolyte for implantable and biodegradable Zinc ion battery. *Advanced Functional Materials*, 32(21), 2111406.

CHAPTER 7

Advanced Soft Robotics for Biomedical Applications

Tiantian Dai and Yanting Liu

7.1 MECHANISM AND DESIGNING OF SOFT ROBOTICS

Soft robotics can convert various external energy to mechanical energy for actuating by materials selection, structural design, and function integration utilizing tethered, untethered, or biohybrid approaches. Figure 7.1 reviewed the popular actuating mechanism of tethered and untethered soft actuators.

For the tethered approach, the fluidic soft actuator is one of the most prevalent soft actuator types. By controlling the fluid pressure inside the hollow channels of the soft body, basic actuating functions such as gripping and locomotion can be achieved (Vasios et al., 2020). Through the dynamic analysis of the soft actuator, the parameters of the robot's mechanical design can be optimized (Luo et al., 2014). Fluidic actuators have the advantages of being highly compliant, easy to fabricate, and able to provide large deformations, but slow and imprecise actuation limits their development (Bell et al., 2021). Electrically driven actuation is also one of the most common tethered soft actuation methods. It utilizes Maxwell stress to induce a mechanical shape change in dielectric soft materials (Ji et al., 2020). For example, dielectric elastomer actuators directly convert electrical energy into mechanical energy upon an applied voltage, which can contract along the direction of the electric field and expand in the area orthogonal to the electric field direction (Ren et al., 2021). Electrothermal actuators are tethered systems that exploit the electrically resistive material to generate Joule heating to achieve thermal expansion and contraction by applying external voltage. Different kinds of materials such as shape-memory polymers (Wei et al., 2022), 2D materials (W. Li et al., 2022a), hydrogels (Zou et al., 2021), etc. can be designed as electrical thermal responsive actuators with the help of metal electrodes and metal nanoparticles. In addition, passive deformation (Choi et al., 2020) caused by tension transmitted through tendons from external motors can be achieved by using multiple motors connected by tendons to different parts of a soft body, which is similar to biological tendons and the supplement of fluidic driven actuator for the soft machines with discontinuous or architected bodies. The complicated connection, large volume, and the requirement of motors, pumps, or cords for tethered soft actuators

DOI: 10.1201/9781003493631-7

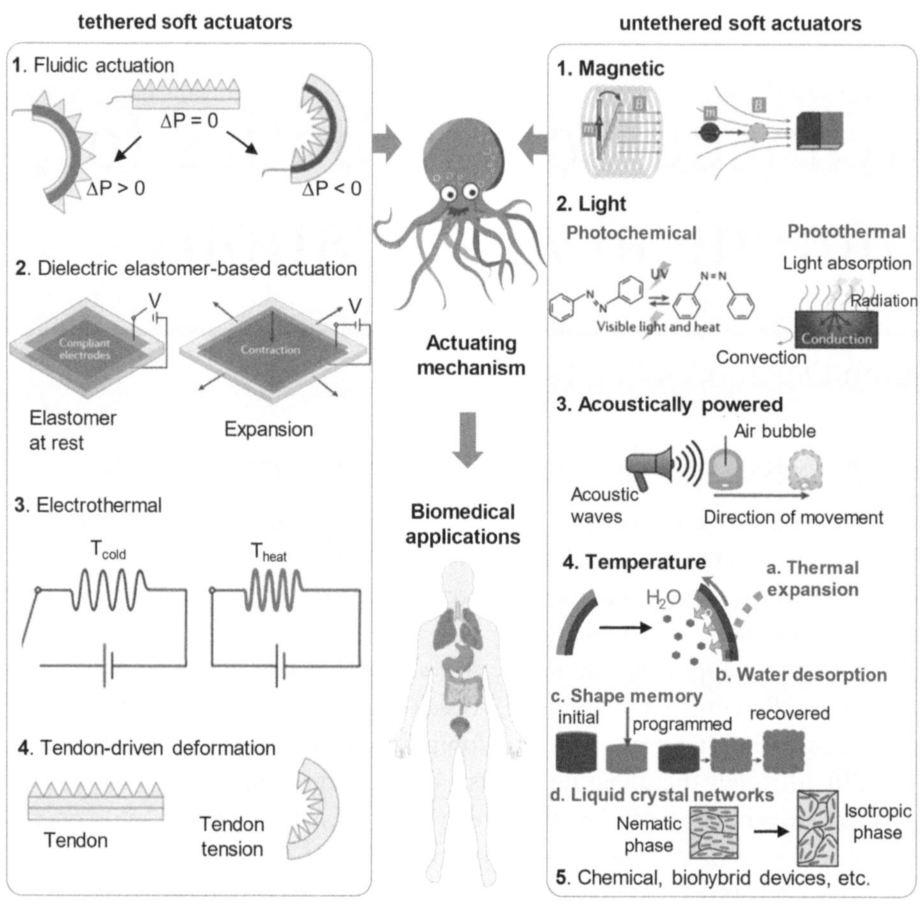

FIGURE 7.1 The actuating mechanism of tethered and untethered soft actuators. (Adapted with permission (Li et al., 2021). Copyright 2021, Springer Nature Limited.)

constrain device miniaturization and mobility. To overcome these challenges, developing untethered soft robots is overwhelming for biomedical applications.

For the untethered approach, the most popular stimuli method is magnetic actuating. Magnetic actuators are actuated by the torques or forces generated by the interaction between controlled external magnetic fields or gradients and the magnetic properties of the actuator. The amplitude, gradient, and direction of the magnetic field can be modulated with high temporal resolution, enabling deep tissue penetration, which is capable of providing both the needed power and precise control of a new generation of medical robotics, especially in miniaturized applications (Ebrahimi et al., 2020; Li et al., 2021). With sophisticated control of external magnetic fields and actuator magnetization profiles, soft robotics with diverse specific structures and sophisticated functions, including metamaterials, programmable/reprogramming deformations, and multimodal locomotion, have been realized (Chung et al., 2020; Wang et al., 2022). Light is also commonly used as a wireless stimulus for soft actuators. The working principle of light-responsive actuators is usually based on photochemical reactions and/ or the photothermal effect. Depending on the chemistry and optical absorptive properties of the light-active components in the actuator, soft actuators can actuate under the irradiation of selective wavelength light or wide-spectrum light (white light). Based on the photochemical effect, the ordering change would occur due to the photoisomerization of azobenzene derivatives (Pang et al., 2019; Zhu et al., 2021) or photothermal conversion caused temperature change would induce actuating (Li et al., 2019). Photothermal conversion is usually realized by using non-radiative transition of electrons and local surface plasma resonance effect (precious metal modification). Under the irradiation of a particular wavelength of light, the photothermal conversion material can quickly change from the ground state to the excited state, dissipate energy in the form of heat, and then return to the ground state (Jin et al., 2022; Yang et al., 2020). The actuating mechanism of photothermal conversion that caused temperature increase is similar to the temperature-induced actuating deformation. By the design of actuating materials, light or temperature change can also trigger mismatch deformation of soft actuator and motion via shape-memory effect (Choi et al., 2020; Jin et al., 2022), inequivalent thermal expansion (Yang et al., 2020; Zhang et al., 2022), water desorption (Duan et al., 2020; J. Li et al., 2022b), phase transition (Meder et al., 2019; Shao et al., 2022), etc. Furthermore, acoustic waves are another viable energy source for mechanical soft actuation, owing to their deep penetration into biological tissues and fluidic media. The acoustic energy can efficiently be converted into motion with the assistance of mechanical resonance by integrating oscillatory elements such as gas bubbles (Kaynak et al., 2022) or sharp, flexible structures (Kaynak et al., 2020) into the robot body to produce propulsion. Other actuating mechanisms like chemical stimuli, such as humidity, ionic strength, and chemical substances, can also actuate stimuli-responsive soft materials as well as biohybrid soft actuators by utilizing biological cells and microorganisms to convert chemical energy into mechanical work.

7.2 SOFT ROBOTS FOR SURGERY AND DRUG DELIVERY

Soft microrobots and nanorobots are small-scale manipulatable devices at the micrometer and nanometer scales which have been noted to be of great interest in biomedical applications such as surgery, targeted drug delivery, and cell manipulation due to their less invasive, biocompatible, and wireless operation. However, many regions inside the body, such as the brain vasculature, remain inaccessible due to the lack of appropriate guidance and precise control technologies. To solve this problem, Pancaldi et al. (2020) introduced a robotic navigation strategy (Figure 7.2a) that relies solely on the ability of the blood flow to transport devices in vessels with arbitrary tortuosity. Tethered ultra-flexible endovascular microscopic probes can be transported through tortuous vascular networks with minimal external intervention by harnessing hydrokinetic energy. The cross-sectional area is orders of magnitude smaller than the most miniature catheter currently available, which enhances the reachability, reduces the risk of iatrogenic damage, significantly increases the

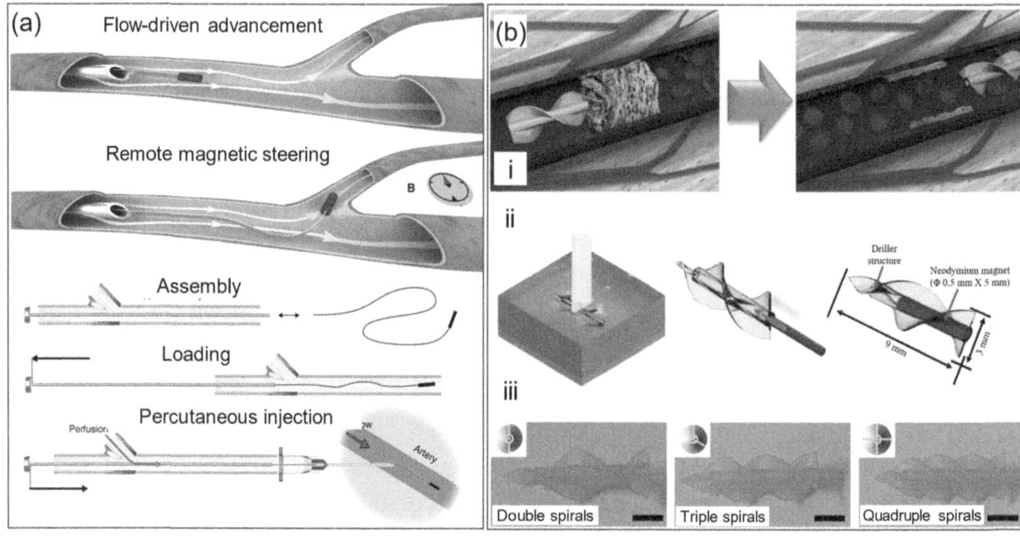

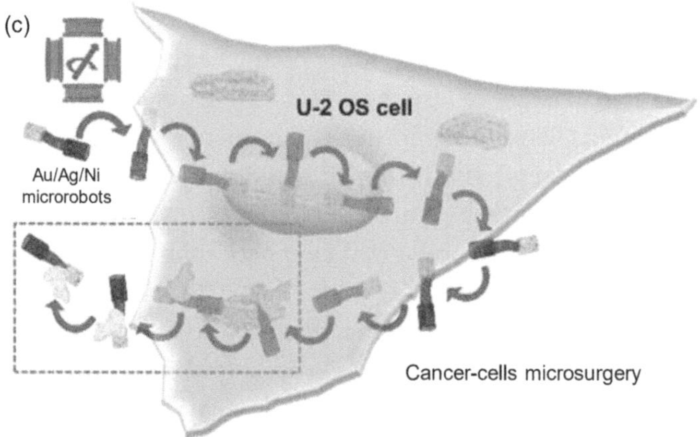

FIGURE 7.2 (a) Tethered ultra-flexible endovascular microscopic probes can be wirelessly navigated in blood vessels. (b) MDAs for navigation in a 3D phantom vascular network. Scale bar represents 2 mm. (c) Cancer cells microsurgery performed transversally upon a rotating magnetic field using asymmetric bent surface Au/Ag/Ni microrobotic scalpels. ([a] Adapted with permission (Pancaldi et al., 2020). Copyright 2018, Springer Nature; [b] Adapted with permission (Lee et al., 2018). Copyright 2018, Springer Nature; [c] Adapted with permission (Vyskočil et al., 2020). Copyright 2018, American Chemical Society.)

speed of robot-assisted interventions, and enables the deployment of multiple leads simultaneously through standard needle injection and saline perfusion. Besides, the demand for miniaturized tools incorporating sensing and actuation for precision surgery is growing. However, the accurate integration and functionalization of chemical and physical sensors are also significant challenges. Barbot et al. (2019) present a micro robotic platform for functionalizing fibers of diameters ranging from 140 to 830 micrometers, with a patterning precision of 5 micrometers and an orientation error below 0.4°. The small size of these soft microrobots allows for much less invasive procedures to be used in place of surgery, which greatly reduces procedure time, associated complications, and recovery time in patients. Lee et al. (2018) fabricated magnetic drilling actuators (MDAs), and the precise manipulation and drilling performance of the developed MDAs in 3D has great potential as intravascular drillers for precise thrombus treatment (Figure 7.2b). Vyskočil et al. (2020) reported a cancer cells microsurgery using asymmetric bent surface Au/Ag/Ni microrobotic scalpels which transversally move in a magnetic field for entering and exiting an individual cancer cell and then cutting a small cellular fragment to manipulate them outside the cell structure (Figure 7.2c).

Besides surgery, microrobots and nanorobots are also crucial for future in vivo biomedical transport and drug delivery applications. The first example of directed delivery of drug-loaded magnetic polymeric particles using magnetically driven flexible nanoswimmers was reported by Gao et al. (2012), as shown in Figure 7.3a. Flexible magnetic nickel–silver nanoswimmers (5–6 μm in length and 200 nm in diameter) can transport micrometer particles at high speeds of more than 10 μm s^{-1} (more than 0.2 body lengths per revolution in dimensionless speed) due to the cargo-towing ability of these magnetic (fuel-free) nanowire motors. In addition, 3D soft micro robotics made of hydrogels that incorporate magnetic particles for drug delivery have also been explored. For example, Fusco et al. (2014) reported an untethered, self-folding, soft microrobotic platform integrating different functionalities to achieve targeted, on-demand delivery of biological agents. The microrobot consists of a group of magnetic alginate microbeads encapsulated by a near-infrared-light (NIR)-responsive hydrogel bilayer structure, which is designed to seal and protect the beads and to open and release them once the surrounding temperature reaches 40 °C (Figure 7.3b). However, accurate implantation of a carrier with a large volume into a specific site in the body in a convenient and safe manner is still challenging, such as in repairing bone defects. Shape-memory materials are competitive candidates to overcome this challenge as shown in Figure 7.3c. Liu et al. (2014) present a porous smart nanocomposite scaffold that consists of chemically cross-linked poly (ε-caprolactone) (c-PCL) and hydroxyapatite nanoparticles with a combination of shape-memory function and controlled delivery of growth factors. The shape-memory function enables the scaffold with a large volume to be deformed into its temporal architecture with a small volume using hot compression and it subsequently recovers its original shape upon exposure to body temperature after it is implanted in the body. Materials like polymers and shape-memory materials have been confirmed to be able to transport and deliver cargos to specific regions locally active. However, the usage of synthetic materials as cargo carriers can result in inferior performance in load-carrying efficiency, biocompatibility, and biodegradability. To address this problem, bacteria-driven microswimmers are reported. Alapan et al. (2018) reported the construction and external guidance of bacteria-driven microswimmers using red blood cells (RBCs; erythrocytes) as autologous cargo carriers for active and guided drug delivery. The biohybrid microswimmer design presented here transforms RBCs from passive cargo carriers into active and guidable cargo carriers toward targeted drug and other cargo delivery applications in medicine.

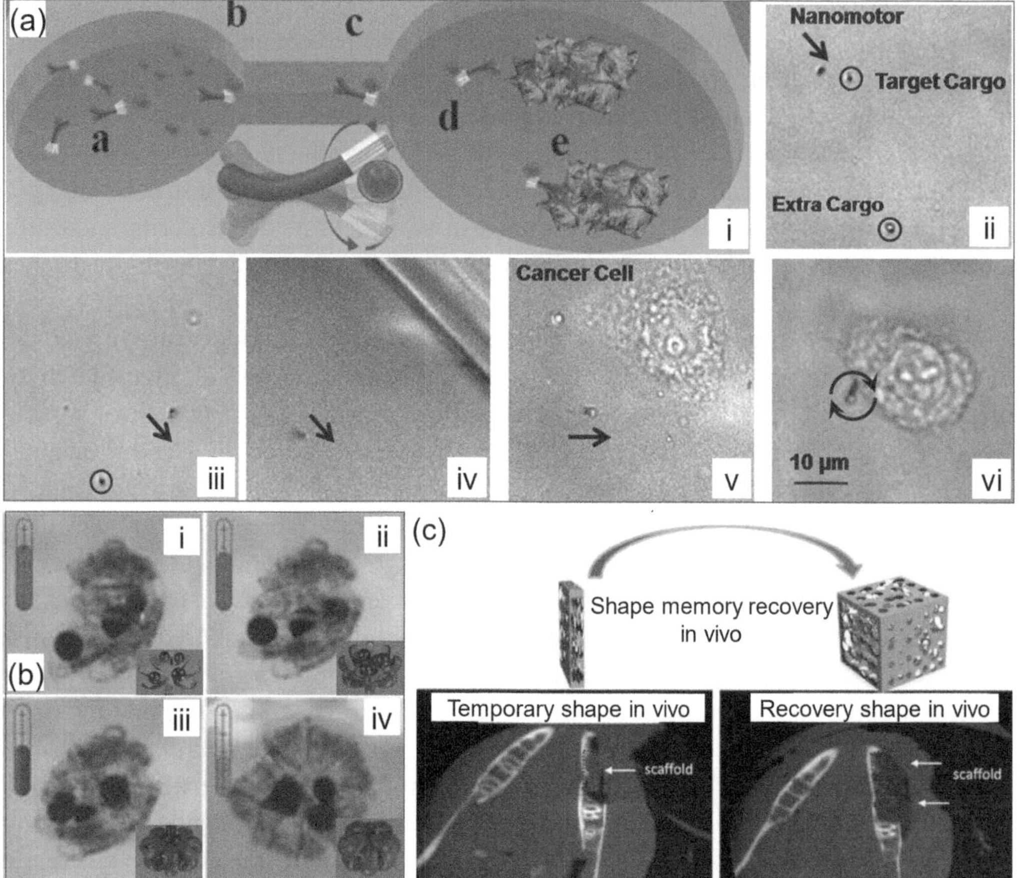

FIGURE 7.3   (a) Drug delivery to HeLa cells using flexible magnetic nanoswimmers in cell-culture media. (b) Magnetic manipulation of platforms and NIR-activated release of microparticles. (c) Delivery of growth factors using a smart porous nanocomposite scaffold to repair a mandibular bone defect. ([a] Adapted with permission (Gao et al., 2012). Copyright 2012, Wiley-VCH; [b] Adapted with permission (Fusco et al., 2014). Copyright 2013, Wiley-VCH; [c] Adapted with permission (Liu et al., 2014). Copyright 2014, American Chemical Society.)

7.3 ARTIFICIAL MUSCLES

The human muscle system is a contractile organ of the human body which consists of regularly repeating functional units, or sarcomeres, which gives them a characteristic striated (or banded) appearance under a light microscope. As illustrated in Figure 7.4a, a fascicle composes bundles of muscle fiber, each of which contains many nuclei and long, parallel myofibrils. In turn, each myofibril is composed of multiple copies of two long proteins, myosin, and actin, together with the proteins that bind them together to form thick and thin filaments, respectively (Sansom, 2022). The chemo-mechanical action of actin and myosin provides the motor for muscle contraction. The variation in action potential generates an electromyography (EMG) signal, myofibrils linearly shorten by adjusting the spatial locations of actin and myosin, whereas the length of the proteins remains constant (Kim et al., 2022).

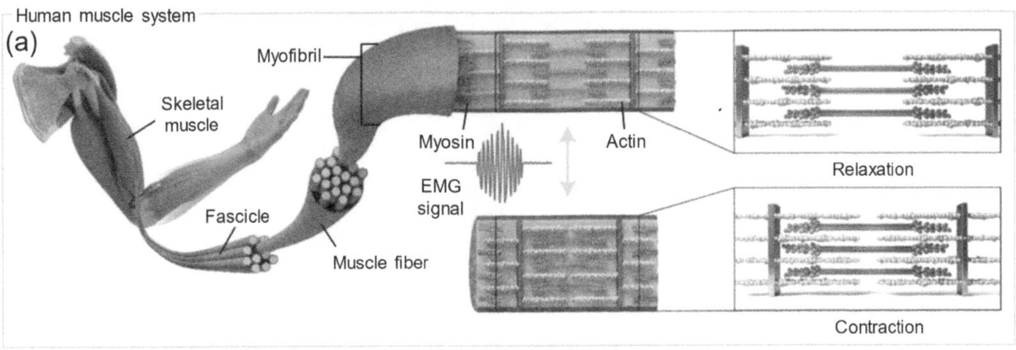

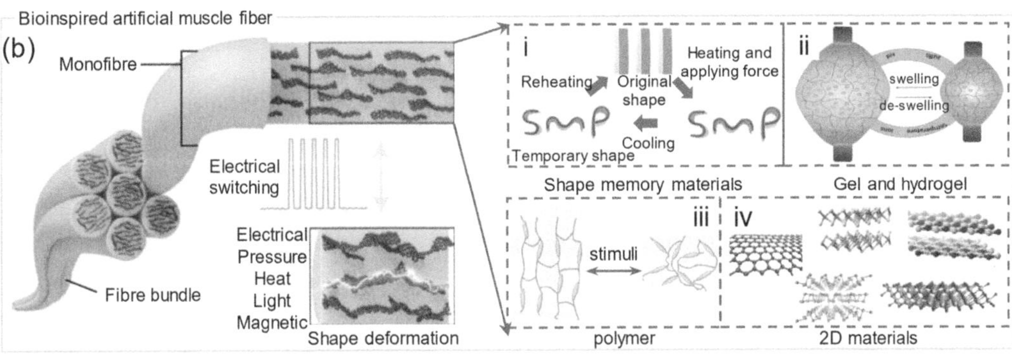

FIGURE 7.4   (a) Structural organization and actuation mechanism of the human skeletal muscle system. [a] Adapted with permission (Kim et al., 2022). Copyright 2022, Springer Nature. (b) Schematic illustrations of the bioinspired artificial muscle fiber based on shape-memory materials. [b] (Adapted with permission (Mora et al., 2019). Copyright 2019, Wiley-VCH), (c) gel and hydrogel (Adapted with permission (Oveissi et al., 2021). Copyright 2021, Elsevier Ltd), polymer (Adapted with permission (Hu et al., 2022). Copyright 2022, American Chemical Society), and 2D materials (Adapted with permission (Sulleiro et al., 2022). Copyright 2022, Elsevier B.V).

On a basic level, muscles can be described as biological actuators, in which energy is supplied by adenosine triphosphate (ATP), and the control is by the nervous system. The growing understanding of the complex structure and mechanism of muscle fibers at the molecular level inspired scientists and engineers to work to develop artificial fiber-like actuators with properties similar to those of skeletal muscles. In biomedical applications, artificial muscles can be defined as a synthetic component that can do for a robot or prosthesis what actual muscles can do for humans. It can exert force to push, pull, lift, bend, or twist. By mimicking the fiber-like structure and function of human muscle (Figure 7.4b) for biomedical applications, different approaches have been explored such as hydraulic systems, servo motors, and other fiber-like soft actuators. However, the high weight and low response time limit the development of hydraulic systems and servo motors. The usually soft actuator materials such as shape-memory materials (Mora et al., 2019), gel and hydrogel (Oveissi et al., 2021), polymer-based soft materials (Hu et al., 2022), and 2D materials (Sulleiro et al., 2022) attract wide attention on the design of lightweight artificial muscle fibers.

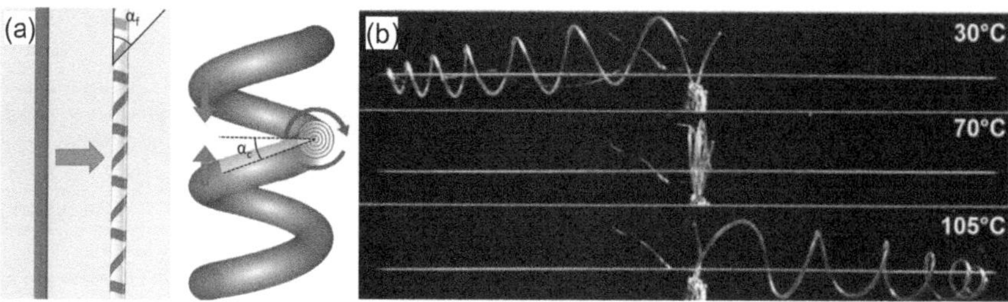

FIGURE 7.5   (a) Schematic diagram of twisted and coiled artificial muscles schematic diagram. (b) Optical pictures of the spiral coil when heated electrically show the progression of actuation. (Adapted with permission (Haines et al., 2016). Copyright 2016, National Academy of Sciences.)

Several typical twisted artificial muscles based on polymers, shape-memory materials, etc, and applications in the biomedical domain are shown in Figure 7.5. Figure 7.5a depicts two normal mechanisms of twisted muscle (left) and coiled muscle (right) (Haines et al., 2016). The left image depicts the transformation from linearly oriented polymer chains in the original fiber to helically oriented chains in the twisted fiber by inserting a twist into an anisotropic fiber. In most aligned fibers, which experience a more significant radial thermal expansion than axial thermal expansion, this causes a reversible untwisting of the fiber as temperature increases, named the thermal torsion effect. The right image demonstrates the writhing of a single coil in a coiled muscle, which is represented as 1 in (α_c), where α_c is the coil angle, defined as the inclination of the coil relative to the plane orthogonal to the coil axis. For a coil tethered at both ends to prevent rotation, when the fiber within a coil untwists, this untwist must be accompanied by an increase in writhe to accommodate a constant linking number. Haines et al. (2016) report a coil formed by a highly twisted nylon 6 fishing line. The spiral structure allows adjacent coils to pass through each other during contraction with increasing temperature (Figure 7.5b). Yuan et al. (2019) reported a kind of twisted shape-memory nanocomposite fibers that combine high torque with large rotation angles, delivering a gravimetric work capacity that is 60 times higher than that of natural skeletal muscles. Mu et al. (2019) described a sheath-run artificial muscle (SRAM) that is made by coating a twisted CNT yarn with a polymer sheath. Sheath-run artificial muscles in this work increase the maximum work capacity by factors of 1.70 to 2.15 for tensile muscles driven electrothermally or by vapor absorption and generate 1.98 watts per gram of average contractile power – 40 times that of human muscle and 9.0 times that of the highest power alternative electrochemical muscle. The excellent actuating properties open new opportunities in biomedical applications such as -assistive movement (Kanık et al., 2019) and artificial skeleton muscles (Suzumori, 2016).

7.4 MICRO SOFT ROBOTICS FOR BIOMEDICAL APPLICATIONS

Microrobots and nanorobots are also widely used for other laboratory-based biomedical applications such as genetic and tissue engineering, imaging, and investigations of biological fluid properties (Koleoso et al., 2020). The design of hollow 3D objects such as capsules and tubes is highly demanded for cell encapsulation, drug delivery, and designing of self-healing materials. The rolling shape and degree can be adjusted by varying the width and length of the bilayer for trapping the cell as shown in Figure 7.6a (Stoychev et al., 2012). Typically, Magdanz et al. (2013) created a micro-bio-robot by combining sperm cells with rolled-up magnetic microtubes, as shown in Figure 7.6b. This micro-bio-robot moves solely based on the flagellar propulsion of the cell and is directed by magnetic micro-tubes with a cavity to trap the cell under the influence of a magnetic field. This biohybrid micro-robot demonstrates the potential of utilizing microtubes driven by motile sperm cells for various applications in medicine, such as micromanipulation and targeted drug delivery. Besides, helical-type microrobots and nanorobots are widely studied because of

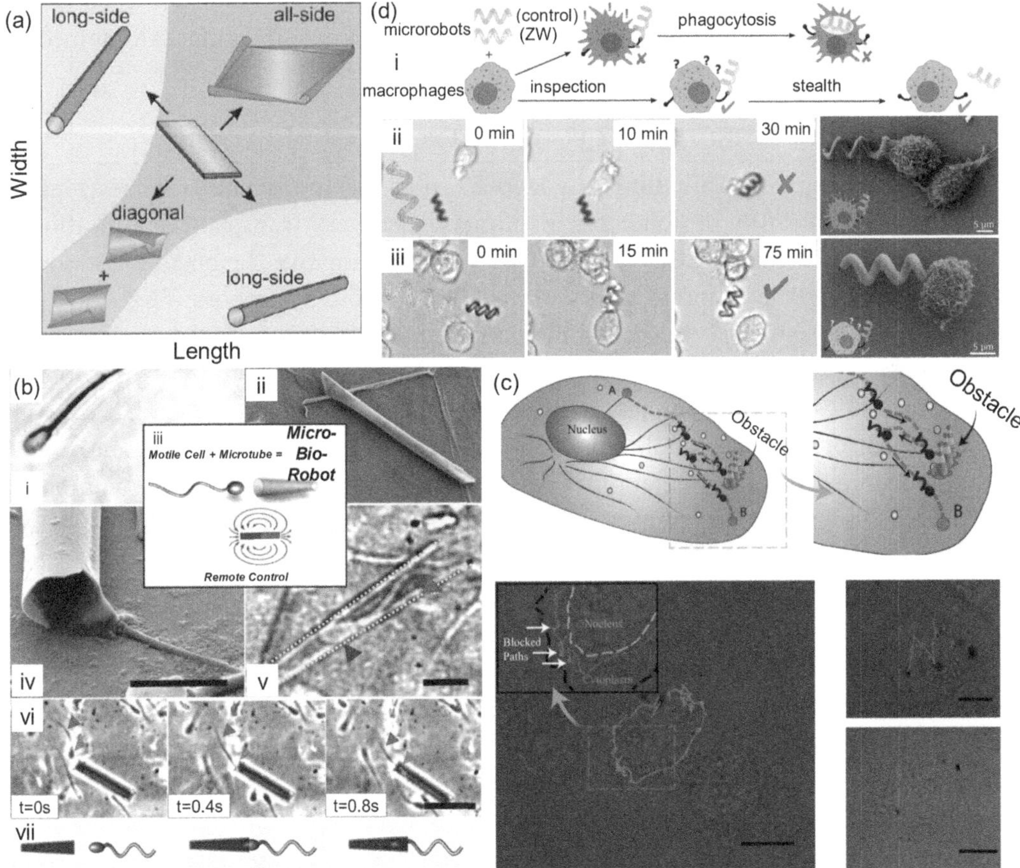

FIGURE 7.6   (a) Adjustable rolling shape by varying the width and length of the bilayer. (b) Flagellar cell combined with a microtube-driven micro-bio-robot which can be guided to defined positions. Scale bar 50 μm. (c) Intracellular controllable manipulation of helical-type hydrogel microrobots driven by small rotating magnetic fields. Scale bar 10 (left) and 15 μm (right), respectively. (d) Inspection and capture of control PEG microrobots as well as inspection and release of stealth micro-robots, respectively. ([a] Adapted with permission (Stoychev et al., 2012). Copyright 2012, American Chemical Society; [b] Adapted with permission (Magdanz et al., 2013). Copyright 2013, Wiley-VCH; [c] Adapted with permission (Pal et al., 2018). Copyright 2018, Wiley-VCH; [d] Adapted with permission (Cabanach et al., 2020). Copyright 2020, Wiley-VCH.)

their proven propulsion abilities. As shown in Figure 7.6c, Pal et al. (2018) achieved cellular internalization and subsequent controllable intracellular manipulation of a system of helical nanomotors driven by small rotating magnetic fields with no adverse effect on the cellular viability, which could be helpful in delivering payloads to specific locations within the cytoplasm. Furthermore, helical-type hydrogel microrobots prepared by two-photon polymerization 3D microprinting are reported by the Cabanach group (2020), which can escape from the recognition of the immune system as a natural protection mechanism against foreign threats. It is first time for non-immunogenic stealth zwitterionic microrobots to avoid detection by the macrophage cells of the innate immune system after exhaustive inspection (>90 hours), which eliminates a major roadblock in the development of biocompatible microrobots and will serve as a toolbox of non-immunogenic materials for medical microrobots and other device technologies for bioengineering and biomedical applications (Figure 7.6d).

7.5 OTHER SOFT ROBOTICS FOR BIOMEDICAL APPLICATIONS

Heart or heart-lung transplantation is a widely accepted therapy for end-stage heart failure (HF), but the availability of donor organs limits the surgery transplant qualification of many patients. Ventricular assist devices (VADs) are alternative therapeutic options for end-stage HF when the donor organ is not available. Previous soft robotic VADs have generally targeted biventricular heart failure and have not engaged the interventricular septum that plays a critical role in blood ejection from the ventricle. To address this problem, Payne et al. (2017) proposed implantable soft robotic devices to augment cardiac function in isolated left or right heart failure by applying rhythmic loading to either ventricle. In addition, inspired by the orientation of the outer two muscle layers of the mammalian heart, Roche et al. (2017) present a soft robotic sleeve implanted around the heart and actively compresses and twists to act as a cardiac VAD. The soft robot mimicked the form and function of the native heart, with a stiffness value of the same order of magnitude as that of the heart tissue, demonstrating the feasibility of supporting heart function in a porcine model of acute HF. Besides, catheters integrated with advanced electronic functionality for minimally invasive forms of cardiac surgery have also been reported (Figure 7.7a) (Han et al., 2020). The catheter-integrated soft multilayer electronic arrays can establish conformal contact with curved tissue surfaces, support high-density spatiotemporal mapping of temperature, pressure, and electrophysiological parameters, and allow for programmable electrical stimulation, radiofrequency ablation, and irreversible electroporation, which can improve surgical performance and patient outcomes. Other applications, such as drug delivery, are also proposed, which differ from those using microrobots and nanorobots that act directly on the cell. Wang et al. (2020) reported a thin magnetic micropump embedded in a contact lens which is capable of on-demand one-directional drug delivery and can be actuated by an external magnetic field (Figure 7.7b). A micro check valve was integrated with a micropump to control drug delivery. By controlling the strength and frequency of the magnetic field pulse, on-demand drug release and controlled dose can be realized. Furthermore, soft robotics can also be reported in applying capsule endoscopy for fine-needle biopsy actuated by magnetic field, which takes biopsy samples

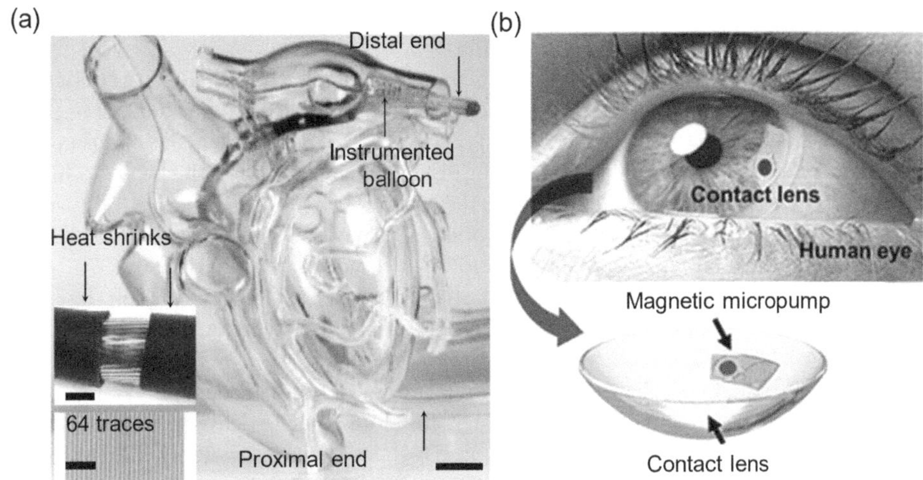

FIGURE 7.7   (a) Image of an inflated, instrumented balloon catheter inserted into a transparent heart model. (b) Magnetic micropump embedded in contact lens for on-demand drug delivery. ([a] Adapted with permission (Han et al., 2020). Copyright 2020, Spring Nature; [b] Adapted with permission (Wang et al., 2020). Copyright 2020, Spring Nature.)

of a deep tissue of the stomach using the fine-needle biopsy technique. Experiments in a porcine stomach show an 85% yield for the biopsy of phantom tumors located underneath the first layers of the stomach wall (Son et al., 2020).

7.6 OUTLOOK

The actuating mechanism of soft robots and biomedical applications in surgery, drug delivery, artificial muscle, and microrobots have been summarized in this chapter. Soft robots, especially microrobots, have the potential to be used to accomplish complex tasks in the human body for real-time control and monitoring, but there are also many challenges including safe contact, adaptability, conformability, navigation in complex 3D environments, biocompatibility, controlled actuation, localization, actuation performance, life cycle, versatility, etc. In recent advances, soft actuators cannot completely replicate biological behaviors and performances. However, the development of new robotic materials will push the limits of current soft robots and help them achieve life-like performance.

REFERENCES

Alapan, Y., Yasa, O., Schauer, O., Giltinan, J., Tabak, A. F., Sourjik, V., & Sitti, M. J. (2018). Soft erythrocyte-based bacterial microswimmers for cargo delivery. *Science Robotics*, 3, 4423(2018).

Barbot, A., Tan, H., Power, M., Seichepine, F., & Yang, G.-Z. J. (2019). Floating magnetic microrobots for fiber functionalization. *Science Robotics*, 4, 8336(2019).

Bell, M. A., Gorissen, B., Bertoldi, K., Weaver, J. C., & Wood, R. J. J. (2021). A modular and self-contained fluidic engine for soft actuators. *Advanced Intelligent Systems*, 4, 2100094.

Cabanach, P., Pena-Francesch, A., Sheehan, D., Bozuyuk, U., Yasa, O., Borrós, S., & Sitti, M. J. (2020). Zwitterionic 3D-printed non-immunogenic stealth microrobots. *Advanced Materials*, 32, 2003013.

Choi, J., Lee, D.-Y., Eo, J.-H., Park, Y.-J., & Cho, K.-J. J. (2020). Tendon-driven jamming mechanism for configurable variable stiffness. *Soft Robotics*, 8(1), 109–118.

Chung, H. J., Parsons, A. M., & Zheng, L. J. (2020). Magnetically controlled soft robotics utilizing elastomers and gels in actuation: A review. *Advanced Intelligent Systems*, 3, 2000186.

Duan, J., Liu, F., Kong, Y., Hao, M., He, J., Wang, J., Sang, Y. (2020). Homogeneous chitosan/graphene oxide nanocomposite hydrogel-based actuator driven by efficient photothermally induced water gradients. *ACS Applied Nano Materials*, 3(2), 1002–1009.

Ebrahimi, N., Bi, C., Cappelleri, D. J., Ciuti, G., Conn, A. T., Faivre, D., Jafari, A. H. J. (2020). Magnetic actuation methods in bio/soft robotics. *Advanced Functional Materials*, 31, 2005137.

Fusco, S., Sakar, M. S., Kennedy, S., Peters, C., Bottani, R., Starsich, F. H. L., Nelson, B. J. J. (2014). An integrated microrobotic platform for on-demand, targeted therapeutic interventions. *Advanced Materials*, 26(6), 952–957.

Gao, W., Kagan, D., Pak, O. S., Clawson, C., Campuzano, S., Chuluun-Erdene, E., Wang, J. J. (2012). Cargo-towing fuel-free magnetic nanoswimmers for targeted drug delivery. *Small*, 8, 460–467.

Haines, C. S., Li, N., Spinks, G. M., Aliev, A. E., Di, J., & Baughman, R. H. (2016). New twist on artificial muscles. *Proceedings of the National Academy of Sciences of the United States of America*, 113(42), 11709–11716.

Han, M., Chen, L., Aras, K. K., Liang, C., Chen, X., Zhao, H., Rogers, J. A. J. (2020). Catheter-integrated soft multilayer electronic arrays for multiplexed sensing and actuation during cardiac surgery. *Nature Biomedical Engineering*, 4, 997–1009.

Hu, J., Yu, M., Wang, M., Choy, K. L., Yu, H. J. (2022). Design, regulation, and applications of soft actuators based on liquid-crystalline polymers and their composites. *ACS Applied Materials & Interfaces*, 14(11), 12951–12963.

Ji, X., Liu, X., Cacucciolo, V., Civet, Y., El Haitami, A., Cantin, S., Shea, H. R. J. (2020). Untethered feel-through haptics using 18-μm thick dielectric elastomer actuators. *Advanced Functional Materials*, 31, 2006639.

Jin, X., Shi, Y., Yuan, Z., Huo, X., Wang, Z. L., & Wu, Z. J. S. E. J. (2022). Bio-inspired soft actuator with contact feedback based on photothermal effect and triboelectric nanogenerator. *Nano Energy*, 99, 107366,

Kanık, M., Orguc, S., Varnavides, G., Varnavides, G., Kim, J., Benavides, T., Anikeeva, P. J. (2019). Strain-programmable fiber-based artificial muscle. *Science*, 365, 145–150.

Kaynak, M., Dirix, P., & Sakar, M. S. J. (2020). Addressable acoustic actuation of 3D printed soft robotic microsystems. *Advanced Science*, 7, 2001120.

Kaynak, M., Dolev, A., & Sakar, M. S. J. (2022). 3D printed acoustically programmable soft microactuators. *Soft Robotics*, 10, 246–257.

Kim, I. H., Choi, S., Lee, J., Jung, J., Yeo, J., Kim, J. T., Kim, S. O. J. (2022). Human-muscle-inspired single fibre actuator with reversible percolation. *Nature Nanotechnology*, 17, 1198–1205.

Koleoso, M., Feng, X., Xue, Y., Li, Q., Munshi, T., & Chen, X. J. (2020). Micro/nanoscale magnetic robots for biomedical applications. *Materials Today Bio*, 8, 100085.

Lee, S., Lee, S., Kim, S., Yoon, C.-H., Park, H. J., Kim, J.-Y., & Choi, H. J. (2018). Fabrication and characterization of a magnetic drilling actuator for navigation in a three-dimensional phantom vascular network. *Science Reports*, 8, 3691.

Li, J., Wang, M., Cui, Z., Liu, S., Feng, D., Mei, G., Liu, Z.-F. J. (2022b). Dual-responsive jumping actuators by light and humidity. *Journal Materials Chemistry A*, 10, 25337–25346.

Li, J., Zhang, R., Mou, L., Jung de Andrade, M., Hu, X., Yu, K., Liu, Z. J. (2019). Photothermal bimorph actuators with in-built cooler for light mills, frequency switches, and soft robots. *Advanced Functional Materials*, 29, 1808995.

Li, M., Pal, A., Aghakhani, A., Pena-Francesch, A., & Sitti, M. J. (2021). Soft actuators for real-world applications. *Nature Reviews Materials*, 7, 235–249.

Li, W., Sang, M., Liu, S., Wang, B., Cao, X., Liu, G., Xuan, S. J. (2022a). Dual-mode biomimetic soft actuator with electrothermal and magneto-responsive performance. *Composites Part B: Engineering*, 238, 109880.

Liu, X., Zhao, K., Gong, T., Song, J., Bao, C., Luo, E., Zhou, S. J. (2014). Delivery of growth factors using a smart porous nanocomposite scaffold to repair a mandibular bone defect. *Biomacromolecules*, 153, 1019–1030.

Luo, M., Tao, W., Chen, F., Khuu, T. K., Ozel, S. (2014). Design improvements and dynamic characterization on fluidic elastomer actuators for a soft robotic snake. *IEEE International Conference on Technologies for Practical Robot Applications (TePRA)*, pp. 1–6.

Magdanz, V., Sánchez, S., & Schmidt, O. G. J. (2013). Development of a sperm-flagella driven micro-bio-robot. *Advanced Materials*, 25, 6581–6588.

Meder, F., Naselli, G. A., Sadeghi, A., & Mazzolai, B. J. (2019). Remotely light-powered soft fluidic actuators based on plasmonic-driven phase transitions in elastic constraint. *Advanced Materials*, 31, 1905671.

Mora, P., Schäfer, H., Jubsilp, C., Rimdusit, S., & Koschek, K. J. (2019). Thermosetting shape memory polymers and composites based on polybenzoxazine blends, alloys and copolymers. *Chemistry-An Asian Journal*, 14, 4129–4139.

Mu, J., Jung de Andrade, M., Fang, S., Wang, X., Gao, E., Li, N., & Baughman, R. H. J. (2019). Sheath-run artificial muscles. *Science*, 365, 150–155.

Oveissi, F., Fletcher, D. F., Dehghani, F., & Naficy, S. J. (2021). Tough hydrogels for soft artificial muscles. *Materials & Design*, 203, 109609.

Pal, M., Somalwar, N., Singh, A., Bhat, R., Eswarappa, S. M., Saini, D. K., & Ghosh, A. J. (2018). Maneuverability of magnetic nanomotors inside living cells. *Advanced Materials*, 30, 1800429.

Pancaldi, L., Dirix, P., Fanelli, A., Lima, A. M., Stergiopulos, N., Mosimann, P. J., Sakar, M. S. J. (2020). Flow driven robotic navigation of microengineered endovascular probes. *Nature Communications*, 11, 6356.

Pang, X., Lv, J. a., Zhu, C., Qin, L., & Yu, Y. J. (2019). Photodeformable azobenzene-containing liquid crystal polymers and soft actuators. *Advanced Materials*, 31, 1904224.

Payne, C. J., Wamala, I., Bautista-Salinas, D., Saeed, M. Y., Van Story, D., Thalhofer, T., Vasilyev, N. V. J. (2017). Soft robotic ventricular assist device with septal bracing for therapy of heart failure. *Science Robotics*, 2, eaan6736.

Ren, Z., Kim, S., Ji, X., Zhu, W., Niroui, F., Kong, J., & Chen, Y. J. (2021). A high-lift micro-aerial-robot powered by low-voltage and long-endurance dielectric elastomer actuators. *Advanced Materials*, 34, 2106757.

Roche, E. T., Horvath, M. A., Wamala, I., Alazmani, A., Song, S.-E., Whyte, W., Walsh, C. J. J. (2017). Soft robotic sleeve supports heart function. *Science Translational Medicine*, 9, eaaf3925.

Sansom, C. (2022). *A test of strength for artificial muscles*. https://www.chemistryworld.com/features/a-test-of-strength-for-artificial-muscles/4015078.article

Shao, Y., Long, F., Zhao, Z., Fang, M., Jing, H., Guo, J., Cheng, Y. J. (2022). 4D printing light-driven soft actuators based on liquid-vapor phase transition composites with inherent sensing capability. *Chemical Engineering Journal*, 454, 140271.

Son, D., Gilbert, H. B., & Sitti, M. J. S.R. (2020). Magnetically actuated soft capsule endoscope for fine-needle biopsy. *IEEE International Conference on Robotics and Automation (ICRA)*, pp. 1132–1139.

Stoychev, G. V., Zakharchenko, S., Turcaud, S. B., Dunlop, J. W. C., & Ionov, L. J. (2012). Shape-programmed folding of stimuli-responsive polymer bilayers. *ACS Nano*, 65, 3925–3934.

Sulleiro, M. V., Dominguez-Alfaro, A., Alegret, N., Silvestri, A., & Gómez, I. J. J. (2022). 2D Materials towards sensing technology: From fundamentals to applications. *Sensing and Bio-Sensing Research*, 38, 100540.

Suzumori, K. (2016). *Pneumatic artificial muscles for orthosis*. https://atlasofthefuture.org/project/pneumatic-artificial-muscles-for-orthosis/

Vasios, N., Gross, A. J., Soifer, S. J., Overvelde, J. T. B., & Bertoldi, K. J. (2020). Harnessing viscous flow to simplify the actuation of fluidic soft robots. *Soft Robot*, 7(1), 1–9.

Vyskočil, J., Mayorga-Martinez, C. C., Jablonská, E., Novotný, F., Ruml, T., & Pumera, M. J. (2020). Cancer cells microsurgery via asymmetric bent surface Au/Ag/Ni microrobotic scalpels through a transversal rotating magnetic field. *ACS Nano*, 14, 7, 8247–8256.

Wang, C., Park, J. J. M., & Letters, N. S. (2020). Magnetic micropump embedded in contact lens for on-demand drug delivery. *Micro and Nano Systems Letters*, 8, 1–6.

Wang, H., Zhu, Z., Jin, H., Wei, R., Bi, L., Zhang, W. J. (2022). Magnetic soft robots: design, actuation, and function. *Journal of Alloys and Compounds*, 922, 166219.

Wei, W., Zhang, P., Cao, F., Liu, J., Qian, K., Pan, D., Li, W. J. (2022). Ultrathin flexible electrospun EVA nanofiber composite with electrothermally-driven shape memory effect for electromagnetic interference shielding. *Chemical Engineering Journal*, 446, 137135.

Yang, Y., Liu, Y., & Shen, Y. J. (2020). Plasmonic-assisted graphene oxide films with enhanced photothermal actuation for soft robots. *Advanced Functional Materials*, 30, 1910172.

Yuan, J., Neri, W., Zakri, C., Merzeau, P., Kratz, K., Lendlein, A., & Poulin, P. J. (2019). Shape memory nanocomposite fibers for untethered high-energy microengines. *Science*, 365, 155–158.

Zhang, D., Yang, K., Liu, X., Luo, M., Li, Z., Liu, C., Zhou, X. J. (2022). Boosting the photothermal conversion efficiency of MXene film by porous wood for light-driven soft actuators. *Chemical Engineering Journal*, 450, 138013.

Zhu, C., Lu, Y., Jiang, L., & Yu, Y. J. (2021). Liquid crystal soft actuators and robots toward mixed reality. *Advanced Functional Materials*, 31, 2009835.

Zou, M., Li, S., Hu, X., Leng, X., Wang, R., Zhou, X., & Liu, Z. J. (2021). Progresses in tensile, torsional, and multifunctional soft actuators. *Advanced Functional Materials*, 31, 2007437.

CHAPTER 8

Advanced Fiber Sensing Technologies in Bio-Integrated Systems

Zhiyuan Meng

8.1 INTRODUCTION

Modern optical fibers technology has revolutionized various fields in recent years, including data communication, medicine, fiber lasers, and sensing. While conventional optical fibers consist of silica cores and claddings, the introduction of photonic crystals has extended the functionality and structure. Microstructured photonic crystal fibers with air holes of varying diameters offer unique control of light propagation within the fibers, enabling the design of optical fibers with specific properties. To further broaden the functionality of optical fibers, multimaterial optical fibers have been developed, integrating insulators, semiconductors, and conductors. The incorporation of plasmonic and metamaterials into optical fibers also opens new frontiers. These novel optoelectronic fibers have been applied in various electronic devices, including light-emitting diodes (LEDs), field-effect transistors (FETs), photodetectors, and solar cells. Compared to rigid and planar optoelectronic devices, fiber-based optoelectronic devices possess individual characteristics such as flexibility, lightweight, and wearability. Moreover, they offer spatial information that is not available from planar devices. Given the unique advantages of advanced optical and optoelectronic fiber devices, they have garnered increasing attention and have been applied in various biologically related systems.

The optimal performance of optical and optoelectronic fibers is dependent on the specific application. For epidermal sensors, flexibility and stretchability are crucial characteristics, as the devices need to conform to the soft skin. However, when these fibers are used as implantable devices, biocompatibility becomes a major challenge. To address this issue, hydrogel-based optical and optoelectronic fibers have gained increasing attention due to their inherent stretchable and biocompatible properties. Nonetheless, their long-term stability, particularly *in vivo*, needs to be thoroughly demonstrated. Therefore, further research is necessary to verify the feasibility and safety of hydrogel optical and

DOI: 10.1201/9781003493631-8

optoelectronic fibers for implantable biomedical applications. Figure 8.1 introduces universal strategies for designing advanced optical and optoelectronic fibers for bio-integrated systems.

This chapter provides a comprehensive overview of the materials commonly adopted in the fabrication of optical and optoelectronic fibers used in bio-integrated systems. In the subsequent sections, we discuss three typical fabrication methods, namely thermal drawing, spinning, and 3D printing technology, which are widely employed in the manufacturing of these fibers. Finally, we highlight the specific applications of optical and optoelectronic fibers in bio-integrated systems, underscoring their potential in advancing biomedical research and healthcare.

8.2 MATERIALS SELECTIONS AND MANUFACTURE TECHNIQUES

8.2.1 Materials Selections in Bio-integrated Systems

Silica glass has been explored to manufacture optical and optoelectronic fibers for long because of its excellently low attenuation and chemical inertness. As the requirements in wearable electronics and implantable devices increase, researchers draw attention from inorganic materials to develop organic polymers due to their higher flexibility, lower Young's modulus, higher strain limits, fracture toughness, lightweight, and impact resistance. Biocompatibility should be considered when optical and optoelectronic fibers are applied in biomedical research and healthcare. Materials selection is a starting to offer the requested functionalities in bio-integrated systems.

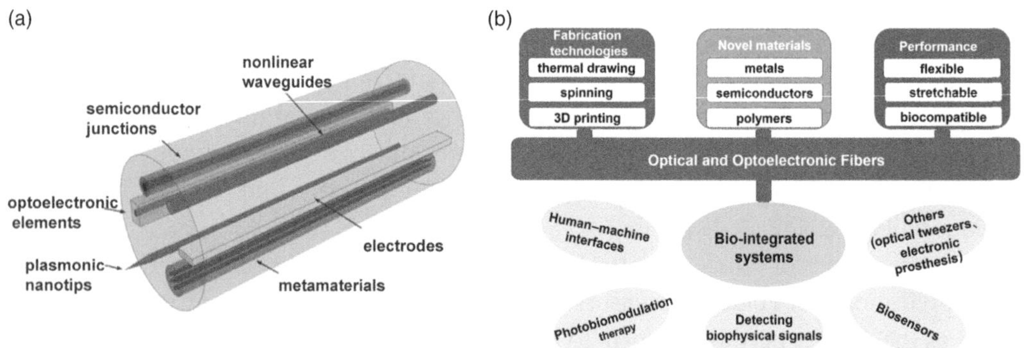

FIGURE 8.1 The schematic of the fiber strategies for bio-integrated systems. (a) Designing of the multifunctional optoelectrical fibers, which are composed of multiple functional components, including nonlinear waveguides, semiconductor junctions, optoelectronic elements, metamaterials, etc. (b) The diagram shows the bio-integrated system elements based on optical and optoelectronic fibers. Material selections, fabrication methods, and expected performances are all important considerations when developing a fiber interface employed in a bio-integrated system, such as detecting biophysical signals, biosensors, human–machine interfaces, photobiomodulation (PBM) therapy, and others. ([a] Adapted with permission. (Alexander Schmidt et al., 2015) Copyright 2015, Wiley.)

8.2.1.1 Materials Selections for Optical Fibers in Bio-Integrated Systems

Optical fibers are traditionally manufactured using silica-based materials. However, their inextensibility and rigidity limit their application in modern electronic devices that aim for miniaturization and integration. For wearable electronics that are closely attached to soft skin, flexibility and stretchability are demanded for monitoring physiological parameters and human–machine interfaces during long-term use. In the case of implantable devices, good biocompatibility of the optical and optoelectronic fibers is crucial to minimize immune reaction with organs. In some studies, hydrogel coatings have been used to improve the biocompatibility of silica-based optical fibers. Additionally, materials that are biodegradable and bioresorbable are preferred to avoid the secondary removal operation. Table 8.1 provides a summary of materials and applications of optical fibers which are utilized in biosystems.

In biomedical applications, both natural and synthetic polymers have been widely used. Nature materials, such as silk protein, cellulose, chitosan, and gelatin, possess intrinsic

TABLE 8.1   Commonly Used Optical Fiber Materials in Bio-integrated System

Category	Materials	Application	Reference
Natural materials	Silk (core)	Waveguide	(Qiao et al., 2017)
	Silk (cladding)	Drug release monitoring	(Liu et al., 2021)
	Cellulose (core)	Temperature sensing	(Skwierczynska et al., 2022)
	Chitosan (cladding)	Breathing monitoring	(Shrivastav et al., 2020)
	Gelatin (cladding)	Breathing monitoring	(Yi et al., 2020)
	PEG (core)	Optogenetic	(Feng et al., 2020)
	PEG-poly(urethane) (PEG-PU) (cladding)	Optogenetics and electrophysiology	(Tabet et al., 2021)
	PAAm	Optogenetics	(Wang et al., 2018)
	Poly(acrylamide-co-poly(ethylene glycol) diacrylate)(core)	Glucose sensing and photomedicine	(Yetisen et al., 2017), (Jiang et al., 2018)
	Poly(ethylene glycol diacrylate-co-acrylamide) (core)	Cancer therapy and brain optogenetic stimulation	(G. Chen et al., 2021a)
Synthetic materials	PLA (core)	Biomarkers and cell apoptosis monitoring, temperature sensing, and photomedicine	(He et al., 2021), (Zhang et al., 2023)
	PLLA and poly(Lactic-co-glycolic acid)(core)	Photobiomodulation	(Jiang et al., 2020)
	Polycarbonate(core)	Photodynamic therapy	(Chin et al., 2021)
	PDMS (cladding)	Human–machine interfaces and temperature and movement monitoring	(Chen et al., 2022)
Synthetic materials (elastomer)	PDMS (coating)	Human–machine interfaces and blood pressure monitoring	(Qiu et al., 2021), (Pang et al., 2022)
	PDMS (core, cladding)	Temperature sensing	(Guo et al., 2019)

biocompatibility and processability, making them a popular choice for monitoring human physiological signals such as temperature and breath when combined with other sensitive materials. Hydrogels, with their high hydrophilicity and similarity in structure and mechanical properties to biological tissues, have garnered significant attention for use in bio-integrated systems. They offer advantages in guiding and manipulating light over solid-state materials due to their low compatibility and refractive index mismatch when integrated with biological tissues (Guimaraes et al., 2021). Hydrogels made from poly(acrylamide) (PAAm), poly(ethylene glycol) (PEG), and their copolymers have been used for strain monitoring, PBM therapy, and biomarkers monitoring. In addition to good biocompatibility and tunable biodegradability, polylactic acid (PLA) or poly(L-lactic acid) (PLLA) have high refractive indices (~1.46) and low extinction for optical waveguides, making them suitable for implantation in PBM therapy and *in vivo* physiological information monitoring. However, bioresorbable materials suffer from transmission and coupling losses due to their time-dependent biodegradability. Polydimethylsiloxane (PDMS), a commonly used elastomer, exhibits excellent optical properties (Prajzler et al., 2018), good elasticity, chemical inertness, and thermosetting property, making it an ideal choice for human–machine interfaces.

8.2.1.2 Materials Selections for Optoelectronic Fibers in Bio-Integrated Systems

Optoelectronic fibers consist of three main parts: cladding, core, and electrode. Table 8.2 summarizes the materials for optoelectronic fibers in bio-integrated systems. The cladding lay, which serves as the protective layer for functional layers, is typically made of insulators. Initially, silica was used as the primary cladding material, but more recently, borate glass as well as functional polymers have been developed. A wide range of semiconductor materials have been used to manufacture the core layer of optoelectronic fibers, which can be divided into five types: (1) IV semiconductors and IV–IV alloys (Si, Ge, Si-Ge, and Sn). (2) III–V compound semiconductors (GaSb and InSb). (3) II–VI compound semiconductors (ZnSe). (4) Chalcogenides. (5) Polymers (polycarbonate (PC)).

TABLE 8.2 Commonly Used Functional Core Materials for Optoelectronic Fibers

Category	Group	Representative Materials	References
Core (semiconductor)	IV semiconductors and IV–IV alloys	Si, Ge, Si-Ge, and Sn	(Ye et al., 2021)
	III–V compound semiconductors	GaSb, InSb	(Yan et al., 2019)
	II–VI compound semiconductors	ZnSe	(Seyedin et al., 2021)
Electrode (conductor)	Chalcogenide	As-Se, As-S-Te, and	(Xu et al., 2018)
	Polymers	polycarbonate	(Park et al., 2017)
	Metals	Ag nanowire, tin, gold, copper	(Ye et al., 2021)
	Polymers and carbon-based fillers	polyethylene (CPE), and 5% graphite	(Park et al., 2017)

Compared to inorganic semiconductors, polymer-based optoelectronic devices offer advantages such as high flexibility, structure tunability, and lightweight, making them suitable for wearable electronics. The conductive electrode layer facilitates signal transmission and power supply to the in-fiber optoelectronic devices. Metals such as gold, copper, tin, and silver are commonly used as electrodes due to their good conductivity and high melting temperatures. However, some metals have low viscosity and surface tension, which makes it difficult to maintain the fiber structure during thermal drawing, leading to mixing with functional semiconductor materials and ultimately damaging the fiber structures and functions (Ye et al., 2021). One potential solution is to introduce conductive polymers which have lower conductivity compared to metals but can be combined with conductive fillers (e.g., carbon-based materials). Another approach is to deposit metallic nanowires on the surface of core fibers via dip-coating or high-pressure chemical vapor deposition.

8.2.2 Fabrication Techniques

Fabrication technologies determine the quality and architecture of optical and optoelectronic fibers. Typical fabrication methods include pressure-assisted filling, high-pressure chemical vapor deposition (HPCVD), spinning, and thermal drawing. Some emerging techniques, like 3D printing, have the potential to achieve large-scale manufacturing and acquire different architectures. Recently, a variety of post-thermal drawing methods to functionalize fiber tips have been utilized, such as pattern transferring, photolithography, and self-assembly. It should be noticed that the adaptation of preparing technology and materials is particularly important. For example, similar thermal and chemical properties are required for thermal drawing technology.

8.2.2.1 Thermal Drawing

Thermal drawing technology is a traditional technology to fabricate optical fibers that enables the integration of materials with optical and photoelectric properties into fibers, enabling efficient preparation for flexible electronic devices with complex structures. The first step in thermal drawing involves preparing a macro preform in which bulk materials are arranged in defined locations in well-defined geometric shapes (Figure 8.2a). Many methods have been adopted to prepare preforms including HPCVD, rod-in-tube approach, sandwich consolidation, and thin-film rolling. After heating the preform in the furnace for a period, the softened melt preform is extended to a length of up to tens of kilometers. The diameter of the resulting fibers can be controlled by adjusting the drawing temperature, feeding speed of the preform, and drawing speed v_{draw} of the blank. By embedding insulators, semiconductors, and conductors into the fiber design (Figure 8.2b), optoelectronic fiber devices can be fabricated. Compared to multi-stage fabrication methods that involve dip-coating or hydrothermal growth of each layer on the core fiber, thermal drawn optoelectronic fibers exhibit higher photoresponsivity (R_λ) and on/off ratio of photocurrent.

The thermal drawing technology offers numerous advantages such as superior uniformity, scalability, and high productivity. However, it is subject to limitations due to differences in the thermal, mechanical, and chemical properties of the various integrated materials. Therefore, not all materials can be combined to fabricate thermal drawn fibers.

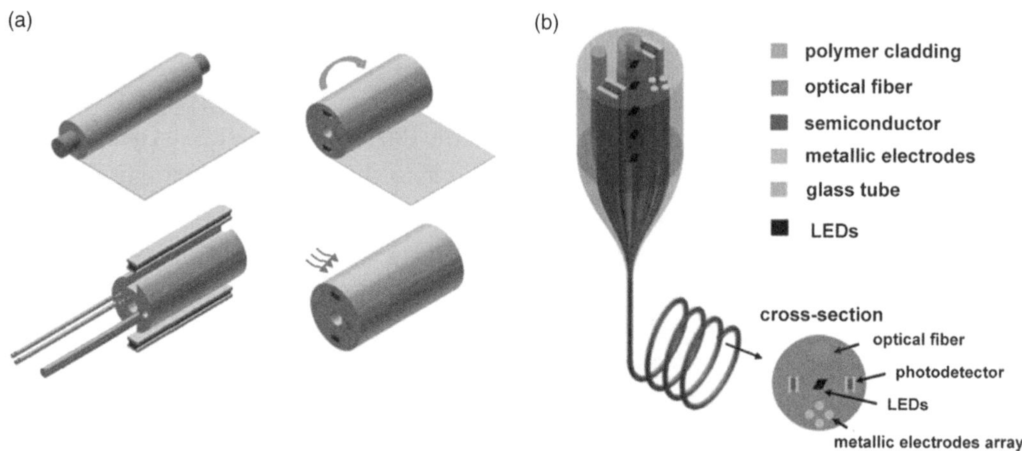

FIGURE 8.2 Thermal drawing technology used to fabricate optical and optoelectronic fibers. (a) Schematic of fabricating the preform. (b) Schematic of thermal drawing process after preform fabrication and resulting optical or optoelectronic fibers containing functional material core and cladding. (Adapted with permission. (Yan et al., 2019) Copyright 2018, Wiley.)

For example, the cladding and core materials must have similar melting temperatures or glass temperatures. Moreover, at least one amorphous material is necessary for thermally drawn fiber, as amorphous materials can resist continuous deformation during the necking process from the preform to the resulting fibers. In addition, materials mismatch in thermal expansion properties and viscosity can result in fiber breakages and cracks.

8.2.2.2 Spinning

Spinning is a widely used method for producing polymer fibers, which are formed through extrusion. Various spinning techniques have been developed, including wet spinning, dry spinning, electrospinning, microfluidic spinning, direct drawing, and direct writing. In a recent study by Doganay et. al. (2023), a wet spinning process was employed to fabricate core-shell optical fibers (Figure 8.3a). The core and shell materials consisted of carbon black (CB)/silver nanowires (Ag NWs)/thermoplastic polyurethane (TPU) and TPU, respectively. TPU/DMF solution and CB-Ag NW-TPU/DMF dispersions were injected into a DI water coagulation bath via two injection pumps. The fibers were subsequently moved directly to another water bath for a duration of 24 hours to enhance the exchange of solvent between DMF and water. Finally, the resulting fibers were collected on a bobbin. The SEM images exhibited the clear core–shell structure of the fibers.

Electrospinning is a widely used method for fabricating nanofibers with smaller diameter fibers and larger surface areas. This technique utilizes a strong electrostatic force to extrude the solution or melt, and factors such as solution viscosity, polymer concentration, voltage values, air humidity, working distance, and surface tension can all impact the manufacturing process and the performance of the resulting fiber. Therefore, the fabrication process is typically carried out in a closed chamber with strict control over air temperature and humidity. Biocompatible polymers, such as PLGA, PLLA, polyvinyl alcohol (PVA),

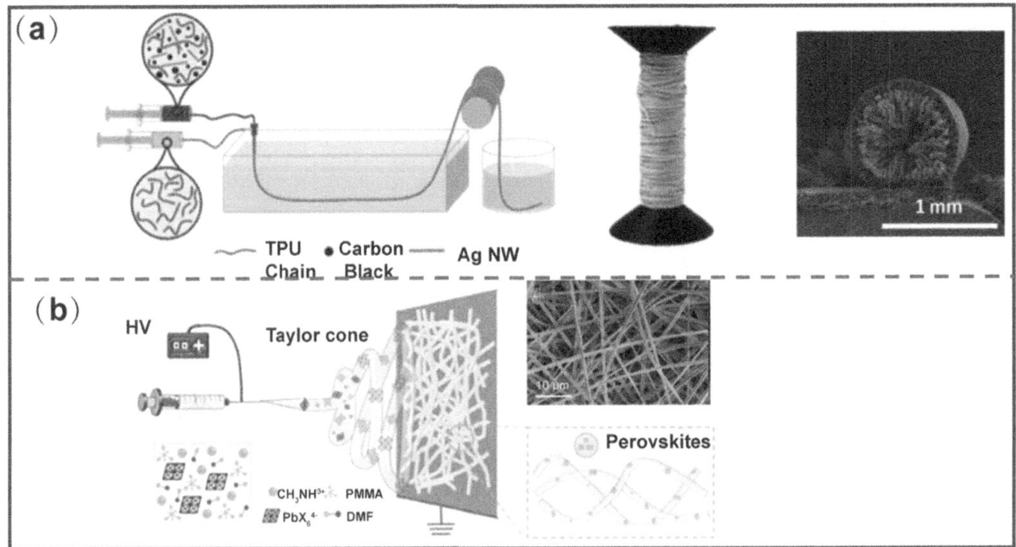

FIGURE 8.3 Spinning technology to prepare the functional fibers. (a) Wet spinning process. The core solution and sheath solution were injected into a coagulating bath and the fibers were formed. The resulting fibers were collected on a bobbin and their morphology was characterized using SEM imaging as shown in the figures. (b) Schematic of the electrospinning process used to fabricate perovskite–polymer fiber membranes, which were subsequently utilized as a large-area display. ([a] Reprinted with permission. (Doganay et al., 2023) Copyright 2023, Elsevier; [b] Reprinted with permission. (Ying Chen et al., 2023b) Copyright 2023, Springer.)

cellulose acetate (CA), and silk, have been electrospun to produce optical and optoelectronic fibers for biomedical applications. Chen and his colleagues (Kim et al., 2022) reported the preparation of stretchable luminescent displays by electrospinning perovskite–polymer composite nanofibers. As depicted in Figure 8.3b, polymethyl methacrylate (PMMA)/methylammonium lead iodide ($MAPbI_3$) nanofibers were obtained using an electrospinning technique. Crystallized $MAPbI_3$ nanocrystals are preferentially embedded in the PMMA fibers because of a high-strength electrical field. The film was then processed to various shapes for display.

8.2.2.3 3D Printing

3D printing is becoming an increasingly popular method for producing optical and optoelectronic fibers due to its rapid prototyping, cost-effectiveness, and ease of use. Various 3D printing technologies, such as fused deposition modeling (FDM), polyjet printing, stereolithography (SLA), direct ink writing (DIW), and two-photon polymerization (2PP), are shown in Figure 8.4a. For sensing applications, Alam and colleagues (2022) utilized a masked stereolithographic apparatus (MSLA) to produce polymer optical fibers. Hydroxyethyl methacrylate (HEMA)/PEGDA, a photocurable resin with good biocompatibility, was chosen, and thermochromic powders were used for temperature sensing. The mixture was mixed under magnetic stirring and poured into the resin vat of

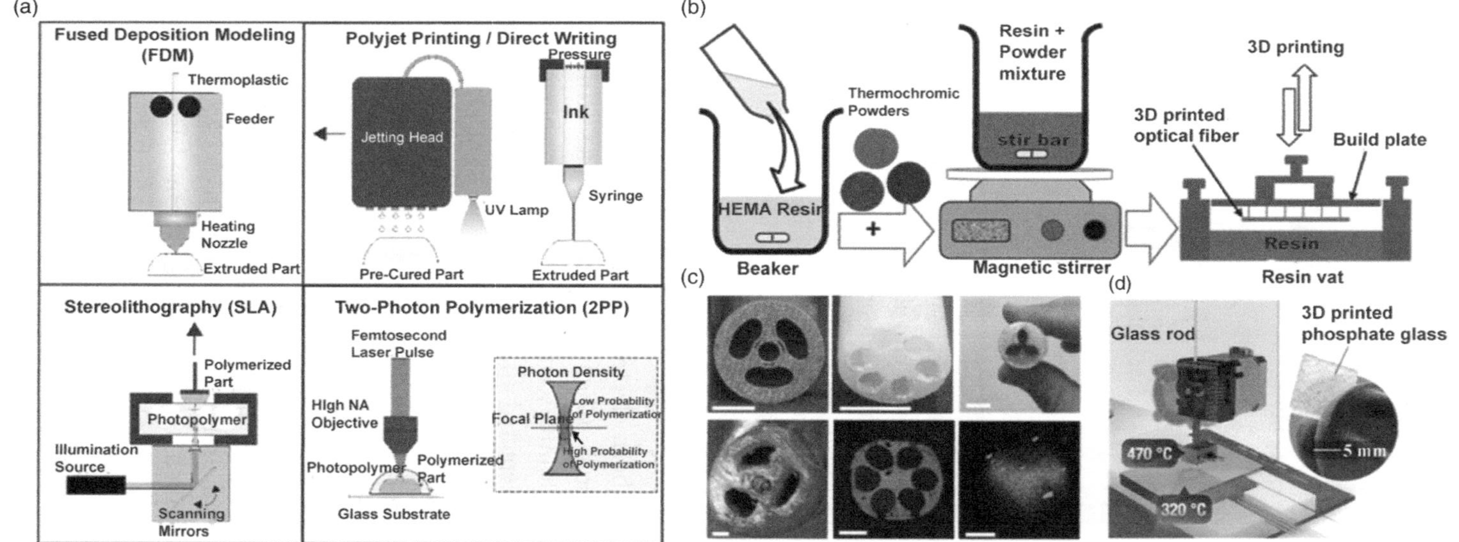

FIGURE 8.4   3D printing technology as an emerging fabrication strategy for optical and optoelectrical fibers. (a) Schematic of four kinds of 3D printing technologies. (b) Schematic of masked stereolithographic apparatus of thermochromic optical fibers. (c) 3D printed preforms with different architectures (scale bar = 1 cm). I: Preform with multiple irregular channels. II: Preform with six equitangentially spaced cylindrical channels. III: Preform with propeller-shaped channels. (d) Thermal drawn glass fiber as the feedback of 3D printing. [a] Reproduced under terms of Optica Publishing Group Open Access Publishing Agreement. (Berglund et al., 2022) Copyright 2022, the Authors, published by Optica Publishing Group; [b] Reproduced with permission. (Alam et al., 2022) Copyright 2022, Elsevier; [c] Reproduced under terms of the CC-BY license (van der Elst et al., 2021) Copyright 2021, the Authors, published by Springer Nature; [d] Reproduced under terms of CC BY-NC-ND license. (Zaki et al., 2020) Copyright 2020, the Authors, Published by Elsevier.

a 3D printer. The 3D-printed optical fibers were produced layer-by-layer under UV light illumination (Figure 8.4b).

The combination of 3D printing and thermal drawing enables the production of functional fibers with arbitrary cross-section structures, as illustrated by the various preform designs shown in Fig 4c. However, the anisotropic porosity inherent to the 3D printing process and the anisotropic thermomechanical and mechanical behavior of the preforms during the thermal drawing process have not been fully addressed. In contrast, a recent study utilized thermally drawn glass fiber as feedstock for FDM 3D printing of optically transparent structures as shown in Figure 8.4d. The results indicated that incorporating a dual material fiber into the 3D printing process can improve the mechanical properties of the materials (Zaki et al., 2020).

8.3 MULTIFUNCTIONAL FIBER-BASED BIOPHYSICAL AND BIOCHEMICAL SENSING SYSTEMS

8.3.1 Detecting Biophysical Signals

Monitoring human body temperature by incorporating thermal-sensitive fluorescent materials into optical fibers has become a common approach. Fan and co-workers (2023) fabricated PU/graphene encapsulated PEDOT:PSS fibers by wet spinning and immersion (Figure 8.5a). The composite fiber sensor demonstrated a temperature sensing range of 30 °C–50 °C and the α value can reach $-1.72\%/°C$ with a linearity of 0.98 (Figure 8.5 b). The composite fiber had a temperature resolution of 0.1 °C, meeting the necessary criteria for accurately measuring slight fluctuations in human body temperature (Figure 8.5c). Figure 8.5d shows a fabric-based flexible temperature sensor. As the temperature sensor integrated into the fabric is designed for prolonged wear, it can continuously monitor human body temperature in real time and transmit the temperature data to a vast database via a mobile phone. However, body movement–induced strain has an adverse effect when stretchable optical fiber sensors are used for wearable applications. Chen and co-workers (2022) reported a stretchable optical fiber temperature sensor based on fluorescent nanoparticles and silicone elastomers. The excitation loss and fluorescence intensity of the sensor showed a linear response to changes in temperature and strain, which were utilized as sensing parameters to decouple the strain from the sensing signal.

Respiratory monitoring is critical, especially for patients with respiratory disorders, heart failure, or health rehabilitation training. Shrivastav and co-workers (2020) reported an optical humidity sensor for human breath monitoring. The sensing material, chitosan, was deposited in the holes of a microstructured optical fiber, creating a Fabry-Pérot (FP) interferometer sensing platform (Figure 8.5e). The working principle of the optical fiber sensor was based on volume changes of hygroscopic chitosan under different humidity conditions, leading to the change in refractive index. Next, evanescent waves at the core–chitosan interface interacted in the FP cavity, resulting in the wavelength and power of reflected light shifting. Thus, the ambient humidity around the probe can be determined by monitoring the wavelength change of a specific tilt angle (Figure 8.5f). From Figure 8.5g, it's clearly seen that the wavelength difference between exhalation and inhalation

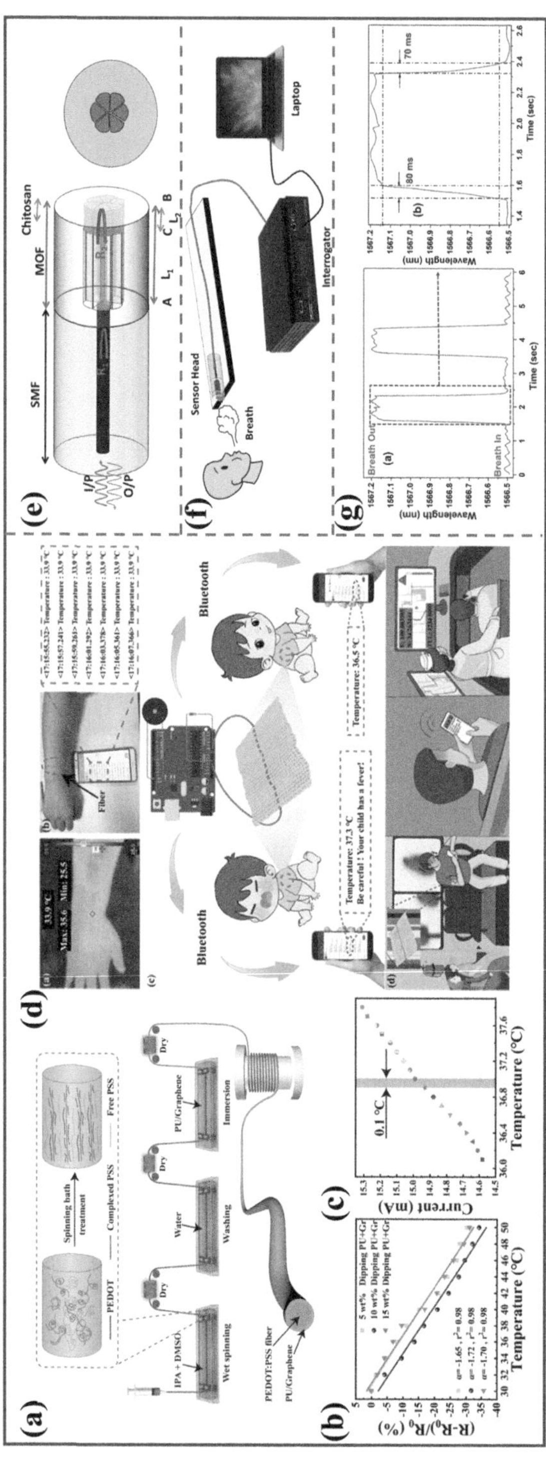

FIGURE 8.5 Advanced fibers applied in temperature monitoring (a–c) and respiratory (d–f) monitoring. (a) Schematic of preparation and characterization of PU/graphene encapsulated PEDOT:PSS fiber. (b) Temperature sensitivity of the composite fibers with different graphene contents. (c) The current curves of the composite fibers when temperature varied from 36.1 to 37.8 °C. (d) A fabric-based flexible temperature sensor and its application. (e) Structural composition of the humidity sensor using a Fabry-Pérot interferometric configuration. (f) Experimental setup for respiratory monitoring. (g) Signal variation of the sensor when humans breathe in and breathe out. [c and d] Adapted with permission. (Fan et al., 2023) Copyright 2023, American Chemical Society; [e–g] Reproduced under terms of Creative Commons CC BY license. (Shrivastav et al., 2020) Copyright 2020, the Authors, published by Springer Nature.

could be distinguished. Additionally, the optical sensor showed ultrafast response and recovery time (80 ms and 70 ms, respectively).

To improve continuity of measurement, Li and co-workers (2023) designed a smart-watch assisted by an optical fiber sensor for continuous and accurate blood pressure monitoring. Figure 8.6a demonstrates the structure of the fiber, including polyethylene (PE) tube, an air core, and two multimode fibers. When the PE tube was under pressure, the deformed shape would change the intensity of the transmitted light. Based on this principle, a flexible optical fiber sensor was fabricated by encapsulating the fiber adapter with PDMS film. The sensor exhibited a sensitivity of −213 µW/kPa within an expansive linear working range of 0–2 kPa. Notably, it exhibited high linearity (R^2 = 0.989) in this range, minimizing distortion in the detection of pulse wave signals. The high coincidence observed in the five cycles indicates that the sensor exhibits strong consistency (Figure 8.6b). Also, the sensor had a fast response time of only 5 ms (Figure 8.6c). To assess free alignment and spatial insensitivity, the proposed sensor was positioned at various locations within the wrist region to detect pulse signals. Clearly, there is no distortion of pulse wave signals resulting from position drift, ensuring accuracy in blood pressure readings (Figure 8.6d). To demonstrate the application of ambulatory blood pressure monitoring, the proposed smartwatch was worn by a female volunteer (Figure 8.6e). It could be observed that the blood pressure data was continuously recorded for one day (Figure 8.6f). By developing an app, real-time blood pressure monitoring becomes more convenient (Figure 8.6g).

Fiber optoelectronics technology has also been utilized to detect physiological signals. The configuration of electrode micropatterns is critical for ensuring that the performance of fiber devices is comparable to that of established planar devices. Kim and co-workers (2020) introduced a fiber organic photodiode (OPD) to monitor the heart rate. As shown in Figure 8.6h, the fiber OPD was composed of Au gate microfiber, Ecoflex elastomer as the protective layer, poly([2,6′-4,8-di(5-ethylhexylthienyl)benzo[1,2-b;3,3-b]-dithiophene]{3-fluoro-2[(2-ethylhexyl)carbonyl]thieno[3,4-b]thiophenediyl) (PTB7-Th) and [6,6]-phenyl-C71-butyric acid methyl ester ($PC_{71}BM$) as the photoactive materials, and CNT microelectrode. The CNT microelectrode, prepared by inkjet printing with a hydrogel template, was spirally wrapped on the fiber surface to ensure tight conformal contact (Figure 8.6i). Figure 8.6j demonstrated that the photoactive layer had high absorbance in the green and red waves, which is the basis of the combination of green and red LEDs as a sensor. The fiber OPD showed a high I_{light}/I_{dark} photocurrent ratio (Figure 8.6k) and bending duration, which was important for wearable electronics. To create a photoplethysmography (PPG) sensor, the fiber OPD as well as a green and a red LED were integrated into a textile bandage (Figure 8.6l). The fiber OPD received the red or green signals after transmission or reflection on the human tissue. Both mode measurements captured PPG signals with repeated systolic and diastolic peaks of the same period as shown in Figure 8.6m. The heart rate of the volunteer was estimably 63 bpm.

8.3.2 Biochemical Signals and Biosensors

Physiologic pH is vital for the normal functioning of tissues and varies in different parts of the body. For example, tumor sites are always acidic, and the changes in pH values

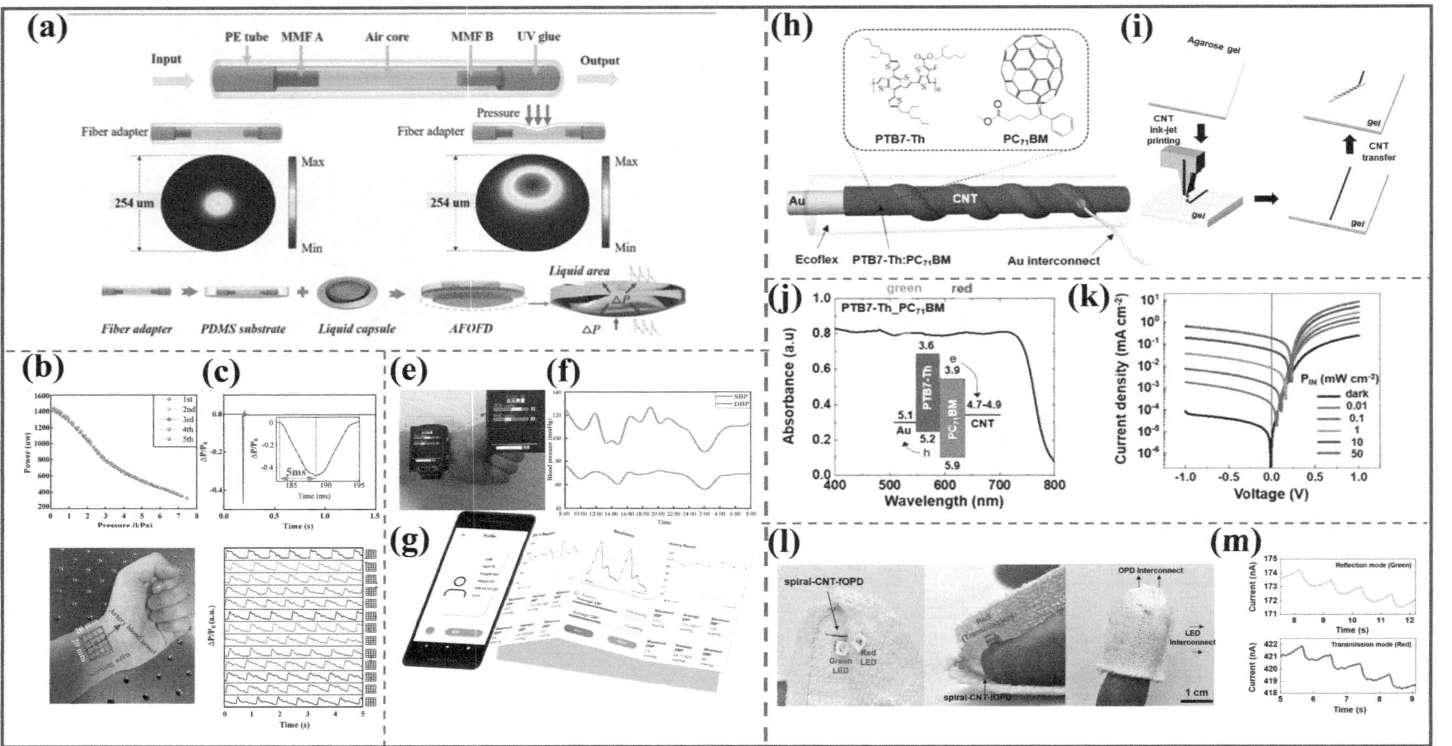

FIGURE 8.6 Optical and optoelectronic fibers used to monitor blood pressure (a–d) and heart rate (e–j). (a) Schematic of the structures of the fiber and corresponding optical fiber sensor. (b) The sensor's optical power–pressure curve over five cycles. (c) Response time of the optical sensor. (d) Pulse signals from various sites of the wrist. (e) The smartwatch worn by a female volunteer. (f) The 24-h blood pressure monitoring. (g) The APP program. Adapted with permission. (Li et al., 2023) Copyright 2023, Springer. (h) Schematic of the device structure and materials composition of the fiber organic photodiode (OPD). (i) Absorption spectrum of PTB7-Th:PC71BM in the range of 400–800 nm. (j) Photograph of the catheter wrapped on a glass rod. (k) Current density–voltage (J–V) curves of the fiber OPD. (l) Photographs of OPD with a red and a green LED as a PPG sensor. (m) PPG signals captured by the fiber OPD from the reflection and transmission modes. Reprinted with permission. (Kim et al., 2020) Copyright 2020, American Chemical Society.

reflect the healing status of a wound. It's typical to measure pH by depositing organic dyes on the tip of the fiber. However, dyes are harmful to human health. Biocompatible coating and pH-sensitive carbon quantum dots were employed to reduce the toxicity to tissues or organs. Another challenge is dye-leaching and photobleaching which lower the sensitivity and stability of the optical sensors (Rezapour Sarabi et al., 2021). Tang and co-workers (2021) reported a dye-free optical fiber pH sensor. The sensor was U-shaped with a coated organic–inorganic composite membrane (Figure 8.7a). The shape of the membrane changed since the hydrogen bonds of the membrane changed when the sensor was in a different pH solution and therefore the refractive index of the film varied. The sensor showed a reversible response from pH 4.5 to 12.5 with an accuracy of ±0.2 pH compared with a commercial probe (Figure 8.7b, c). For biomedical applications, the sensor was employed to monitor the pH of human serum (Figure 8.7d), which demonstrated that the proposed sensor could record the dynamic changes while adjusting the pH value of serum from about 7.7 to 6.4.

Various glucose monitoring systems have been utilized for short-term glucose detection, including implantable electrochemical sensors, but they come with certain limitations, such as signal drift due to enzymatic reactions and accuracy constraints (Gupta et al., 2022). Hydrogel-based optical fibers show good potential because of their biocompatibility, flexibility, and capability to be combined with functional groups for glucose sensing. In a study by Mohamed Elsherif and co-workers (Yetisen et al., 2017), hydrogel optical fibers were prepared using poly(acrylamide-co-poly(ethylene glycol) diacrylate) functionalized with phenylboronic acid as the core layer and Ca alginate as the cladding layer (Figure 8.7e). The complexation of phenylboronic acid and the cis-diol groups of glucose allowed the diameter of the hydrogel fiber to change reversibly (Figure 8.7f). Gelatin matrices were utilized as phantom tissues *in vitro* to visualize the propagation of light throughout the hydrogel optical fibers (Figure 8.7g). Results showed that light attenuation was less than 10% when the optical fibers were inserted into gelatin matrices under laser lamination. Moreover, the fabricated hydrogel fiber could deliver light into the targeted area when it was injected into porcine tissue *ex vivo* (Figure 8.7h). However, despite these promising results, few optical sensors have been implanted *in vivo* for long-term glucose monitoring. Designing effective implantable optical sensors for glucose monitoring requires careful consideration of device configuration, especially the configuration of electrode micropatterns, to ensure that the performance of fiber devices is comparable to established planar devices.

The global pandemic of Corona Virus Disease 2019 (COVID-19) has brought significant challenges to the field of medical diagnosis. Although reverse transcription polymerase chain reaction (RT-PCR) is widely used to detect SARS-CoV-2 infection, it has limitations including high false-negative rates and complexity. As an alternative solution, biosensors and spectroscopy based on optical fibers have been proposed for virus detection. Chen and co-workers (2023a) developed a surface plasmon resonance (SPR)-based fiber tip biosensor for amplification-free monkeypox virus detection and genotyping. The fabrication process of the biosensor is shown in Figure 8.7i. The proposed CRISPR-SPR-FT biosensor was modified with AuNPs via partially complementary DNA, in which an ssDNA reporter

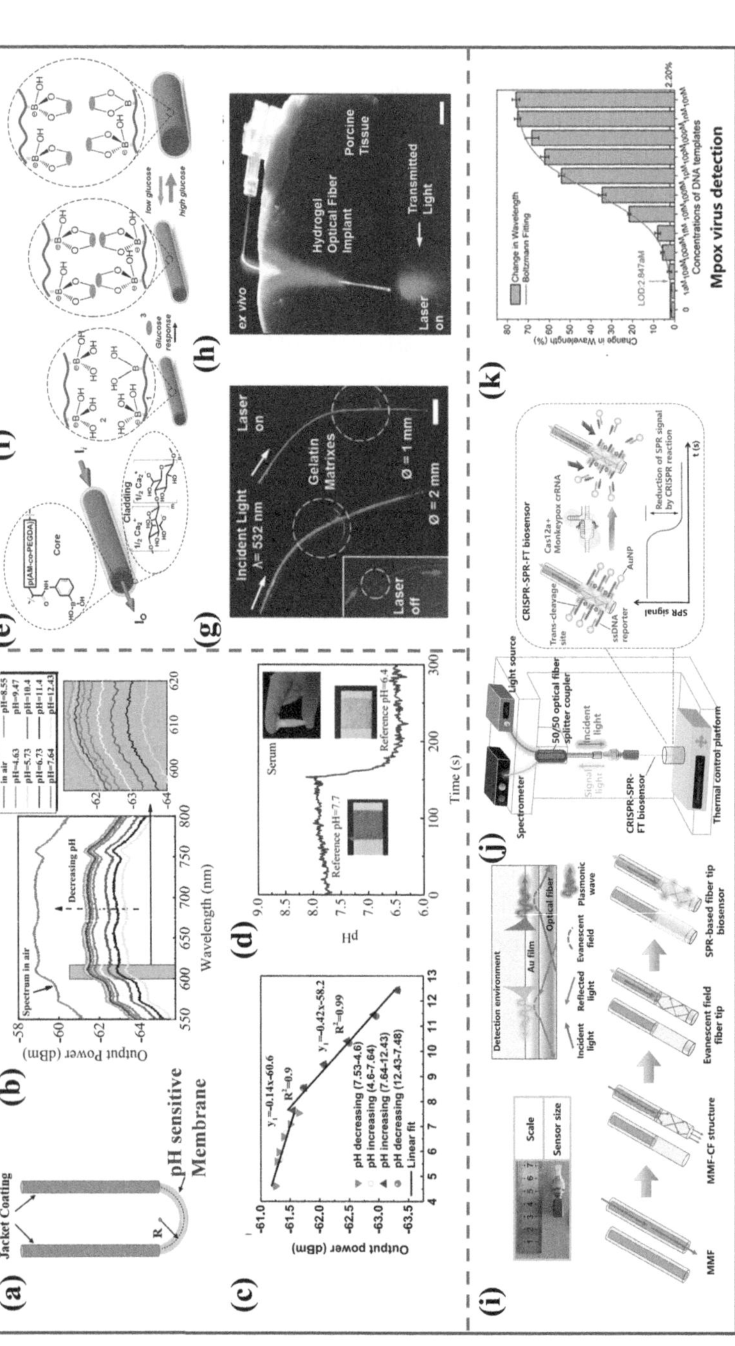

FIGURE 8.7 Optical and optoelectronic fibers applied in biosensors. (a)–(d): Optical fibers in pH sensing. (a) Schematic of the U-shaped optical fiber sensor with a pH-sensitive membrane. (b) The spectral response of the optical fiber sensor at different pH levels. (c) Linear fitting curves. (d) pH measurement of human serum with the sensor. Reproduced under terms of Creative Commons Attribution 4.0 License (Tang et al., 2021) Copyright 2021, the Authors, published by IEEE Xplore. (e)–(h): Hydrogel-based optical fibers in glucose monitoring. (e) Schematic of the structural composition of hydrogel optical fibers. (f) Mechanism of glucose sensitivity of the sensor. (g) Light transmission of hydrogel optical fibers through gelatin matrices. Scale bar = 1 cm. The inset showed the hydrogel optical fiber was sandwiched in gelatin when the laser was off. (h) Light-guiding in porcine tissue. Scale bar = 3 mm. Reproduced under the terms of the Creative Commons CC BY license. (Yetisen et al., 2017) Copyright 2017, the Authors, published by Wiley. (i)–(k): Virus detection. (i) Schematic of the fabrication process of the biosensor. (j) Schematic of the design of the CRISPR-SPR-FT biosensing platform for monkeypox virus detection. (k) Surface plasmon resonance (SPR) signals with different concentrations of target dsDNA template. Reproduced with permission. (Y. Chen et al., 2023a) Copyright 2023, American Chemical Society.

with a critical trans-cleavage site is designed on the biosensor. Target DNA–activated Cas12a–crRNA causes transcleavage of the ssDNA reporter gene. During CRISPR/Cas12a sensing, spectral signals are transmitted and recorded in real time via an optical fiber-based biosensing system. The loss of AuNPs on the sensor surface resulted in corresponding changes in the SPR signals (Figure 8.7j). As shown in Figure 8.7k, the limit of detection of the biosensor was calculated to be 2.847 aM, which could detect samples with virus concentrations below 1.8 copies/µL without the need for a pre-amplification step. Meanwhile, Wu and his team (2022) developed a portable smartphone-based optical fiber that integrates an immunosensing system for diagnosing COVID-19. The device is approximately 108 × 158 × 150 mm in size and can analyze serum samples from clinically diagnosed COVID-19 patients and healthy volunteers. The device showed a sensitivity of 72% and a specificity of 100%, which was highly correlated with those obtained using commercial ELISA kits and simple Western analysis. These optical fiber–based biosensors offer a promising platform for fast, accurate, and cost-effective COVID-19 detection, which could significantly improve the current state of diagnostics.

8.4 OTHER ADVANCED FIBER TECHNOLOGIES IN BIO-INTEGRATED SYSTEMS

8.4.1 Human–Machine Interfaces

The field of human–machine interaction has become increasingly important in many areas, including human healthcare, robots, and virtual reality. Optical and optoelectronic fibers offer several advantages as human–machine interfaces, including immunity to electromagnetic interference, high performance in humid environments, and the ability to sense multiple parameters simultaneously. Compared to other wearable electronic sensors that are based on resistance, capacitance, or piezoelectricity, optical and optoelectronic fibers are particularly well-suited to large-area sensing applications. To enable this, Ma et al. (2022) integrated an optical fiber array with flexible PDMS films to create a smart textile for human–machine interaction (Figure 8.8a). The thick textile layer was made of coarse twill fabric with a warp and weft structure that converted finger sliding into periodic vibrations of the optical fibers. The feasibility of intelligent textiles supporting optical fibers for human–machine interaction was demonstrated by using a five-optical fiber array to control the fingers of a robotic hand (Figure 8.8b). The robotic hand was able to perform various gestures including flexing individual fingers or more complex gestures such as OK sign and fist pump (Figure 8.8c). In addition to a static tactile response, the smart textiles were tested to detect dynamic finger slippage for complex human–machine interaction using machine learning. Textiles adhered to a doll were used to collect time–domain signals, each corresponding to an emotional expression (Figure 8.8d). Different touch manners produced different emotional expressions on the doll's face (Figure 8.8e) and the recognition accuracy of the optical sensors was as high as 98.1% (Figure 8.8f). These findings demonstrate the potential of optical fibers in smart textiles for advanced human–machine interactions.

In recent research on human–machine interaction, electronic readers have been a major focus. However, they may not always be accessible to the naked eye. To address this issue,

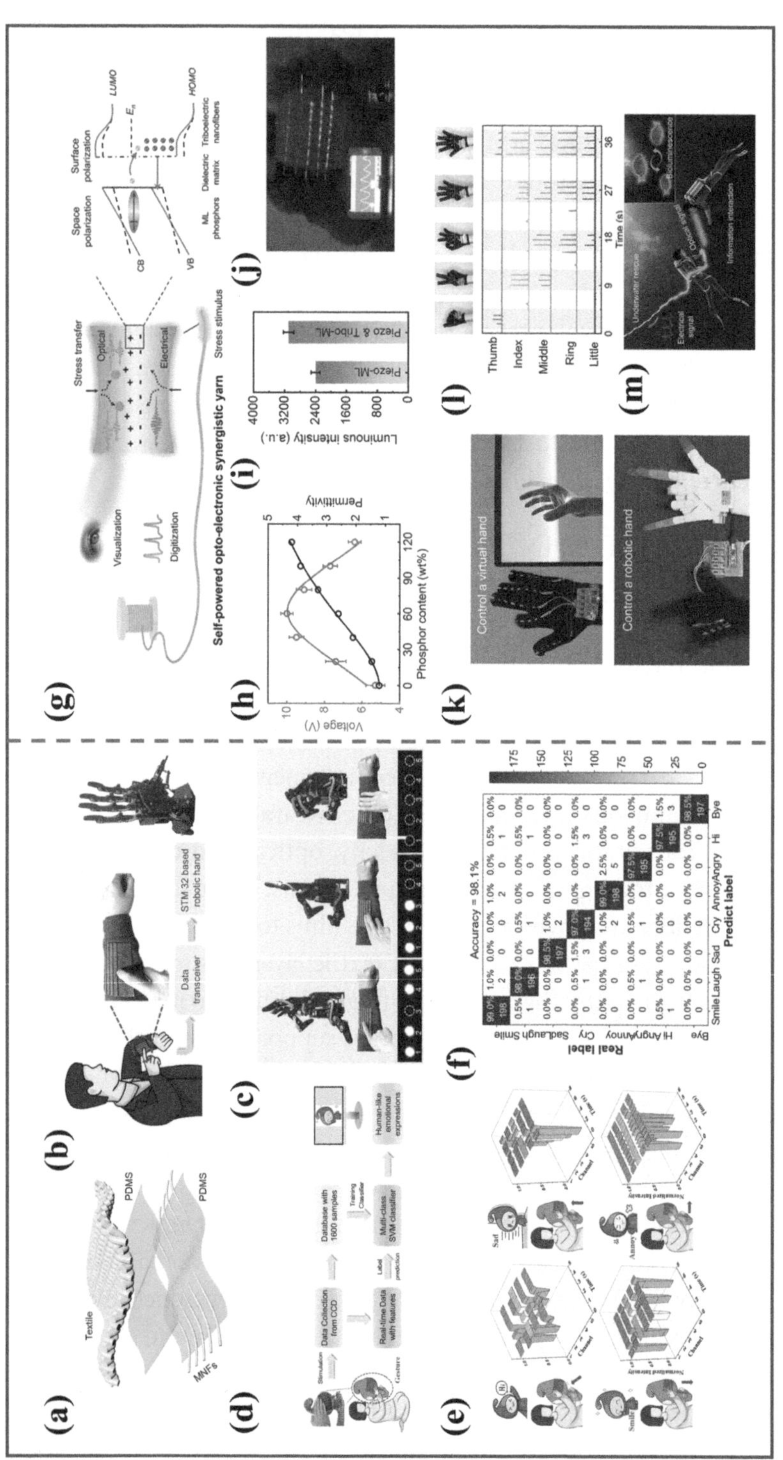

FIGURE 8.8 Novel fiber devices used in human–machine interfaces. (a)–(f): Optical fiber–integrated smart textiles for human–machine interface. (a) Schematic of the structure of optical smart textiles. (b)–(c) Schematic of the logic control process by smart textiles. (d) Schematic of emotional virtual interaction. (e) Emotional expressions in different time-domain signals. (f) Confusion matrix. Reproduced with permission. (Ma et al., 2022) Copyright 2022, Springer Nature. (g)–(m): Optoelectronic intelligent fiber sensor with visual–digital synergies. (g) The design of the SOEFS and optoelectronic synergy mechanism. (h) Voltage and permittivity under different contents of phosphor. (i) Enhancement of luminescent intensity. (j) SOEFS-enabled textiles with visual–digital synergies during stretching. SOEFS applied to AR interaction, robotic manipulation (k), gesture recognition (l), and underwater information interaction (m). Adapted with permission. (Y. Chen et al., 2021b) Copyright 2021, Wiley.

Yang and co-workers (Y. Chen et al.,2021b) reported the development of an optoelectronic intelligent fiber sensor (SOEFS) that is self-powered and provides feedback through both visible and electrical signals based on the mechanoluminescent (ML)-triboelectric synergistic effect (Figure 8.8g). The SOEFS is composed of a core of poly(vinylidene fluoride-trifluoroethylamine) (P(VDF-TrFE)) nanofibers and a sheath of elastomer poly(styrene-b-(ethylene-co-butylene)-b-styrene (SEBS) and ML phosphors. This optoelectronic device exhibited significantly enhanced electrical output (100%) and optical output (30%) (Figure 8.8h, i). When integrated into textiles, the optoelectronic bimodal SOEFS can create a synergy between vision and digital information during the stretching process (Figure 8.8j). Furthermore, the SOEFS has been applied to various applications such as gesture recognition, AR interaction, robotic manipulation, and underwater information interaction (Figure 8.8k, l, m).

8.4.2 Photobiomodulation (PBM) Therapy

Photobiomodulation (PBM) therapy has emerged as a promising treatment modality for tissue regeneration, photodynamic therapy, and optogenetics by enabling light delivery to targeted areas *in vivo*. Optogenetics technology utilizes genetic and optical techniques to control the excitatory or inhibitory state of neurons and record electrophysiological signals from the targeted regions. By utilizing transgene technology, photosensitive proteins can be specifically expressed on the membrane of neurons and they can respond to different wavelengths to influence neuron states. Park and colleagues (2017) have developed a flexible optoelectronic device that achieves one-step optogenetics. This thermal drawn fiber device comprises an optical waveguide made of PC (core)/cyclic olefin copolymer (COC) (cladding), six electrodes made of conductive polyethylene (CPE) and 5% graphite (gCPE), and two microfluidic channels (Figure 8.9a). The opsin genes were delivered into specific sites of a mouse's brain through the microfluidic channels, thus avoiding a second surgery. After two weeks of implantation, the optoelectronic device enabled the expression of the CHR2 photosensitive protein (protein to excite neurons) (Figure 8.9b). Subsequently, the device captured the electrophysiological signals of optically evoked potentials via light transmission of the PC/COC waveguide (Figure 8.9c). The device's stable optical stimulation capability was demonstrated for up to three months by recording the potentials (Figure 8.9d). Due to its all-polymer composition, the optoelectronic fiber device has superior biocompatibility compared to steel microwire (Figure 8.9e).

Jiang and co-workers (2020) developed biodegradable polymer optical fibers to transmit green light to regulate bone regeneration. The optical fibers effectively delivered green light into deeper tissues for PBM as shown in Figure 8.9f. Micro-CT and quantitative analysis shown in Figures 8.9g–i clearly demonstrate that green light irradiation using these optical fibers accelerated bone regeneration. The results of western blots suggested that green light activated P-ERK and RUNX2, leading to osteogenesis (Figure 8.9j). Biocompatible optical fibers have been used to transmit light to the surface of tissues. However, it's still a constraint to deliver light to deeper tissues. Researchers introduced bioabsorbable photonic waveguides for light delivery to deeper tissues. PLLA waveguides were inserted in the full-thickness skin incision for photochemical tissue bonding. Finally, a wound of thickness

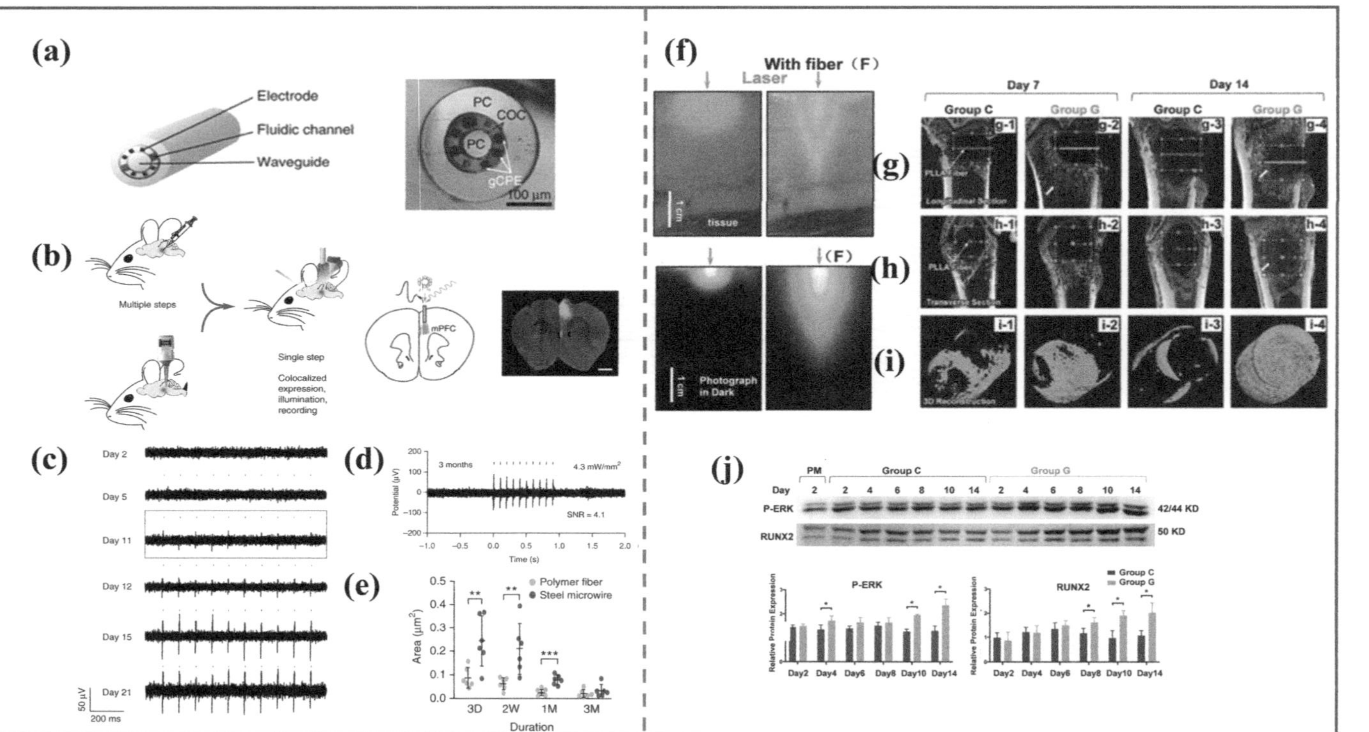

FIGURE 8.9 Optical and optoelectronic fibers in PBM therapy. (a)–(e): an implantable optoelectronic fiber device for optogenetics. (a) A schematic and cross-sectional microscope image of the multifunctional optoelectronic fiber. (b) Left: a schematic comparison between traditional two-step surgery and one-step surgery in this research for optogenetics. Middle: a working process illustration of the fiber probe including viral delivery, optical stimulation, and electrical recording. Right: fluorescent image of the expression of ChR2-eYFP for two weeks after implantation. (c) Optically evoked potential recording from day 2 to day 21 by the fiber. (d) Optically evoked potential recording after three months. (e) Average fluorescence area of glial scarring of the polymer fiber and steel microwire. Reproduced with permission. (Park et al., 2017) Copyright 2017, Springer Nature. (f)–(j): Green light-based PBM with an optical fiber for bone regeneration. (f) Schematic diagrams of green light transmission in the tissue without or with the optical fiber. (g)–(h) 3D micro-CT images of bone growth under green light (Group G) or no illumination (Group C) on day 7 and day 14. (i) Quantitative analysis of micro-CT. (j) Western blots of the protein expression level of P-ERK and RUNX2 at different time. Adapted with permission. (Jiang et al., 2020) Copyright 2020, Wiley.

over 10 mm of porcine skin was healed. Importantly, PLLA could be resorbed by the tissues eliminating the need for removing the optical fiber after implantation (Nizamoglu et al., 2016).

By inserting optical fibers into the cavity of human organs, photodynamic therapy has been used clinically for the non-invasive treatment of local tumors. To improve therapy efficiency and reduce the side effects of photosensitizers, researchers have opted for intra-tumoral injection instead of intravenous injection. However, instillation into targeted cancer sites does not prevent photosensitizers from spreading to distant organs. To achieve local controlled release, researchers have explored coating photosensitizers on the surface of implantable optical fibers. This approach has proven effective in prolonging the retention of immunotherapeutics, thereby enhancing anti-tumor efficacy when combined with immunotherapy (Chin et al., 2021).

8.4.3 Others

In addition to the technologies discussed above, advanced fiber technology has enabled the development of several other innovative tools. Among these, optical tweezers have become an invaluable tool for optical trapping and manipulation in a range of applications, including cell trapping, labeling, and analysis, as well as cell assembly for studying cell–cell interactions. The ability to assemble randomly distributed cells into regular structures and arrays under optical forces provides inspiration for other biomedical fields, such as targeted therapy, drug delivery, and microfluidic chip driving. Deng et al. (2022) recently reported the development of a capillary optical fiber tweezer (COFT) for the ballistic transport and trapping of yeast cells (Figure 8.10a). The COFT is capable of capturing over two cells simultaneously during the trapping process (Figure 8.10b). However, biocompatibility is a crucial consideration for optical tweezers as they can cause mechanical damage when they are implanted into an organism.

An optoelectronic device that converts optical stimulation into electronic signals shows promise for the development of electronic prosthetics. (Ceron et al. 2021)recently reported an artificial optoelectronic sensorimotor synapse based on a stretchable organic transistor. The self-powered photodetector generated voltage pulses in response to ambient optical signals including infrared, visible, and ultraviolet light, which drove the organic transistor as the presynaptic spikes. Excitatory postsynaptic current signals were subsequently formed, enabling the principle of optical wireless communication. Furthermore, the presynaptic spikes were transmitted to organic nanowires, which generated postsynaptic electrical signals capable of controlling artificial muscles (Figure 8.10c, d). This system therefore constitutes an artificial muscle actuator with light-interactive actuation.

8.5 CONCLUSION AND OUTLOOK

By employing proper fabrication methods and materials, optical and optoelectronic fibers have exhibited great potential for wearable sensors, human–machine interfaces, and implantable devices. However, there still remain some challenges for optical and optoelectronic fibers to face in bio-integrated systems. First, besides their biocompatibility, the main requirements placed on biomaterials-based optical and optoelectronic fibers are their

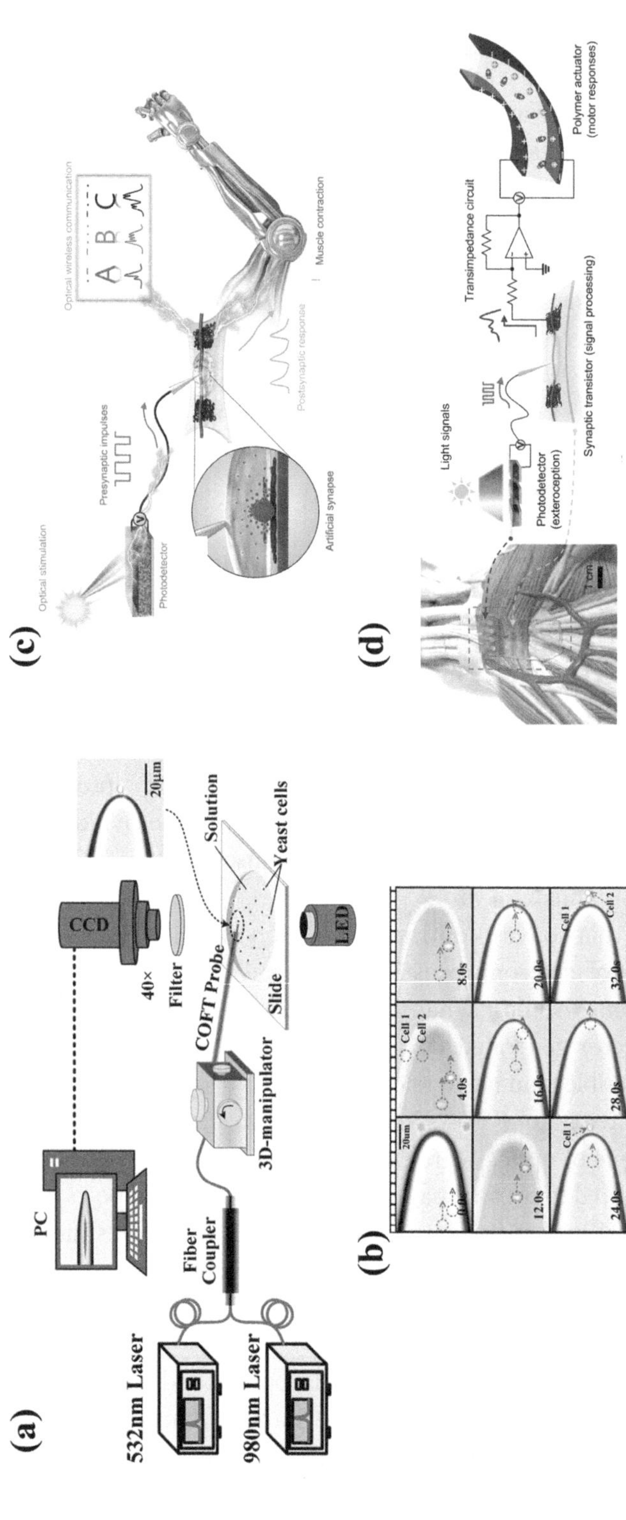

FIGURE 8.10 Optical and optoelectronic fiber-based devices for optical tweezers and electronic prosthetics. (a) Schematic of the COFT system for optical manipulation. The inset shows a trapped yeast cell by the COFT probe. (b) Optical microscopy images of the micromanipulation of two cells. Reproduced with permission (Deng et al., 2022) Copyright 2022, Royal Society of Chemistry. (c) Schematic of the organic optoelectronic sensorimotor synapse. (d) Photography of optoelectronic synapse on the model of human internal structure and neuromuscular electronic system. Reproduced under a Creative Commons Attribution NonCommercial License 4.0. Copyright 2018, The authors, published by American Association for the Advancement of Science.

ability to match the required mechanical properties and their adaptable degradation time for a given specific application. Second, optical and optoelectronic fibers have higher optical attenuation due to bending, which limits their application in short distance. Third, achieving miniaturization effectively is difficult, especially for implantable devices integrated with other electronic elements. So, future research of optical and optoelectronic fibers should exploit or improve materials and fabrication methods based on the needs of optical transmission and adaptability with tissues. Furthermore, AI techniques can be utilized to solve the above problems; for example, materials library selection and outcome prediction, data analysis, and translating the data from optical signals into meaningful parameters.

REFERENCES

Alam, F., Elsherif, M., Salih, A. E., & Butt, H. (2022). 3D printed polymer composite optical fiber for sensing applications. *Additive Manufacturing*, 58, 102996.

Alexander Schmidt, M., Argyros, A., & Sorin, F. (2015). Hybrid optical fibers – an innovative platform for in-fiber photonic devices. *Advanced Optical Materials*, 4(1), 13–36.

Berglund, G., Wisniowiecki, A., Gawedzinski, J., Applegate, B., & Tkaczyk, T. S. (2022). Additive manufacturing for the development of optical/photonic systems and components. *Optica*, 9(6), 623–638.

Ceron, S., Kimmel, M. A., Nilles, A., Petersen, K. J. I. R., & Letters, A. (2021). Soft robotic oscillators with strain-based coordination. *IEEE Robotics and Automation Letters*, 6(4), 7557–7563.

Chen, G., Wang, G., Tan, X., Hou, K., Meng, Q., Zhao, P., &. Zhu, M. (2021a). Integrated dynamic wet spinning of core-sheath hydrogel fibers for optical-to-brain/tissue communications. *National Science Review*, 8(9), nwaa209.

Chen, M., He, Y., Liang, H., Zhou, H., Wang, X., Heng, X., & Yang, Z. (2022). Stretchable and strain-decoupled fluorescent optical fiber sensor for body temperature and movement monitoring. *ACS Photonics*, 9(4), 1415–1424.

Chen, Y., Chen, Z., Li, T., Qiu, M., Zhang, J., Wang, Y., & Zhang, H. (2023a). Ultrasensitive and specific clustered regularly interspaced short palindromic repeats empowered a plasmonic fiber tip system for amplification-free monkeypox virus detection and genotyping. *ACS Nano*, 17(13), 12903–12914.

Chen, Y., Yang, J., Zhang, X., Feng, Y., Zeng, H., Wang, L., & Feng, W. (2021b). Light-driven bimorph soft actuators: design, fabrication, and properties. *Materials Horizons*, 8(3), 728–757.

Chen, Y., Zhang, Z., Sun, Y., & Wang, G. (2023b). Waterproof, self-adhesive, and large-area luminescent perovskite–polymer fiber membranes. *Advanced Fiber Materials*, 5(5), 1737–1748.

Chin, A. L., Jiang, S., Jang, E., Niu, L., Li, L., Jia, X., & Tong, R. (2021). Implantable optical fibers for immunotherapeutics delivery and tumor impedance measurement. *Nature Communications*, 12(1), 5138.

Deng, H., Chen, D., Wang, R., Li, F., Luo, Z., Deng, S., & Yuan, L. (2022). Fiber-integrated optical tweezers for ballistic transport and trapping yeast cells. *Nanoscale*, 14(18), 6941–6948.

Doganay, D., Demircioglu, O., Cugunlular, M., Cicek, M. O., Cakir, O., Kayaci, H. U., & Unalan, H. E. (2023). Wet spun core-shell fibers for wearable triboelectric nanogenerators. *Nano Energy*, 116.

Fan, W., Liu, T., Wu, F., Wang, S., Ge, S., Li, Y., & Li, Y. (2023). An antisweat interference and highly sensitive temperature sensor based on poly(3,4-ethylenedioxythiophene)-poly(styrenesulfonate) fiber coated with polyurethane/graphene for real-Time monitoring of body temperature. *ACS Nano*, 17(21), 21073–21082.

Feng, J., Zheng, Y., Bhusari, S., Villiou, M., Pearson, S., & Campo, A. (2020). Printed degradable optical waveguides for guiding light into tissue. *Advanced Functional Materials*, 30(45), 2004327.

Guimaraes, C. F., Ahmed, R., Marques, A. P., Reis, R. L., & Demirci, U. (2021). Engineering hydrogel-based biomedical photonics: Design, fabrication, and applications. *Advanced Materials*, 33(23), 2006582.

Guo, J., Zhou, B., Yang, C., Dai, Q., & Kong, L. (2019). Stretchable and temperature-sensitive polymer optical fibers for wearable health monitoring. *Advanced Functional Materials*, 29(33), 1902898.

Gupta, B. D., Pathak, A., & Shrivastav, A. M. (2022). Optical biomedical diagnostics using lab-on-fiber technology: A review. *Photonics*, 9(2), 86.

He, J., Lu, C., Jiang, H., Han, F., Shi, X., Wu, J., & Peng, H. (2021). Scalable production of high-performing woven lithium-ion fibre batteries. *Nature*, 597(7874), 57–63.

Jiang, N., Ahmed, R., Rifat, A. A., Guo, J., Yin, Y., Montelongo, Y., & Yetisen, A. K. (2018). Functionalized flexible soft polymer optical fibers for laser photomedicine. *Advanced Optical Materials*, 6(3), 1701118.

Jiang, Y., Qi, W., Zhang, Q., Liu, H., Zhang, J., Du, N., & Wang, Y. (2020). Green light-based photobiomodulation with an implantable and biodegradable fiber for bone regeneration. *Small Methods*, 4(7), 1900879.

Kim, H., Kang, T. H., Ahn, J., Han, H., Park, S., Kim, S. J., & Lim, J. A. (2020). Spirally wrapped carbon nanotube microelectrodes for fiber optoelectronic devices beyond geometrical limitations toward smart wearable E-Textile applications. *ACS Nano*, 14(12), 17213–17223.

Kim, H.-J., Oh, H., Kim, T., Kim, D., & Park, M. (2022). Stretchable photodetectors based on electrospun polymer/perovskite composite nanofibers. *ACS Applied Nano Materials*, 5(1), 1308–1316.

Li, L., Sheng, S., Liu, Y., Wen, J., Song, C., Chen, Z., & Shum, P.-P. (2023). Automatic and continuous blood pressure monitoring via an optical-fiber-sensor-assisted smartwatch. *PhotoniX*, 4(1), 21.

Liu, M., Zhang, Y., Liu, K., Zhang, G., Mao, Y., Chen, L., & Tao, T. H. (2021). Biomimicking antibacterial Opto-Electro sensing sutures made of regenerated silk proteins. *Advanced Materials*, 33(1), 2004733.

Ma, S., Wang, X., Li, P., Yao, N., Xiao, J., Liu, H., & Zhang, L. (2022). Optical micro/nano fibers enabled smart textiles for human–machine interface. *Advanced Fiber Materials*, 4(5), 1108–1117.

Nizamoglu, S., Gather, M. C., Humar, M., Choi, M., Kim, S., Kim, K. S., & Yun, S. H. (2016). Bioabsorbable polymer optical waveguides for deep-tissue photomedicine. *Nature Communications* 7, 10374.

Pang, Y.-N., Liu, B., Liu, J., Wan, S.-P., Wu, T., Yuan, J., & Wu, Q. (2022). Singlemode-multimode-singlemode optical fiber sensor for accurate blood pressure monitoring. *Journal of Lightwave Technology*, 40(13), 4443–4450.

Park, S., Guo, Y., Jia, X., Choe, H. K., Grena, B., Kang, J., & Anikeeva, P. (2017). One-step optogenetics with multifunctional flexible polymer fibers. *Nature Neuroscience*, 20(4), 612–619.

Prajzler, V., Neruda, M., & Nekvindová, P. (2018). Flexible multimode polydimethyl-diphenylsiloxane optical planar waveguides. *Journal of Materials Science: Materials in Electronics*, 29(7), 5878–5884.

Qiao, X., Qian, Z., Li, J., Sun, H., Han, Y., Xia, X., & Wang, C. (2017). Synthetic engineering of spider silk fiber as implantable optical waveguides for low-loss light guiding. *ACS Applied Materials & Interfaces*, 9(17), 14665–14676.

Qiu, Y., Wang, C., Lu, X., Wu, H., Ma, X., Hu, J., & Liu, A. (2021). A biomimetic *Drosera capensis* with adaptive decision-predation behavior based on multifunctional sensing and fast actuating capability. *Advanced Functional Materials*, 32(13), 2110296.

Rezapour Sarabi, M., Jiang, N., Ozturk, E., Yetisen, A. K., & Tasoglu, S. (2021). Biomedical optical fibers. *Lab Chip*, 21(4), 627–640.

Seyedin, S., Carey, T., Arbab, A., Eskandarian, L., Bohm, S., Kim, J. M., & Torrisi, F. (2021). Fibre electronics: towards scaled-up manufacturing of integrated e-textile systems. *Nanoscale*, 13(30), 12818–12847.

Shrivastav, A. M., Gunawardena, D. S., Liu, Z., & Tam, H. Y. (2020). Microstructured optical fiber based Fabry-Perot interferometer as a humidity sensor utilizing chitosan polymeric matrix for breath monitoring. *Scientific Reports*, 10(1), 6002.

Skwierczynska, M., Stopikowska, N., Kulpinski, P., Klonowska, M., Lis, S., & Runowski, M. (2022). Ratiometric upconversion temperature sensor based on cellulose fibers modified with yttrium fluoride nanoparticles. *Nanomaterials (Basel)*, 12(11), 1926.

Tabet, A., Antonini, M. J., Sahasrabudhe, A., Park, J., Rosenfeld, D., Koehler, F., & Anikeeva, P. (2021). Modular integration of hydrogel neural interfaces. *ACS Central Science*, 7(9), 1516–1523.

Tang, Z., Gomez, D., He, C., Korposh, S., Morgan, S. P., Correia, R., & Liu, L. (2021). A U-shape fibre-optic pH sensor based on hydrogen bonding of ethyl cellulose with a sol-gel matrix. *Journal of Lightwave Technology*, 39(5), 1557–1564.

van der Elst, L., Faccini de Lima, C., Gokce Kurtoglu, M., Koraganji, V. N., Zheng, M., & Gumennik, A. (2021). 3D printing in fiber-device technology. *Advanced Fiber Materials*, 3(2), 59–75.

Wang, L., Zhong, C., Ke, D., Ye, F., Tu, J., Wang, L., & Lu, Y. (2018). Ultrasoft and highly stretchable hydrogel optical fibers for in vivo optogenetic modulations. *Advanced Optical Materials*, 6(16), 1800427.

Wu, Z., Wang, C., Liu, B., Liang, C., Lu, J., Li, J., & Li, T. (2022). Smartphone-based high-throughput fiber-integrated immunosensing system for point-of-care testing of the SARS-CoV-2 nucleocapsid protein. *ACS Sensors*, 7(7), 1985–1995.

Xu, H., Yin, L., Liu, C., Sheng, X., & Zhao, N. (2018). Recent advances in biointegrated optoelectronic devices. *Advanced Materials*, 30, 1800156.

Yan, W., Page, A., Nguyen-Dang, T., Qu, Y., Sordo, F., Wei, L., & Sorin, F. (2019). Advanced multimaterial electronic and optoelectronic fibers and textiles. *Advanced Materials*, 31(1), 1802348.

Ye, T., Wang, J., Jiao, Y., Li, L., He, E., Wang, L., & Zhang, Y. (2021). A tissue-like soft all-hydrogel battery. *Advanced Materials*, 34(4), 2105120.

Yetisen, A. K., Jiang, N., Fallahi, A., Montelongo, Y., Ruiz-Esparza, G. U., Tamayol, A., & Yun, S. H. (2017). Glucose-sensitive hydrogel optical fibers functionalized with phenylboronic acid. *Advanced Materials*, 29(15), 1606380.

Yi, Y., Jiang, Y., Zhao, H., Brambilla, G., Fan, Y., & Wang, P. (2020). High-performance ultrafast humidity sensor based on microknot resonator-assisted mach-zehnder for monitoring human breath. *ACS Sensors*, 5(11), 3404–3410.

Zaki, R. M., Strutynski, C., Kaser, S., Bernard, D., Hauss, G., Faessel, M., & Cardinal, T. (2020). Direct 3D-printing of phosphate glass by fused deposition modeling. *Materials & Design*, 194, 108957.

Zhang, W., Huang, X., Liu, W., Gao, Z., Zhong, L., Qin, Y., & Li, J. (2023). Semiconductor plasmon enhanced upconversion toward a flexible temperature sensor. *ACS Applied Materials & Interfaces*, 15(3), 4469–4476.

Optimizing Power Strategies and Circuit Designs for Soft Electronics in Bio-Integrated Systems

Yuhan Bian and Xiandi Wang

9.1 SELF-POWER TECHNOLOGIES

Current energy generation strategies for flexible electronics include solar, thermal, piezoelectric, and biochemical energy harvesting. However, these strategies have some limitations, such as low efficiency, intermittent availability, complex fabrication, or compatibility issues. One of the emerging energy generation strategies for flexible electronics is the triboelectric nanogenerator (TENG), which can convert various mechanical energy, such as friction, vibration, or human motion, into electricity.

By using the contact electrification and electrostatic induction principles, TENG is especially suitable in the field of soft electronics. It can adopt various flexible materials as electrodes and friction layers, such as conductive polymers, carbon nanotubes, metal nanowires, silicone rubber, etc., and can use different structural designs, such as planar, vertical, spherical, fibrous, coaxial, etc., to adapt to different mechanical stimuli and application scenarios. As shown in Figure 9.1, when two different materials in a TENG come into contact and then separate, they develop opposite electrical charges due to the triboelectric effect – one becomes positively charged and the other negatively charged. As they separate, this charge imbalance leads to electrostatic induction, causing a redistribution of charge on nearby conductors and generating an electric current. TENG can operate in four fundamental modes: vertical contact-separation, lateral sliding, single-electrode, and freestanding triboelectric layer. In this chapter, we will describe the advantages and disadvantages of these four modes in soft applications.

The vertical contact-separation working mode has facile and scalable fabrications, simple design strategy, high instantaneous output power, and is easy to scale up with multiple layer integrations. The TENGs in this working mode are usually driven by an external

DOI: 10.1201/9781003493631-9

mechanical impact, and a critical factor affecting its output voltage is the amplitude of the separation distance between the two triboelectric layers (or contact surfaces), while the output current is dictated by the speed at which the two surfaces are being contacted or separated. Hence, most of the advanced designs are focused on the way to realize spontaneous separation by introducing a spacer or taking advantage of the elastic resilience of the materials. As shown in Figure 9.1, a spring-assisted separation structure is developed (Zhu et al., 2013). The TENG had a layered structure with two substrates and polymethyl methacrylate (PMMA) was selected as the material for substrates. The two substrates are connected by four springs installed at the corners, leaving a narrow spacing between the contact electrode and the polydimethylsiloxane (PDMS).

While the vertical mode is ideal for capturing energy from vertical movements and generating higher output voltages, the sliding mode is more suited for scenarios with lateral or sliding movements and requires efficient area utilization. The basic structure for sliding-mode TENG is shown in Figure 9.1. The structure is very similar to the contact-separation mode discussed before, and the only difference is the separation direction of the tribo-charges parallel to the triboelectric surfaces. To further increase the charge generation capability and decrease surface wear, some researchers decided to couple the vertical contact-separation mode and the lateral sliding mode (Yu et al., 2023). In terms of structure, this TENG consists of two triboelectric layers made of polyamide (PA) and fluorinated ethylene propylene (FEP) films, respectively. The two layers are separated by a conductive layer made of copper foil. The PA and FEP films are attached to a flexible substrate made of polyethylene terephthalate (PET) film. When the PA and FEP films come into contact and then slide against each other, triboelectric charges are generated and transferred to the copper electrode. The charges can then be collected and used to power electronic devices. This TENG exhibited a 35.6 times increase in output power compared to traditional TENGs. It also retains 99.8% of its output after 200,000 cycles, demonstrating remarkable durability. The CSS-TENG is also able to generate a direct current of 3.7 mA after power management, which is enough to light ten 30 W lamps.

The single-electrode mode of TENGs requires just one active triboelectric layer and an electrode, making it lightweight and easy to fabricate, which is ideal for integrating into flexible and wearable technology. As depicted in Figure 9.1 (Wang et al., 2018), the TENG described in this work consists of two layers of PDMS elastomer with a layer of silver nanowires (Ag NWs) sandwiched in between. The Ag NWs serve as the triboelectric material, while the PDMS layers provide mechanical flexibility and durability. When the TENG is subjected to mechanical deformation, such as bending or stretching, the Ag NWs come into contact with the PDMS layers and generate an electrical charge through the triboelectric effect. This charge can then be collected and used to power the triboelectric tactile sensor (TETS). This sensor has a number of potential applications in the field of healthcare, including monitoring vital signs, detecting skin diseases, and providing feedback for prosthetic limbs. It can also be used in robotics and virtual reality applications to provide a more realistic and immersive experience.

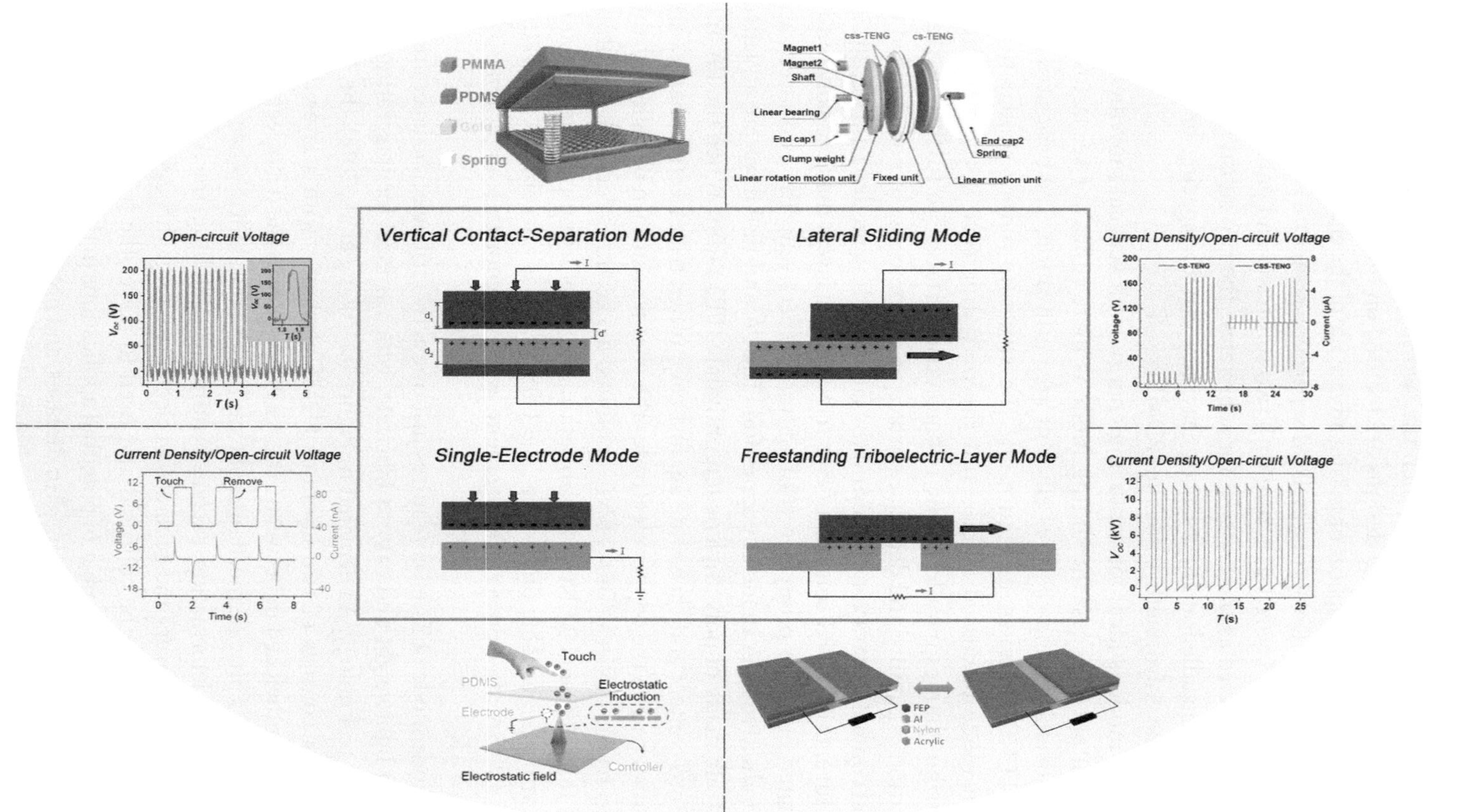

FIGURE 9.1 Internal: The fundamental four modes of TENGs: vertical contact-separation mode, contact-sliding mode, single-electrode mode, and freestanding triboelectric layer mode. External: Typical applications of four modes of TENGs with their current density/open-circuit voltage curves. Adapted with permission. (Yu et al., 2023) Copyright 2023, Royal Society of Chemistry. Adapted with permission, (Zhu et al., 2013) Copyright 2013, American Chemical Society. Adapted with permission, (Wang et al., 2014) Copyright 2014, Wiley. Adapted with permission, (Wang et al., 2018) Copyright 2018, Wiley.

Despite its advantages in simplicity and efficiency, the single-electrode mode of TENGs still faces several limitations such as limited durability as well as flexibility, unstable electrical output, etc. The freestanding triboelectric nanogenerator (F-TENG) also does not require electrode deposition on the moving part, thus keeping the convenience of fabrications and operations. Furthermore, this working mode could deliver a much higher efficiency of charge transfer than that of the single-electrode mode. F-TENG usually consists of a layer and a pair of stationary electrodes. The triboelectric layer is driven to move between the two electrodes to induce a periodical change in the potential difference between them. The potential difference then drives the cyclic electrons to flow between the two electrodes to complete the power generation process. The F-TENG depicted in Figure 9.1 had a pre-charged triboelectric layer (Wang et al., 2014). The movement of the triboelectric layer between the electrodes induces an alternating current due to the electrostatic induction at contact and non-contact modes. The F-TENG was fabricated using acrylic sheets and ICP-treated FEP film, while Cr and Al were deposited using an e-beam evaporator for the electrodes. The F-TENG can generate an extremely high open-circuit voltage over 10 kV and achieve effective charge transfer, equal to the tribo-charges in each sliding motion and can also deliver a maximum power density of approximately 6.7 W/m^2 on an external load.

9.2 FLEXIBLE SOLAR CELLS

Solar power-related technologies have attracted considerable attention as ideal alternatives to conventional energy sources due to the merits of being green, renewable, and inexpensive. However, despite the fact that mankind can gain all its required energy/power from sunlight, the contribution of solar energy as a global energy source is still negligible compared with conventional non-renewable energy sources. Among the developed devices for harvesting sunlight, flexible and wearable solar cells have become ideal candidates for the next generation of practical photovoltaic devices due to their flexibility, lightweight, facile processability, potential integration into curved surfaces, adaptability to roll-to-roll production procedures, and facile transportation and storage. Generally, solar cells can be divided into flexible organic solar cells (OSCs), inorganic flexible solar cells, and hybrid flexible solar cells. In particular, the organic nature of the materials used in OSCs enables flexibility, making them suitable for applications requiring bendable and lightweight solar panels, and ongoing research focuses on improving the efficiency, stability, and scalability of the OSC technology.

In OSCs, polymers or small molecules absorb the sunlight and the generation of electron–hole pairs. OSCs involve a flexible substrate, a transparent electrode, and the active layers. These layers are sandwiched between the front electrode and a back electrode, typically made of aluminum or another conductive material, forming a heterojunction. The resulting potential difference induces the flow of electrons through the external circuit, thus creating an electric current. As shown in Figure 9.2, when exposed to sunlight, the organic active layer absorbs photons, leading to the creation of electron–hole pairs. These charges then separate, with electrons moving toward the electron acceptor material and the holes moving toward the electron donor material, creating a built-in electric field. This

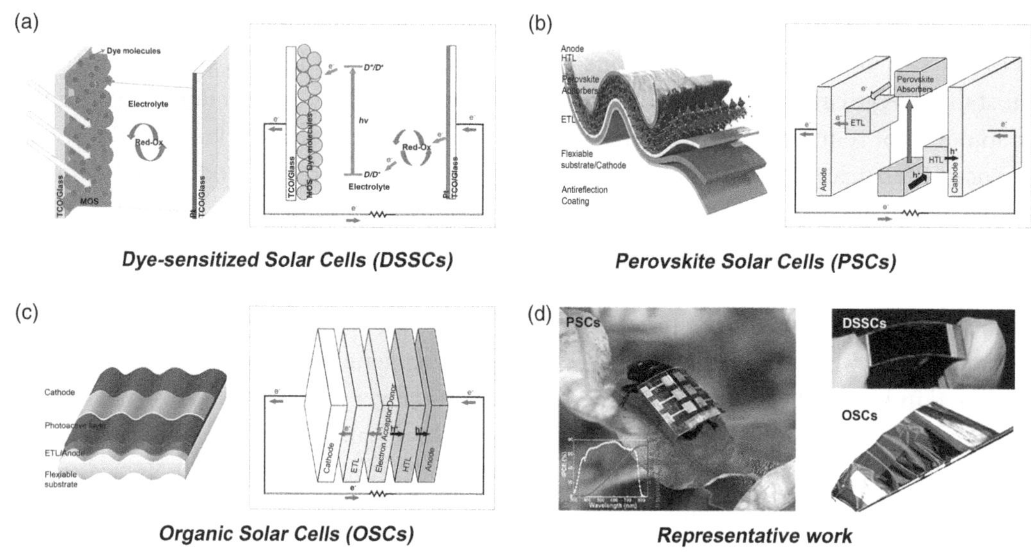

FIGURE 9.2 (a–c) Structures and principles of three types of solar cells. (d) Typical applications of three types of solar cells. (Adapted with permission, (Feng et al., 2018) Copyright 2018, Wiley. Adapted with permission, (Kaltenbrunner et al., 2012) Copyright 2012, Spring Nature. Adapted with permission, (Li et al., 2019) Copyright 2019, Elsevier. Adapted with permission, (Zhang et al., 2019) Copyright 2019, American Chemical Society.)

potential difference prompts the flow of electrons through an external circuit, generating an electric current.

One of the OSCs, as shown in Figure 9.3, is constructed on plastic foil substrates that are less than 2 micrometers thick (Kaltenbrunner et al., 2012). It is ultrathin and lightweight, making it highly flexible. The substrate provides structural support, while the transparent conductive oxide (TCO) layer acts as an anode, allowing light to pass through and extract holes from the active layer. The PEDOT:PSS layer serves as a hole transport layer (HTL), facilitating the movement of positive charge carriers (holes) from the active layer to the anode. The active layer, composed of a blend of regioregular poly(3-hexylthiophene-2,5-diyl) (P3HT) and phenyl-C61-butyric acid methyl ester (PCBM), absorbs sunlight and generates excitons, with P3HT acting as the donor material and PCBM acting as the acceptor material. The cathode buffer layer enhances electron extraction from the active layer and improves contact with the cathode, which collects electrons from the active layer and completes the electrical circuit. In particular, this device has a power conversion efficiency (PCE) equal to that of glass-based solar cells, indicating that it is capable of converting a significant portion of sunlight into electrical energy. Additionally, the OSC has a specific weight ■ value of 10 W g^{-1}, making it over ten times thinner, lighter, and more flexible than any other solar cell technology to date.

Capturing the sunlight with dye-sensitized TiO_2 layer, dye-sensitized solar cells (DSSCs) are another type of OSCs with low cost. As depicted in figure, a typical DSSC consists of a TCO layer which serves as the transparent electrode, allowing light to pass through and reach the active layers of the solar cell, and is typically coated on the flexible substrate.

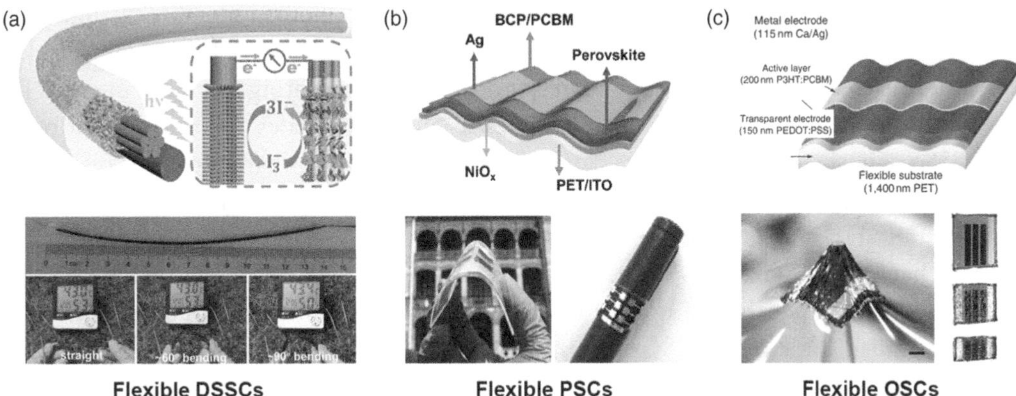

FIGURE 9.3 (a) Schematic illustration of flexible DSSCs structure. DSSC devices power up commercial electronics under bending. (b) Schematic illustration of flexible PSC structure. Digital photographs showing the flexible PSCs under bending and folding conditions. (c) Scheme of the ultra-light and flexible organic solar cell. Digital photographs of the device attached to the elastomeric support. (Adapted with permission (Zhang et al., 2019) Copyright 2019, American Chemical Society. Adapted with permission, (Li et al., 2019) Copyright 2019, Elsevier. Adapted with permission, (Kaltenbrunner et al., 2012) Copyright 2012, Spring Nature.)

Besides, a layer of wide-bandgap nanocrystalline metal oxide semiconductors (MOS) such as SnO_2, ZnO, and TiO_2 with mesoporous structure is applied on top of the TCO layer. This layer acts as the semiconductor and provides a large surface area for the absorption of dye molecules. On the surface of the mesoporous MOS layer are adsorbed organic dye molecules, also known as sensitizers. These dyes capture photons from sunlight, promoting the excitation of electrons and generating electron–hole pairs. The dye-sensitized TiO_2 layer is sandwiched between two electrolyte layers. The electrolyte typically contains a redox couple (e.g., iodide/triiodide) that facilitates the regeneration of the dye molecules by accepting electrons. Finally, a counter electrode, often made of platinum or another conductive material, is placed opposite to the dye-sensitized layer. This electrode catalyzes the reduction of the redox couple in the electrolyte.

The mechanism of a DSSC is based on three phenomena: (1) the absorption of light and separation of charges, (2) the transportation and collection of the newly generated charges, and (3) regeneration of the oxidized dye molecules. In the first step, dye molecules are excited through the absorption of light and generate excitons (i.e., electron–hole pairs). In the second part, the excitons are separated from each other and the metal oxides transfer the electrons to the dye. In the third part, the electrons pass the mesoporous layer composed of porous metal oxides and return to the cathode. Next, a catalytic interaction occurs between the platinized TCO substrate and iodide-based electrolyte along with a redox reaction within the electrolyte, leading to the regeneration of excited dye molecules.

The DSSC discussed in the study is a flexible fiber-shaped DSSC with a high conversion efficiency of 10.28% (Zhang et al., 2019). The cell consists of a photoanode, a counter electrode, and an electrolyte. The photoanode is composed of TiO_2 nanotubes, while the counter electrode is made up of a composite material consisting of polyaniline (PANI) and

Co0.85Se nanosheets. Under illumination, the dye in the photoanode absorbs light and generates electrons, which are then transferred to the counter electrode through the electrolyte. This electron flow creates a current and voltage, generating electrical energy. The use of PANI in the counter electrode serves as nucleation sites for the deposition of Co0.85Se nanosheets and enhances catalytic activity, reducing charge transfer resistance. The Co0.85Se nanosheets further enhance the electrocatalytic activity of transition metal ions, resulting in improved photovoltaic performance.

Another special part of OSCs is perovskite solar cells (PSCs) which use perovskite materials as the light-absorbing layer (Feng et al., 2018). Specifically, not all the PSCs are OSCs, because some of the PSCs use inorganic–organic hybrid materials as the active layer. In most cases, PSCs are comprised of flexible substrates, often plastic or metal foil, upon which layers of TCO, an HTL, a perovskite absorber layer, and an electron transport layer (ETL) are successively deposited. The TCO layer acts as the front electrode, allowing sunlight to penetrate, while the HTL and ETL facilitate the movement of positive and negative charge carriers, respectively. Incident light is absorbed by the perovskite absorber layer, composed of materials like methylammonium lead iodide, inducing the generation of electron–hole pairs. These carriers then separate, with electrons moving through the ETL and holes through the HTL. The resulting potential difference creates an electric current. The TCO layers serve as electrodes, collecting the charge carriers. The PSC's tunable perovskite composition and solution-based fabrication methods contribute to their efficiency, while their flexibility allows integration into diverse applications. Ongoing research aims to improve stability and further optimize the performance of PSCs.

The PSC shown in Figure 9.3 is composed of an ITO/PET substrate and a bulk heterostructure composed of Ag/BCP/PCBM/MA1–yFAyPbI3–xClx (perovskite)/NiOx/ITO/PET (Li et al., 2019). The NiOx layer was deposited on the ITO/PET substrate via e-beam evaporation. And the perovskite layer was prepared by a two-step spin-coating route following the reported recipe. The PSC can be directly worn on a live beetle, demonstrating favorable wearability. This PSC demonstrates an overall efficiency of 14.01% and a high output voltage of 1.05 V. Four flexible PSC devices connected in series can deliver a remarkable voltage output of 3.95 V and a high PCE of 10.20%. The PSC–LIC integrated system delivers an overall efficiency of 8.41% and a high output voltage of 3 V at a discharge current density of 0.1 A g^{-1}. It could still achieve a remarkable overall efficiency exceeding 6%, even at the high current density of 1 A g^{-1}, outperforming the state-of-the-art photocharging power sources.

9.3 FLEXIBLE WIRELESS ENERGY TRANSMISSION

Despite the merits of flexible solar cells, their relatively poor efficiency, durability, and life span have limited their use in daily scenarios. Compared with these flexible energy strategies, wireless energy transmission can provide continuous and reliable power supply for bendable and lightweight devices, such as wearable electronics, sensors, and displays, without the need for batteries, which are bulky, heavy, and have limited lifetimes. It can also reduce the fabrication cost and complexity, as well as enhance the performance and functionality of flexible devices, by allowing for dynamic and adaptive power management, remote control, and data communication.

Wireless energy transmission is the process of transferring electrical energy without using wires or cables. As shown in Figure 9.4, the transmission system typically consists of four main elements: a power source, compensation circuits, coils, and loads. The power source, such as a signal generator, provides electrical energy to the transmitter coil, which generates a magnetic field. It determines the input power and the frequency of the wireless transmission. The compensation circuits, such as capacitors or inductors, adjust the impedance and resonance of the coils, which improve the efficiency and power transfer. The electromagnetic induction uses two coils of wire to transfer power across an air gap by generating and receiving a time-varying magnetic field. For now, flexible coils can be made by fractal design (Xu et al., 2013), ink printing (Zhao et al., 2023), nanomaterial integration (Zhang et al., 2020), and liquid metal injection (Qusba et al., 2014) to achieve high efficiency and flexibility. They determine the coupling coefficient and the mutual inductance of the wireless transmission. Load, such as a battery or a device, determines the output power and the load resistance of the wireless transmission. Recently, researchers have developed a series of stretchable antennas integrated into flexible systems.

Body fluid monitoring is an important component of smart medical systems, and wireless energy transmission brings convenience to real-time monitoring of body fluids. Tears contain many biomolecules; therefore, research is currently being conducted for the

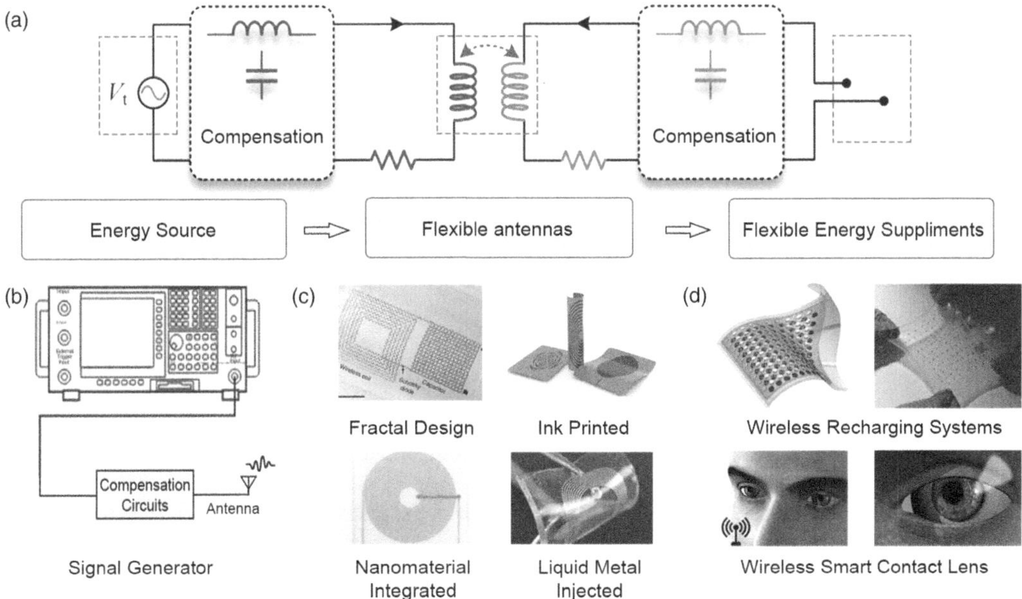

FIGURE 9.4   (a, b) Schematic illustration of wireless power transmission system. (c) Different kinds of stretchable antennas. (d) Two classic applications for wireless power transfer. (Adapted with permission, Copyright 2023 (Xu et al., 2013) Spring Nature. Copyright 2023 (Zhao et al., 2023) Spring Nature. Copyright 2020 (Zhang et al., 2020) Spring Nature. Copyright 2014 (Qusba et al., 2014) IEEE. Copyright 2018 (Park et al., 2018) AAAS.)

development of smart contact lenses, which represent wearable electronics with functions such as diagnosing ophthalmic diseases and detecting biomolecules in tears. The contact lens receives power from the antenna attached around the patient's eye and transfers the strain gauge information back to the attached antenna. This information is sent to a portable recorder and is then transferred to a computer via Bluetooth. Park et al. reported a smart contact lens that monitors glucose levels through the operation of LEDs (2018). Transparent antennas were fabricated with metal nanowires to ensure visibility and the rigid components required for wireless driving (rectifiers, LED, and glucose sensor) were placed and protected on flexible hybrid substrates (Figure 9.5). This design provides elasticity to the

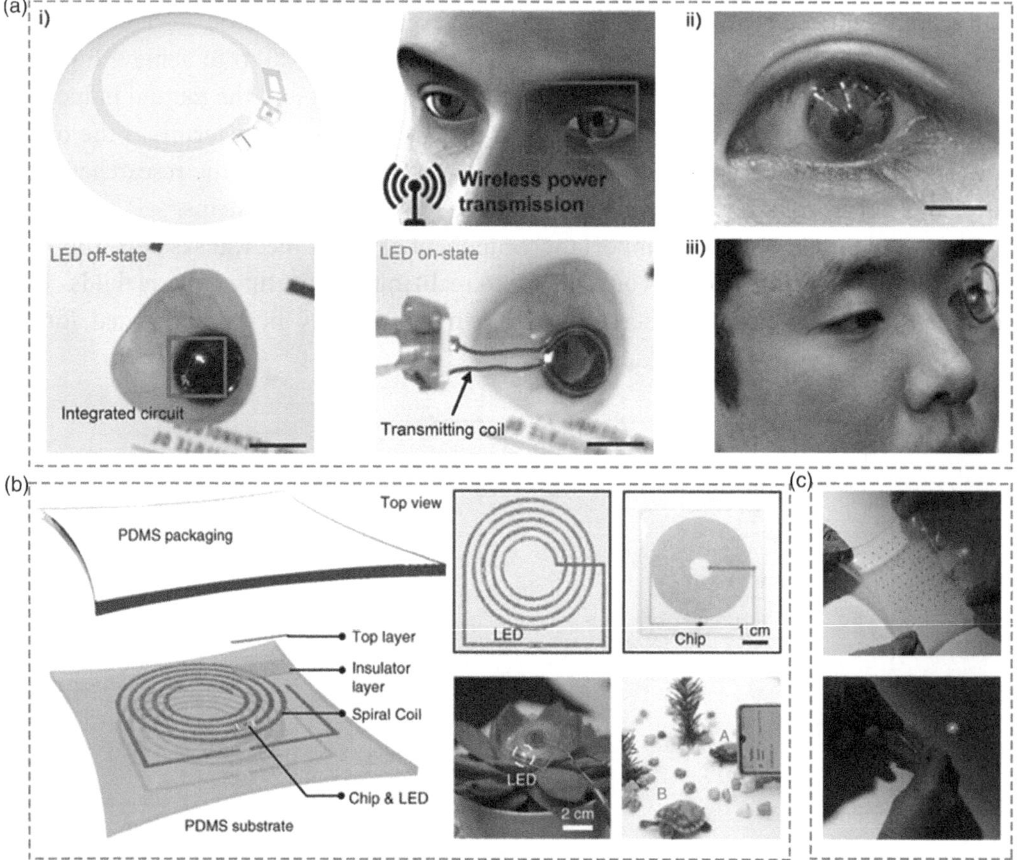

FIGURE 9.5 (a) Schematic illustration and operation of soft, smart contact lens. i) Smart contact lenses for glucose detection. ii) Smart contact lenses for quantitative monitoring of intraocular pressure. iii) Smart contact lenses with supercapacitors under wireless charging conditions. (b) Schematic illustration of the exploded view of stretchable transparent devices. Digital photos of NFC tags and NFC tags attached to tortoises for identification. (c) Flexible battery with red light-emitting diodes stretched to 300% and folded. (Adapted with permission, (Park et al., 2018) Copyright 2018, AAAS. Adapted with permission, Copyright 2021 (Kim et al., 2021) Spring Nature. Adapted with permission, (Park et al., 2019) Copyright 2019, AAAS. Adapted with permission, Copyright 2020 (Zhang et al., 2020) Spring Nature. Adapted with permission, Copyright 2013 (Xu et al., 2013) Spring Nature.)

entire smart contact lens system. By wirelessly transmitting power using inductive coupling, the concentration of glucose can be determined by dimming the LED light as the resistance of the glucose sensor decreases as the glucose concentration increases. Figure 9.5 also shows other smart contact lenses used for quantitative monitoring of intraocular pressure and those integrated with supercapacitors (Kim et al., 2021; Park et al., 2019).

Combining stretchable antennas with content recognition, Wang et al. designed a stretchable transparent Ag NF spiral coil that can be assembled into more complex functional wireless electronics for data communication (Zhang et al., 2020). PDMS was employed as the substrate, the insulator layer, and the encapsulation layer, which were transparent and stretchable to absorb the strain energy. Tiny electronic components with high effective stiffness adhered to the stretchable substrate, which could withstand less stress when the device was under strain. The Ag NF spiral coil tags can operate in a battery-free mode via an external reader, with data and power transmission by magnetic inductive coupling based on NFC protocols. Images of a representative device and its applications (identification of tortoise A) are shown in Figure 9.5. Besides, the audio signal (music or sound) can be modulated onto the carrier wave via an FM generator, which is then received by a stretchable spiral coil and fed into a spectrum analyzer for auditory and visual monitoring.

Integrated stretchable antenna can also help provide the means to charge stretchable batteries, without direct physical contact, realizing the next generation of portable devices. Rogers et al. designed a rechargeable lithium-ion battery technology that exploits thin, low-modulus silicone elastomers as substrates (Xu et al., 2013). A secondary coil couples the electromagnetic flux from a primary coil and a Schottky diode provides rectification. In this case, the output power from the primary coil was 187 mW. With a working distance of 1 mm between the primary and secondary coils, the power received on the secondary coil is 9.2 mW, corresponding to an efficiency of 4.9%. The charging curves of a small-scale battery using the wireless coil appear in Figure 9.5. The battery voltage rises to 2.5 V in about 6 min.

REFERENCES

Feng, J., Zhu, X., Yang, Z., Zhang, X., Niu, J., Wang, Z., Yang, D. (2018). Record efficiency stable flexible perovskite solar cell using effective additive assistant strategy. *Advanced Materials*, 30(35), 1801418.

Kaltenbrunner, M., White, M. S., Głowacki, E. D., Sekitani, T., Someya, T., Sariciftci, N. S., Bauer, S. (2012). Ultrathin and lightweight organic solar cells with high flexibility. *Nature Communications*, 3(1), 770.

Kim, J., Park, J., Park, Y. G., Cha, E., Ku, M., An, H. S., Park, J. U. (2021). A soft and transparent contact lens for the wireless quantitative monitoring of intraocular pressure. *Nature Biomedical Engineering*, 5(7), 772–782.

Li, C., Cong, S., Tian, Z., Song, Y., Yu, L., Lu, C., Liu, Z. (2019). Flexible perovskite solar cell-driven photo-rechargeable lithium-ion capacitor for self-powered wearable strain sensors. *Nano Energy*, 60, 247–256.

Park, J., Ahn, D. B., Kim, J., Cha, E., Bae, B. S., Lee, S. Y., Park, J. U. (2019). Printing of wirelessly rechargeable solid-state supercapacitors for soft, smart contact lenses with continuous operations. *Science Advances*, 5(12), 2375–2548.

Park, J., Kim, J., Kim, S. Y., Cheong, W. H., Jang, J., Park, Y. G., Park, J. U. (2018). Soft, smart contact lenses with integrations of wireless circuits, glucose sensors, and displays. *Science Advances*, 4(1), 9841.

Qusba, A., RamRakhyani, A. K., So, J. H., Hayes, G. J., Dickey, M. D., Lazzi, G. (2014). On the design of microfluidic implant coil for flexible telemetry system. *IEEE Sensors Journal*, 14(4), 1074–1080.

Wang, S., Xie, Y., Niu, S., Lin, L., Wang, Z. L. (2014). Freestanding triboelectric-layer-based nanogenerators for harvesting energy from a moving object or human motion in contact and non-contact modes. *Advanced Materials*, 26(18), 2818–2824.

Wang, X., Zhang, Y., Zhang, X., Huo, Z., Li, X., Que, M., Pan, C. (2018). A highly stretchable transparent self-powered triboelectric tactile sensor with metallized nanofibers for wearable electronics. *Advanced Materials*, 30(12), 1706738.

Xu, S., Zhang, Y., Cho, J., Lee, J., Huang, X., Jia, L., Rogers, J. A. (2013). Stretchable batteries with self-similar serpentine interconnects and integrated wireless recharging systems. *Nature Communications*, 4(1), 1543.

Yu, Y., Gao, Q., Zhang, X. S., Zhao, D., Xia, X., Wang, J. L., Cheng, T. H. (2023). Contact-sliding-separation mode triboelectric nanogenerator. *Energy & Environmental Science*, 16(9), 3932–3941.

Zhang, J., Wang, Z., Li, X., Yang, J., Song, C., Li, Y., … Wang, B. (2019). Flexible platinum-free fiber-shaped dye sensitized solar cell with 10.28% efficiency. *ACS Applied Energy Materials*, 2(4), 2870–2877.

Zhang, Y., Huo, Z., Wang, X., Han, X., Wu, W., Wan, B., Wang, Z. L. (2020). High precision epidermal radio frequency antenna via nanofiber network for wireless stretchable multifunction electronics. *Nature Communications*, 11(1), 5629.

Zhao, W., Ni, H., Ding, C., Liu, L., Fu, Q., Lin, F., Zhao, Q. (2023). 2D Titanium carbide printed flexible ultrawideband monopole antenna for wireless communications. *Nature Communications*, 14(1), 278.

Zhu, G., Lin, Z. H., Jing, Q. S., Bai, P., Pan, C. F., Yang, Y., Wang, Z. L. (2013). Toward large-scale energy harvesting by a nanoparticle-enhanced triboelectric nanogenerator. *Nano Letters*, 13(2), 847–853.

International Standardization Activities

Zhiyuan Meng

10.1 INTERNATIONAL STANDARDIZATION FOR WEARABLE TECHNOLOGIES

Recent technological advancements have allowed wearable devices to come in many different forms. For example, the trend toward increasingly smaller, thinner, and more flexible devices is possible due to advances in miniaturization and a shift from touch to new interfaces activated by voice or motion. As a result, wearable devices become unobtrusive and almost invisible.

This development is beneficial to medical devices. For example, electronic thin patches could be used to help deal with diabetes. They can be applied to the skin to continuously monitor glucose levels and, in some cases, pump insulin into the bloodstream. In a research by Steven R. Steinhubl and Eric J. Topol (2018), a wearable ultrasound patch can continuously monitor cardiovascular performance (blood pressure) outside the intensive care unit. This is part of a move toward patient monitoring that can be used for both hospital inpatient supervision (e.g. enhancing the quality of neonatal and pediatric critical care in a research by John A. Rogers (Chung et al., 2020) as well as part of outpatient care. Another medical advancement suggests the integration of wearable technology to enhance and evaluate human movement during the process of physical rehabilitation. In collaboration with a New York City hospital, a VR electronics company has designed a full-body suit that offers customized, real-time diagnoses along with physical therapy for patients. This is achieved through the use of sensors that gather biometric data, capture movement, and provide haptic feedback. IEC is developing standards for AR and VR as well as smart glasses displays. ISO/IEC JTC 1/Subcommittee 24 is dedicated to interfaces with information technology–based applications related to computer graphics and virtual reality, image processing, environmental data representation, mixed and augmented reality support, and information interaction and visual presentation. IEC TC 110 sets standards for electronic displays, including organic light-emitting diodes, three dimensional (3D), holographic, and flexible screens. For example, it published IEC 62341-2-1 on organic light-emitting

DOI: 10.1201/9781003493631-10

diode displays, which specifies the basic ratings and characteristics of organic light-emitting diode display modules. It also released the technical report (TR) IEC 62629-41-1 on 3D and holographic display equipment.

As the most common form in wearable devices, electronic skin sensors are manufactured to monitor human movement and physiological parameters. By being attached to different parts of the human body (Nappi et al., 2021; Tseghai et al., 2022; Zhao et al., 2022), electronic skin can monitor parameters such as electromyography, ECG, and EEG. Electronic textiles (e-textiles), designed based on simply attaching conventional electronic components to clothing (Wohnsdorf et al., 2022), have gained significant attention in recent years. E-textiles can inherit the advantages of traditional fabrics such as lightweight, flexibility, breathability, and a certain degree of ductility while having electronic functions. Currently, fabric-based electronic devices have been widely studied and used in the Internet of Things (IoT), artificial intelligence (AI), body motion tracking, pressure mapping, rehabilitation, and healthcare. When sensors are embedded with bandages, gloves, shoes, sockets, and diapers, they can achieve monitoring the wound status, identifying objects, assessing over-pronated/over-supinated foot, and assisting prosthetists in designing comfortable sockets and wireless healthcare and monitoring special needs, respectively (Abbass et al., 2021; Ali et al., 2023; Huang et al., 2021; Lu et al., 2022; Lv et al., 2022). The emerging research focus on biodegradable transient electronics, characterized by devices that readily break down into safe components at the end of their lifespan, holds significance in addressing electronic waste challenges. This research direction also opens avenues for innovative applications, including wearable health monitors that can be effortlessly washed off the body when no longer needed (Cook et al., 2023). As skin wounds are often susceptible to bacterial attack, an electronic patch with an antibacterial effect is more preferred (Eskandari et al., 2022).

In March 2017, the International Electrotechnical Committee (IEC) established Technical Committee 124 (TC 124), which aims to develop and provide standards specifically for wearable electronic devices and technologies. TC 124 provides standardization in the field of wearable electronic devices and technologies which include patchable materials and devices, implantable materials and devices, ingestible materials and devices, and electronic textile materials and devices. IEC 63203-101-1 provides terminology frequently used in literature related to wearable electronic devices and technologies in the IEC 63203 series thus ensuring a common basis for the discussion of key concepts. This list includes wearable electronic devices and technologies, near-body wearable electronics, on-body wearable electronics, in-body wearable electronics, and electronic textiles. The IEC 63203-2 series relates mainly to measurement methods for e-textiles in wearable electronics, such as electrical resistance and washing durability. Also, the relative components including fabrics, insulation materials used for electronic textiles, and connectors are provisioned. The detailed description is shown in Table 10.1.

Wearable sensors play an important role in the field of real-time monitoring of human physiological health parameters, such as blood pressure, breathing, metabolites, or wound healing. The integration of wearable devices into the body in a seamless manner requires careful consideration of not only the composition (materials) and structure (design) of the

TABLE 10.1 Standardization in the Field of Wearable Electronic Devices and Technologies

IEC Standards	Scope	Normative References
IEC 63203-101-1:2021	Terminology frequently used in the literature related to wearable electronic devices and technologies in the IEC 63203 series.	
IEC 63203-201-1	Provisions and test methods for measurement of properties of conductive yarns.	IEC 60468:1974 ISO 105-E04 ISO 139 ISO 6330 EN 16812:2016
IEC 63203-201-2	Provisions for conductive fabrics and insulation materials used for electronic textiles and measurement methods for their properties.	IEC 60243-1:2013 IEC 60468:1974 IEC 62631-3-1:2016 ISO 105-E04 ISO 139 ISO 6330 EN 16812:2016
IEC 63203-201-3:2021	A test method for determination of the electrical resistance of conductive fabrics under simulated microclimate within clothing.	ISO 139, Textiles – Standard atmospheres for conditioning and testing ISO 11092:2014 ISO 21232:2018 EN 16812:2016
IEC 63203-201-4 ED1	Electronic textile – Test method for determining sheet resistance of conductive fabrics after abrasion.	
IEC 63203-203-1 ED1	Test method for measuring performance of fabric-based triboelectric nanogenerators.	
IEC 63203-203-2 ED1	Test method for measuring performance of fabric-based piezoelectric nanogenerators.	
IEC 63203-204-1:2023	A household washing durability test method for e-textile products.	ISO 139 ISO 6330:2012
IEC 63203-204-2-ED1	Test method to characterize electrical resistance change in the knee and elbow bending test of e-textile system.	
IEC TR 63203-250-1:2021(E)	The use cases of conductive snap fasteners applied as electrical connectors for e-textile products available on the market and guidance on future standardization works.	
IEC 63203-301-1 ED1	Test method of electrochromic films for wearable equipment.	
IEC 63203-401-1:2023	A measurement method of tensile strain for stretchable, resistive strain sensors.	IEC 62899-202-4:2021 ISO 291:2008 ISO/TS 12901-2:2014
IEC 63203-402-1:2022	Test methods for wearable glove-type motion sensors to measure finger movements.	IEC 62047-6 IEC 62951-1 ISO 291 ISO 21420:2020
IEC 63203-402-2 ED1	Performance measurement of fitness wearables – Step counting.	

(Continued)

TABLE 10.1 (Continued)

IEC Standards	Scope	Normative References
IEC 63203-402-3 ED1	Performance measurement of fitness wearables – Test methods for the determination of the accuracy of heart rate.	
IEC 63203-403-1 ED1	Test methods of surface electromyography sensors for wearable applications.	
IEC 63203-801-1:2022	The ultra-low power physical layer (PHY) of SmartBAN.	
IEC 63203-801-2:2022	Low complexity medium access control (MAC) for SmartBAN.	IEC 63203-801-1:2022
IEC 63203-406-1:2021	Defines the terms, definitions, symbols, configurations, and test methods to be used to specify the standard measurement conditions and methods for determining the contact-surface temperature of wrist-worn wearable electronic devices intended to be worn directly on a human wrist and that can be worn continuously during use.	IEC 62368-1:2018
IEC 63517 ED1	Test methods for the performance of heating products – Heating temperature and power consumption.	
IEC 60601-2-10:2012 ED2	Particular requirements for the basic safety and essential performance of nerve and muscle stimulators.	

device itself but also the specific requirements and interactions at the device/body interface. IEC 63203-401-1 describes the characterization procedures for evaluating the gauge factor, linearity, response characteristics, and hysteresis of unimodal tension sensors. Test methods for wearable glove-type motion sensors and wrist-worn wearable electronic devices are also specified in IEC 63203-402-1 and IEC 63203-406-1, respectively.

Soft electronics always require large deformation. Therefore, devices with high stretchability are preferred. A stretchable multifunctional sensing device that simulates the characteristics of human skin in a large area array has been successfully developed and has broad application prospects in the fields of artificial skin, prosthetics, personal healthcare, and human activity monitoring. Among the current manufacturing methods of electronic devices, printed electronics is a new way to manufacture low-cost, flexible electronics utilizing an old manufacturing method combined with novel materials. IEC Technical Committee 119 provides international standards that cover terminology, materials, processes, equipment, products, and health, safety, and sustainability of printed electronics (Table 10.2).

Printed electronics are produced on various printing substrates with the use of various printing techniques. IEC 62899-201-2 defines the measurement methods for the properties of stretchable substrates in order to evaluate stretchable functional layers (conductive, semiconducting, and insulating) formed by printing technologies. IEC 62899-202:2023 defines the terms and specifies the standard test methods for characterization and evaluation of conductive inks. This document also provides measurement methods for evaluating

TABLE 10.2 Standardization in the Field of Printed Electronics

IEC Standards	Scope	Normative References
IEC 62899-201	Defines the terms and specifies the evaluation method for substrates used in the printing process to form electronic components/devices.	
IEC 62899-201-2:2021(E)	Measurement methods for the properties of stretchable substrates.	IEC 60243-1 IEC 62631-3-1 IEC 62631-3-2 IEC 62899-201 ISO 3801 ISO 5084 ISO 13934-1 ISO 22198
IEC 62899-202:2023	Defines the terms and specifies the standard test methods for the characterization and evaluation of conductive inks.	
IEC 62899-202-3:2019(E)	Defines the terms and specifies a standard method for the measurement of the sheet resistance of printed conductive films using a contactless eddy-current method.	IEC 62899-202
IEC 62899-202-4:2021(E)	Defines the terminology and measurement methods for the properties of stretchable printed layers.	IEC 60243-1 IEC 61557-2 IEC 62631-3-1 IEC 62899-202 ISO 105-C10 ISO 105-E04 ISO 291
IEC 62899-202-5:2018(E)	A mechanical bending test for evaluating the electrical properties of a printed conductive layer on an insulating substrate under repeated mechanical deformation.	
IEC 62899-202-6:2020(E)	A method of *in situ* measurement for the resistance change of a conductive layer formed by printing methods on a flexible substrate under specified temperature and humidity conditions.	IEC 62899-202-5
IEC 62899-202-7:2021(E)	A test method to measure the peel strength of a printed layer on a flexible substrate.	
IEC 62899-202-9:2023	Describes basic patterns to evaluate the electrical reliability of a conductive layer under mechanical deformation.	IEC 62899-502-1
IEC 62899-202-10:2023	Defines terminology and measurement methods for the resistance change of conductive ink layer(s) as a function of thermoplastic elongation.	
IEC 62899-203:2018(E)	Defines terms and specifies standard methods for characterization and evaluation.	
IEC 62899-204:2019(E)	Defines the terms and specifies the standard methods for characterization and evaluation.	
IEC TR 62899-250:2016(E)	A technical report (TR) that explores a new technological field to establish standardization activities in TC 119 (Printed electronics), in particular, and to contribute to the development and market expansion of wearable smart device (WSD) technology.	
IEC 62899-301-1:2017(E)	Measurement terms and methods related to the external dimension of a rigid plate master.	

(Continued)

TABLE 10.2   (Continued)

IEC Standards	Scope	Normative References
IEC 62899-301-2:2017(E)	Measurement terms and methods related to the critical dimensions of the features and the registration accuracy of the features on rigid plate masters.	
IEC 62899-302-1:2017(E)	The method for determining the inkjet drop speed is based on visualized droplet images obtained by a drop analysis system.	
IEC 62899-302-2:2018€	The method for determining the accurate inkjet droplet volume is based on images obtained by drop-in-flight measurement systems.	
IEC 62899-302-3:2021(E)	In-flight imaging methods for the measurement of the direction of ink drops jetted from inkjet printheads using drop watchers.	
IEC TR 62899-302-5:2023	Provides the significant characteristics, parameters, and system properties that are relevant for functional inkjet printing for printed electronics.	
IEC 62899-303-1:2018(E)	Standard mechanical dimensions (especially related to the web size) of equipment for printed electronics.	
The IEC 62899-4XX series	Requirements for the printability of printed electronics.	IEC 60050
IEC 62899-501-1:2019(E)	Failure modes and mechanical stress test methods for the determination of reliability characteristics of bendable or flexible printed primary cells and secondary cells and batteries	IEC 60050-482:2004, 482-01-01, IEC 60050-482:2004, 482-01-02, IEC 60050-482:2004, 482-01-03, IEC 60050-482:2004, 482-01-04 and IEC 60050-482:2004, 482-01-05
IEC 62899-502-1:2017(E)	The quality assessment methods, especially the mechanical stress test methods, for reliability assessment.	IEC 62715-6-1 IEC 62341-5:2009 IEC 62341-6-1 IEC 62595-2-1:2016 IEC 62922
IEC 62899-502-2:2019(E)	Combined mechanical and environmental stress test methods for flexible OLED (organic light emitting diode) elements fabricated using the printing method. Mechanical stress tests include the static and cycling vending test and the dynamic and static rolling test.	IEC 60068-1:2013 IEC 60068-2-2 IEC 62341-6-1 IEC 62341-6-2 IEC 62341-6-3 IEC 62715-5-1 IEC 62715-5-3 IEC 62715-6-1 IEC 62899-502-1 IEC 62922
IEC 62899-503-1:2020(E)	A test method for displacement current measurement (DCM) of printed thin film transistors (TFTs) or organic thin film transistors (OTFTs).	ISO 291
IEC 62899-503-3:2021(E)	A measuring method of contact resistance for printed thin film transistors (TFTs) by the transfer length method (TLM).	

(Continued)

TABLE 10.2 (Continued)

IEC Standards	Scope	Normative References
IEC 62899-505:2020(E)	Mechanical and thermal test methods for the determination of the reliability characteristics of a printed flexible gas sensor, which is operated at a relatively low temperature and is composed of a flexible substrate, electrode, and gas sensing layer.	IEC 60068-2-14 IEC 60721-3-7 IEC 62899-201 IEC 62899-501-1 IEC 62899-502-1 ISO 11999-3
IEC TR 62899-550-1:2022(E)	A technical report provides a framework for evaluating the mechanical and thermal durability of printed and/or flexible electronic components and products.	
IEC 62899-101:2019(E)	Defines terms used in the field of printed electronics, addressing topics including, but not limited to, materials, printing processes, and print characterization.	

the properties of conductive layers made both from an additive process using conductive inks and from a subtractive process used in printed electronics including the sheet resistance, electrical properties, peel strength of a printed layer, and electrical reliability. The formation of stretchable wiring and functional devices is one of the most promising themes for printed electronics. Stretchable wiring, made by this type of printing, has given rise to printed e-textiles used in wearable electronics. Until now, the main focus has been on the conductivity of textiles, which traditionally have been used mostly to make garments. If a wire were to break within the embedded printed electronics, then the item may no longer function. However, now IEC 62899-202-4 offers methods for evaluating these types of stretchable layers, including the insulating layers used with the conductive layers, which is important from a safety point of view, to avoid potentially dangerous electric shocks.

The quality of devices shouldn't be ignored. IEC 62899-501-1, IEC 62899-502-1, and IEC 62899-502-2 specify failure modes and mechanical stress test methods for the determination of the reliability characteristics of bendable or flexible printed primary cells and secondary cells and batteries. IEC TR 62899-550-1:2022(E), which is a TR, provides a framework for evaluating the mechanical and thermal durability of printed and/or flexible electronics components and products. This includes the bending test, torsion test, stretching test, steady heat test as well as the thermal cycle test. These are typical conditions that are easily encountered in daily life for printed and/or flexible electronics components and products. Besides, IEC 62899-505:2020(E) specifies mechanical and thermal test methods for the determination of the reliability characteristics of a printed flexible gas sensor.

TC47 is to prepare international standards for the design, manufacture, use, and reuse of discrete semiconductor devices, integrated circuits, display devices, sensors, electronic component assemblies, interface requirements, and microelectromechanical devices using environmentally sound practices. Activities include wafer-level reliability, package outlines, terms and definitions, quality issues, physical environmental testing, device-specific test methods, device specifications and minimum content, pinouts, interface requirements, and applications. Specially, emerging neuromorphic devices like memristors are considered in some still going projects of TC47. It's helpful for companies and research centers to provide evaluation methods for memristors before the devices are made into products. According to plans in TC47, the evaluation method of basic characteristics, linearity, spike-dependent plasticity, and asymmetry in memristor devices will be deliberated.

On-body power-supply devices are indispensable for diverse bioelectronic applications and have garnered extensive research attention in the past decade. To address the need for both high safety and flexibility in biomedical applications, Bentley and co-workers (2022) have developed a fabric-based, biocompatible Ag/AgCl-zinc flexible battery tailored for wearable biomedical devices. The Ag/AgCl and zinc electrodes, measuring 14 mm x 8 mm, were screen-printed onto a habotai silk fabric in a planar single-cell configuration. IEC TR 63071:2016(E) provides models and frameworks for the power-supplying scheme for wearable systems and equipment. To date, the battery has remained the conventional powering solution for wearable devices; yet, it falls short of meeting the escalated demand for a lightweight, conformal, and seamless energy solution that future wearable technology demands. Specifically, the existing battery is rigid and bulky, making it unsuitable for applications in biomedical engineering. Furthermore, the current battery technology contributes to environmental pollution, which exacerbates the need for alternative solutions. However, it is heartening to observe that significant advancements have been made in clean and renewable energy technologies over the past decade, paving the way for potentially better power solutions for wearable devices. Different wearable powering solutions, such as solar cells and batteries, thermoelectrically powered devices, piezoelectric devices, and TENGs, have been widely studied. IEC 62830-6:2019(E) defines the terms, definitions, and symbols and specifies the configurations and test methods to be used to evaluate and determine the performance characteristics of vertical contact-mode triboelectric energy–harvesting devices for practical use. This document is applicable to energy-harvesting devices such as power sources for wearable devices and wireless sensors used in healthcare monitoring, consumer electronics, general industries, military, and aerospace applications without any limitations on device technology and size.

10.2 INTERNATIONAL STANDARDIZATION FOR IMPLANTABLE BIOELECTRONICS

Unlike wearable therapeutics, implantable bioelectronics are directly interfaced with specific organs and tissues *in vivo*, allowing for efficient feedback stimulation. To date, a plethora of implantable bioelectronics with tailored functionalities have been designed to tackle complex medical conditions in a patient-friendly approach. The ISO 14708 series specifies the therapeutic usages of implantable bioelectronics for treating typical diseases, including bradyarrhythmias, tachyarrhythmia, hearing impairment, neurological disorders, and others. The specific description is shown in Table 10.3. The tests that are specified in these documents are type tests and are to be carried out on a sample of a device to assess the device's behavioral responses and are not intended to be used for routine testing of manufactured products.

Over the past few decades, brain–machine interfacing technologies have been extensively researched for their ability to gather crucial information from the brain, provide feedback signals to the brain, and, more recently, for their potential in treating neurological

TABLE 10.3 Standardization in the Field of Implantable Electronics

IEC Standards	Scope	Normative References
ISO 14708-1:2014	Requirements that are generally applicable to active implantable medical devices.	
ISO 14708-2:2019	Requirements that are applicable to those active implantable medical devices intended to treat bradyarrhythmias and devices that provide therapies for cardiac resynchronization.	
ISO 14708-3:2017	Electrical stimulation of the central or peripheral nervous systems	
ISO 14708-4:2022	Delivers a medicinal substance to site-specific locations within the human body to provide the basic assurance of safety for both patients and users.	ISO 14708-1:2014
ISO 14708-5:2020	Requirements for safety and performance of active implantable circulatory support devices, including type tests, animal studies, and clinical evaluation requirements.	
ISO 14708-6:2019	Requirements that are applicable to implantable cardioverter defibrillators and CRT-Ds and the functions of active implantable medical devices intended to treat tachyarrhythmia.	
ISO 14708-7:2019	Requirements that are applicable to those active implantable medical devices that are intended to treat hearing impairment via electrical stimulation of the auditory pathways.	
ISO 12189:2008	Methods for fatigue testing of spinal implant assemblies (for fusion or motion preservation) using an anterior support.	
ISO 27186:2020	A four-pole connector system for implantable cardiac rhythm management (CRM) devices which have pacing, electrogram sensing, and/or defibrillation functions.	
ISO 14117:2019	Test methodologies for the evaluation of the electromagnetic compatibility (EMC) of active implantable cardiovascular devices that provide one or more therapies for bradycardia, tachycardia, and cardiac resynchronization in conjunction with transvenous lead systems.	

disorders. However, traditional brain–machine interfacing devices suffer from significant limitations due to the mechanical mismatch between the brain and the devices, leading to inefficient interfacing and compromised sustainability. Current research efforts are focused on (i) developing electrodes with compliant mechanical properties that can conform to the brain's surface, ensuring high signal-to-noise ratios (SNRs) and minimizing tissue damage, even in the presence of brain micromotion; (ii) reducing the size and spacing of electrodes and incorporating multiplexed array designs to achieve enhanced spatial and temporal resolutions in brain mapping; and (iii) creating a high-quality interface characterized by low impedance for improved SNR, enhanced biocompatibility, and reduced biofouling.

Gu and co-workers (2023) present a flexible 3D optoelectronic array featuring 512 electrophysiological recording channels, utilizing a silk-based shuttle-free implantation technique. This shuttle-free implantation method offered minimal invasiveness and high efficiency in the implantation of 3D neural electrode arrays with extensive coverage and high electrode density. Consequently, they achieved stable chronic recordings spanning one month *in vivo*. Additionally, they integrated a silk fiber, characterized by its high transparency and low optical loss, into a neural electrode array to facilitate optogenetic stimulation. Wang and her colleagues (2023) report a real-time functional brain mapping technique that relies on high-channel-count, ultra-conformal electrocorticographic (ECoG) electrodes. The MEMS-based 64-channel ECoG electrodes exhibit excellent conformance to the curvilinear surface of the cortex, ensuring superior neural signal recording quality. This neural interface was employed in Labrador dogs to delineate cortical regions associated with eyelid, nose, and limb motor functions. The obtained results demonstrated strong agreement with those obtained through electrical cortical stimulation (ECS) mapping, which was widely recognized as the gold standard for mapping the eloquent cortex. Their research offered an instantaneous functional map, holding tremendous potential for real-time passive functional mapping of the eloquent cortex.

Research in brain–machine interfaces, utilizing electronic implants, has primarily aimed to minimize the risks associated with the surgical removal of the implanted devices from the brain. Transient electronic devices, which have the capability to naturally dissolve within the in vivo environment, have been recently highlighted as a potential solution. These devices are composed of materials possessing well-established *in vivo* dissolution rates, such as single-crystal silicon, silicon dioxide, silicon nitride, magnesium, and magnesium oxide nanomaterials, such that the lifespan of the electronic implants can be deliberately controlled. Huang et al. introduced a method for creating microelectrode arrays (MEAs) that are biodegradable, adhesive, and compliant with soft tissue. The MEAs are fabricated using photolithography in a batch process, with tunable photoresist/developer composition, and consist of polylactic acid (PLA) biodegradable insulation layers and Pt/PLA hybrid electrodes. The use of an adhesive hydrogel facilitates the dissolution of sacrificial layers and promotes interfacial adhesion, allowing for the direct transfer printing of Pt-PLA MEAs stacks. This integrated approach offers, for the first time, the possibility of batch-producing implanted hydrogel MEAs that combine metal/organic composites as conformal electrodes with fully biodegradable insulation layers. These devices exhibit significantly lower impedance (ranging from 0.1 to 2.5 kΩ at 1 kHz) compared to values reported in most literature.

The peripheral nervous system, which is composed of sensory and motor nerves, serves a dual purpose in communication. It conveys external information gathered by mechanoreceptors to the spinal cord and also prompts muscular action to mobilize limbs. Despite advancements, several challenges persist. Firstly, due to the cylindrical and slender shape of nerves, it is challenging to securely affix standard rigid bioelectronics to peripheral nerves. Secondly, unlike the relatively static nature of brain tissues, peripheral nerves undergo constant deformation because of the surrounding muscles' movements. These mechanical distortions can cause device fatigue and trigger electrical or mechanical failures. Furthermore, the mismatch in modulus between the tissue and the device results in shear stress at the point of contact, which can lead to inflammatory responses. Zhang et al. developed a 3D neural electrode by integrating a nano-gold film onto a flexible shape memory polymer (SMP) substrate, transforming it from a 2D planar state (2018). When exposed to normal saline at 50°C, these flattened neural electrodes could spontaneously conform to the 3D shape of peripheral nerves, leveraging the shape memory effect. To showcase its clinical applicability, they conducted two *in vivo* animal experiments: vagus nerve stimulation (VNS) to regulate heart rate and sciatic nerve stimulation to control leg movements. This technology exemplified a novel approach where 3D bioelectronics was initially fabricated in a 2D state but could adapt to match 3D biological tissues using smart materials, presenting significant potential for clinical applications. Other implantable electronics in IEEE conferences are described in Table 10.4.

TABLE 10.4   Implantable Electronics in IEEE Conferences

IEEE Conferences	Title	Main Content	References
2022 European Microelectronics and Packaging Conference	Implantable Interface for an Arm Neuroprosthesis	An arm neuroprosthesis implantable interface.	
2022 35th International Conference on Micro Electro Mechanical Systems (MEMS)	A Fully-Implantable MEMS-Based Autonomous Cochlear Implant	A fully implantable, MEMS-based, low-power, energy-harvesting, next-generation cochlear implant (CI)	(Kulah et al., 2022)
2022 35th International Conference on Micro Electro Mechanical Systems (MEMS)	Low-Voltage Flexible Interdigital Electrode for Pulsed Field Ablation with Effect Evaluation	A novel flexible interdigital electrode (FIE) for pulsed-field ablation of atrial fibrillation.	(Xu et al., 2022)
2022 35th International Conference on Micro Electro Mechanical Systems (MEMS)	Assembly and Parallel Implantation of a Penetrating Flexible Probe with Thousands of Microelectrodes	A method of packaging and parallel implantation of a single probe with over 2,000 channels, which can be used in the simultaneous real-time multi-brain region neural activity recording.	(Wang et al., 2022)
2023 36th International Conference on Micro Electro Mechanical Systems (MEMS)	Three-Dimensional Flexible Neural Opto-Electronic Array With Silk-Based Shuttle-Free Implantation	A flexible three-dimensional (3D) optoelectronic array of 512 electrophysiological recording channels with the silk-based shuttle-free implantation method.	(Gu et al., 2023)
2023 36th International Conference on Micro Electro Mechanical Systems (MEMS)	Silk-Enabled Foldable and Conformal Neural Interface with In-Plane Shielding for High-Quality Electrophysiological Recordings	A flexible, foldable, and conformal neural interface with in-plane shielding fabricated by the MEMS process.	(Liang et al., 2023)
2023 36th International Conference on Micro Electro Mechanical Systems (MEMS)	Real-Time Functional Brain Mapping Based on High-Channel-Count, Ultra-Conformal Neural Interface	A real-time functional brain mapping technique based on high-channel-count, ultra-conformal electrocorticographic (ECoG) electrodes to record neural signals	(Wang et al., 2023)
2023 36th International Conference on Micro Electro Mechanical Systems (MEMS)	Fabrication of Biodegradable Soft Tissue-Mimicked Microelectrode Arrays for Implanted Neural Interfacing	Biodegradable, adhesive, and soft tissue-compliant microelectrode arrays (MEAs) to achieve *in vivo* site-specific neural stimulation and recording.	(Huang et al., 2023)

(*Continued*)

TABLE 10.4 (Continued)

IEEE Conferences	Title	Main Content	References
2022 International Electron Devices Meeting	Optogenetic Neural Probes: Fiberless, High-Density, Artifact-Free Neuromodulation	Micro-LED optoelectrode with 256 recording electrodes and 128 stimulation microLEDs in four silicon micro-needle shanks for optogenetic probes.	(Ko et al., 2022)
2022 International Electron Devices Meeting	Bio-inspired 3D Neural Electrodes for Peripheral Nerve Stimulation using Shape memory Polymers	A 3D neural electrode with shape memory effect for peripheral nerve stimulation.	Zhang et al., 2018)
2022 International Electron Devices Meeting	Soft Wireless Optogenetic and Hybrid Implants for Advanced Neural Interfacing	Presents soft wireless optogenetic and hybrid implants to enable highly precise, target-specific neuromodulation and neural activity monitoring for advanced neural interfacing.	(Jeong, 2022)

10.3 INTERNATIONAL STANDARDIZATION FOR SYSTEMS

Typically, functional electronic devices in biomedical engineering combine hardware, software, and mobile applications that connect to the cloud to collect, transmit, and analyze personal health data. TC 62 aims to prepare international standards, and other publications, with the focus on the safety and performance of medical equipment, software, and systems. ISO/DIS 9241-920 provides guidance on the design and selection of hardware, software, and combinations of hardware and software interactions, including 1) the design/use of tactile/haptic inputs, outputs, and/or combinations of inputs and outputs, with general guidance on their design/use as well as on designing/using combinations of tactile and haptic interactions for use in combination with other modalities or as the exclusive mode of interaction, 2) the tactile/haptic encoding of information, including textual data, graphical data, and controls, 3) the design of tactile/haptic objects, 4) the layout of tactile/haptic space, and 5) interaction techniques. For guidance and recommendations on the accessibility of tactile/haptic interactions, including information on the use of Braille, see ISO 9241-971. The recommendations given in this part of ISO 9241 are applicable to a variety of tactile/haptic devices, representing the real world or virtual or mixed realities (e.g. exoskeletons, wearables, force feedback devices, touchables, and tangibles) and stimulation types (e.g. acoustic radiation pressure and electrical muscle stimulation) and they can also be found in virtual and augmented environments. The use of gestures (e.g. multitouch) can be found in ISO 9241-960. Information on gesture-based interfaces can be found in the multipart standard ISO/IEC 30113. Information on contactless gestures can be found in ISO TS 9241-430.

Wearables can generate continuous streams of data to make the patient the point of care. Technology, based on AI algorithms, can analyze the condition of the patient and enable the clinician to devise an accurate treatment plan exactly when required by the patient. In specific areas of digital healthcare, the IEC 63203-801 series provides a standardized communication interface and protocols for wireless connectivity between the edge computing device or hub coordinator and the sensing nodes. The caveat exists that medical data generated by technology can potentially be vulnerable to hacking. Challenges in the wearable technology field encompass data security, trust concerns, and regulatory obstacles. To promote safety, security, privacy, and cross-vendor interoperability for active assisted living (AAL) services, IEC SyC AAL publishes standards. AAL refers to systems and equipment that assist senior citizens or individuals with disabilities in living independently at home. An example of this is IEC TR 60601-4-5:2021, which offers comprehensive guidance on tailoring IEC 62443 to address the particular requirements of the healthcare sector.

Another important standards series is IEC 80001, which provides guidance on risk management for the use of medical devices in networked environments. These standards define a risk management process that covers the entire life cycle of networked medical devices, from design and development to decommissioning. They focus on identifying and mitigating potential risks associated with connected medical devices, including cybersecurity threats and communication failures between devices.

10.4 CONCLUSION AND OUTLOOK

Soft electronics is the future trend of electronic devices used in the field of biomedical engineering. In this chapter, we review the international standard activities on soft electronics applied in BME, including IEEE conferences, IEC standards, and ISO standards. Wearable electronics and implantable electronics and systems are discussed. We note that the international standards for flexible electronics are still being developed, for example, some new devices such as TENGs, memristors, transient electronics, hydrogel, etc. These standardization work can help provide some guidance in the absence of a broader consensus. Successful standardization frameworks will recognize shifts in access to healthcare, not just in hospitals and healthcare settings but also in homes, workplaces, leisure settings, and mobile phones. The development of new and revised standards needs to be complemented by methodologies designed to help organizations acquire, navigate, and make the most of them. Methods for defining and measuring the benefits of standardization activities need to be included to ensure that these benefits are realized and opportunities are exploited.

REFERENCES

Abbass, Y., Seminara, L., Saleh, M., & Valle, M. (2021). Novel wearable tactile feedback system for post-stroke rehabilitation. *2021 IEEE Biomedical Circuits and Systems Conference (BioCAS)*.

Ali, S., Khan, A., & Bermak, A. (2023). Smart diaper embedded with fully printed sensors for wireless healthcare and monitoring. *2023 IEEE International Conference on Flexible and Printable Sensors and Systems (FLEPS)*.

Bentley, D. M., Heald, R., & Prakash, S. (2022). Fabrication and evaluation of a flexible battery for wearable biomedical applications. *2022 IEEE 35th International Conference on Micro Electro Mechanical Systems Conference (MEMS)*.

Chung, H. U., Rwei, A. Y., Hourlier-Fargette, A., Xu, S., Lee, K., Dunne, E. C., Xie, Z., Liu, C., Carlini, A., Kim, D. H., Ryu, D., Kulikova, E., Cao, J., Odland, I. C., Fields, K. B., Hopkins, B., Banks, A., Ogle, C., Grande, D., … Rogers, J. A. (2020). Skin-interfaced biosensors for advanced wireless physiological monitoring in neonatal and pediatric intensive-care units. *Nature Medicine*, 26(3), 418–429.

Cook, A., Goodwin, K., Taylor, P. S., Balaban, E., Alfredsson, M., Horne, R. J., Bird, D., Batchelor, J. C., & Casson, A. J. (2023). Sputtered zinc electrodes on pullulan substrates for flexible biodegradable transient electronics. *2023 IEEE International Conference on Flexible and Printable Sensors and Systems (FLEPS)*.

Eskandari, P., Beaver, C. L., Rossbach, S., Maddipatla, D., & Atashbar, M. (2022). Flexible microplasma discharge device for treating burn wound injuries against fungal infections. *2022 IEEE International Conference on Flexible and Printable Sensors and Systems (FLEPS)*.

Gu, C., Yang, H., Zhang, B., Zhou, Z., Sun, L., Li, M., Wei, X., & Tao, T. H. (2023). Three-dimensional flexible neural opto-electronic array with silk-based shuttle-free implantation. *2023 IEEE 36th International Conference on Micro Electro Mechanical Systems (MEMS)*.

Huang, C., Wang, Z., Fukushi, K., Nihey, F., Kajitani, H., & Nakahara, K. (2021). Assessment of over-pronated/over-supinated foot using foot-motion measured by an in-shoe motion sensor. *2021 IEEE Biomedical Circuits and Systems Conference (BioCAS)*.

Huang, W.-C., Lei, W.-L., & Peng, C.-W. (2023). Fabrication of biodegradable soft tissue-mimicked microelectrode arrays for implanted neural interfacing. *2023 IEEE 36th International Conference on Micro Electro Mechanical Systems (MEMS)*.

Jeong, J. W. (2022). Soft wireless optogenetic and hybrid implants for advanced neural interfacing. *2022 International Electron Devices Meeting (IEDM)*.

Ko, E., Kim, K., Voroslakos, M., Oh, S., Buzsaki, G., Wise, K. D., & Yoon, E. (2022). Optogenetic neural probes: fiberless, high-density, artifact-free neuromodulation. *2022 International Electron Devices Meeting (IEDM)*.

Kulah, H., Ulusah, H., Chamanian, S., Batu, A., Ugur, M. B., Yuksel, M. B., Yilmaz, A. M., Yigit, H. A., Koyuncuoglu, A., Topcu, O., & Soydan, A. K. (2022). A fully-implantable mems-based autonomous cochlear implant. *2022 IEEE 35th International Conference on Micro Electro Mechanical Systems Conference (MEMS)*.

Liang, J., Chen, Z., Wang, X., Xu, F., Wei, X., Sun, L., Li, M., Tao, T. H., & Zhou, Z. (2023). Silk-enabled foldable and conformal neural interface with in-plane shielding for high-quality electrophysiological recordings. *2023 IEEE 36th International Conference on Micro Electro Mechanical Systems (MEMS)*.

Lu, Z., Zhu, W., Chen, Y., Charnley, J., Dejke, V., Pomazanskyi, A., Ko, S.-T., Zeybek, B., Mehryar, P., Ali, Z., Karamousadakis, M., & Chen, D. (2022). Wearable pressure sensing for lower limb amputees. *2022 IEEE Biomedical Circuits and Systems Conference (BioCAS)*.

Lv, W., Chen, X., Zhang, Y., Quan, W., Chen, X., Fan, C., Shi, J., Yang, J., Zeng, M., & Yang, Z. (2022). A wireless flexible smart bandage for wound monitoring. *2022 IEEE 35th International Conference on Micro Electro Mechanical Systems Conference (MEMS)*.

Nappi, S., Miozzi, C., Mazzaracchio, V., Fiore, L., Camera, F., D'Uva, N., Amendola, S., Occhiuzzi, C., Arduini, F., & Marrocco, G. (2021). A plug& play flexible skin sensor for the wireless monitoring of pandemics. *2021 IEEE International Conference on Flexible and Printable Sensors and Systems (FLEPS)*.

Steinhubl, S. R., & Topol, E. J. (2018). A skin patch for sensing blood pressures. *Nature Biomedical Engineering*, 2(9), 633–634.

Tseghai, G. B., Malengier, B., Fante, K. A., & Van Langenhove, L. (2022). Velcro hook electroencephalogram textrode for brain activity monitoring. *2022 IEEE International Conference on Flexible and Printable Sensors and Systems (FLEPS)*.

Wang, X., Chen, Z., Liang, J., Wei, X., Sun, L., Li, M., Zhou, Z., & Tao, T. H. (2023). Real-time functional brain mapping based on high-channel-count, ultra-conformal neural interface. *2023 IEEE 36th International Conference on Micro Electro Mechanical Systems (MEMS)*.

Wang, X., Yang, H., Zhu, Z., Li, H., Gu, C., Zhang, B., Wei, S., Yu, H., Zhou, Z., Sun, L., Tao, T. H., & Wei, X. (2022). Assembly and parallel implantation of a penetrating flexible probe with thousands of microelectrodes. *2022 IEEE 35th International Conference on Micro Electro Mechanical Systems Conference (MEMS)*.

Wohnsdorf, S., Simon, J., & Klapper, U. (2022). Opportunities and challenges of smart textile systems for occupational safety of electricians. *2022 IEEE International Conference on Flexible and Printable Sensors and Systems (FLEPS)*.

Xu, M., Hong, W., Qin, M., Song, Z., Shi, Y., Yang, B., & Liu, J. (2022). Low-voltage flexible interdigital electrode for pulsed field ablation with effect evaluation. *2022 IEEE 35th International Conference on Micro Electro Mechanical Systems Conference (MEMS)*.

Zhang, Y., Zheng, N., Ma, Y., Xie, T., Feng, Y. (2018). Bio-inspired 3D neural electrodes for the peripheral nerves stimulation using shape memory polymers. *2018 IEEE International Electron Devices Meeting (IEDM)*.

Zhao, Y., Li, Y., Zhou, J., He, G., Liu, Y., Zhao, J., Zhao, B., Lin, M., Wang, X., Qian, Z., Chen, S., Wan, T., & Lian, Y. (2022). An event-driven system architecture for smart flexible sensors in healthcare applications. *2022 IEEE International Flexible Electronics Technology Conference (IFETC)*.

Index

Pages in *italics* refer to figures and pages in **bold** refer to tables.